RELIGIOUS AND SPIRITUAL ISSUES IN PSYCHIATRIC DIAGNOSIS

A Research Agenda for DSM-V

RELIGIOUS AND SPIRITUAL ISSUES IN PSYCHIATRIC DIAGNOSIS

A Research Agenda for DSM-V

Edited by

John R. Peteet, M.D.
Francis G. Lu, M.D.
William E. Narrow, M.D., M.P.H.

Published by the
American Psychiatric Association
Arlington, Virginia

Note: The authors have worked to ensure that all information in this book is accurate at the time of publication and consistent with general psychiatric and medical standards, and that information concerning drug dosages, schedules, and routes of administration is accurate at the time of publication and consistent with standards set by the U.S. Food and Drug Administration and the general medical community. As medical research and practice continue to advance, however, therapeutic standards may change. Moreover, specific situations may require a specific therapeutic response not included in this book. For these reasons and because human and mechanical errors sometimes occur, we recommend that readers follow the advice of physicians directly involved in their care or the care of a member of their family.

The findings, opinions, and conclusions of this report do not necessarily represent the views of the officers, trustees, or all members of the American Psychiatric Association. The views expressed are those of the authors of the individual chapters.

Copyright © 2011 American Psychiatric Association
ALL RIGHTS RESERVED

Manufactured in the United States of America on acid-free paper
14   13   12   11   10   5   4   3   2   1
First Edition

Typeset in AGaramond and Frutiger.

American Psychiatric Publishing, Inc.
1000 Wilson Boulevard
Arlington, VA 22209-3901
www.appi.org

Library of Congress Cataloging-in-Publication Data
Religious and spiritual issues in psychiatric diagnosis : a research agenda for
DSM-V / edited by John R. Peteet, Francis G. Lu, William E. Narrow. — 1st ed.
    p. ; cm.
Includes bibliographical references and index.
ISBN 978-0-89042-658-6 (pbk. : alk. paper)
1. Psychiatry and religion. 2. Diagnostic and statistical manual of mental
disorders. I. Peteet, John R., 1947– II. Lu, Francis G. III. Narrow, William E.,
1957–
    [DNLM: 1. Diagnostic and statistical manual of mental disorders. 2. Mental
Disorders—diagnosis. 3. Religion and Psychology. 4. Spirituality. WM 141 R383
2011]
    RC455.4.R4R454 2011
    616.89′075—dc22

                                                                    2010015522

British Library Cataloguing in Publication Data
A CIP record is available from the British Library.

CONTENTS

CONTRIBUTORS

Dan G. Blazer, M.D., Ph.D.
J. P. Gibbons Professor of Psychiatry and Behavioral Sciences, Duke University Medical Center, Durham, North Carolina

Derek Bolton, Ph.D.
Professor of Philosophy and Psychopathology, King's College London, Institute of Psychiatry, and Centre for Humanities and Health, London, England

C. R. Cloninger, M.D.
Wallace Renard Professor of Psychiatry, Genetics, and Psychology, Washington University School of Medicine, St. Louis, Missouri

Mary Lynn Dell, M.D., D.Min.
Associate Professor of Psychiatry and Pediatrics and Bioethics, Division of Child and Adolescent Psychiatry, Case Western Reserve University School of Medicine, Cleveland, Ohio

Armando R. Favazza, M.D., M.P.H.
Emeritus Professor of Psychiatry, University of Missouri-Columbia School of Medicine, Columbia, Missouri

Richard J. Frances, M.D.
Clinical Professor of Psychiatry, New York University Medical School, New York, New York

K. W. M. (Bill) Fulford, D.Phil., FRCP, FRCPsych
Emeritus Professor of Philosophy and Mental Health, University of Warwick; Member of the Faculty of Philosophy and Honorary Consultant Psychiatrist, University of Oxford; Special Adviser for Values-Based Practice, Department of Health, United Kingdom; and Founder Editor PPP; and Fellow, St. Cross College, Oxford, England

Marc Galanter, M.D.
Professor and Director, Division of Alcoholism and Drug Abuse, Department of Psychiatry, New York University School of Medicine; and Research Scientist, Nathan Kline Institute for Psychiatric Research, New York, New York

David M. Gellerman, M.D., Ph.D.
Staff Psychiatrist, Sacramento VA Medical Center, Mather; and Assistant Clinical Professor, Department of Psychiatry and Behavioral Sciences, University of California at Davis Medical Center, Sacramento, California

Gerrit Glas, M.D., Ph.D.
Professor of Philosophy and Psychiatry, Leiden University Medical Centre and Department of Philosophy Leiden University, Leiden; and Director of Residency Training and Psychiatrist, Dimence, Zwolle, The Netherlands

Linda Glickman, Ph.D.
Research Assistant Professor, Division of Alcoholism and Drug Abuse, Department of Psychiatry, New York University School of Medicine, New York, New York

Philippe Huguelet, M.D.
Lecturer and Head of Sector of Adult Psychiatry, University Hospital of Geneva and University of Geneva, Geneva, Switzerland

Allan M. Josephson, M.D.
Professor and Chief, Division of Child and Adolescent Psychiatry, Department of Psychiatry and Behavioral Sciences, University of Louisville, Louisville, Kentucky, and, CEO, Bingham Clinic, Louisville, Kentucky

Paramjit T. Joshi, M.D.
Endowed Professor and Chair, Department of Psychiatry and Behavioral Sciences, Children's National Medical Center, and Professor of Psychiatry, Department of Behavioral Sciences and Pediatrics, George Washington University School of Medicine, Washington, D.C.

Jocelyn A. Kilgore, M.D.
Assistant Professor, Department of Psychiatry, and Scientist, Center for the Study of Traumatic Stress, Uniformed Services University of the Health Sciences, Bethesda, Maryland

Harold G. Koenig, M.D.
Professor of Psychiatry and Behavioral Sciences, Associate Professor of Medicine, and Director, Center for Spirituality, Theology and Health, Duke University Medical Center, Geriatric Research, Education and Clinical Center, Durham VA Medical Center, Durham, North Carolina

James W. Lomax, M.D.
Associate Chairman and Director of Educational Programs and Karl Menninger Chair of Psychiatric Education, Menninger Department of Psychiatry and Behavioral Sciences, Baylor College of Medicine, Houston, Texas

Francis G. Lu, M.D.
Luke and Grace Kim Endowed Professor in Cultural Psychiatry, Director of Cultural Psychiatry, and Associate Director of Residency Training, Department of Psychiatry and Behavioral Sciences, University of California, Davis Health System, Sacramento, California

David Lukoff, Ph.D.
Professor of Psychology, Institute of Transpersonal Psychology, Palo Alto, California

P. Alex Mabe, Ph.D.
Professor, Department of Psychiatry and Health Behavior, Medical College of Georgia, Augusta, Georgia

William E. Narrow, M.D., M.P.H.
Associate Director, Division of Research, American Psychiatric Association, Arlington, Virginia; Research Director, DSM-V Task Force

Carol S. North, M.D., M.P.E.
The Nancy and Ray L. Hunt Chair in Crisis Psychiatry, Professor of Psychiatry, and Director, Program in Trauma and Disaster, VA North Texas Health Care System, Dallas, Texas; and Professor, Departments of Psychiatry and Surgery/Division of Emergency Medicine, The University of Texas Southwestern Medical Center, Dallas, Texas

John R. Peteet, M.D.
Associate Professor of Psychiatry, Harvard Medical School, Boston, Massachusetts; former Chair, American Psychiatric Association Corresponding Committee on Spirituality, Religion and Psychiatry

Philip A. Quanbeck II, Ph.D.
Associate Professor and Chair, Department of Religion, Augsburg College, Minneapolis, Minnesota

Jennifer Radden, D.Phil.
Professor of Philosophy, University of Massachusetts, Boston, Massachusetts; Consultant in Medical Ethics, McLean Hospital, Belmont, Massachusetts

Teresa A. Rummans, M.D.
Professor of Psychiatry, Mayo Clinic College of Medicine, Rochester, Minnesota;
Chair, Department of Psychiatry and Psychology, Mayo Clinic Florida, Jackson-
ville, Florida

John Z. Sadler, M.D.
Daniel W. Foster Professor of Medical Ethics, and Professor of Psychiatry and of Clinical Sciences, The University of Texas Southwestern Medical Center, Dallas, Texas

Bruce W. Scotton, M.D.
Clinical Professor of Psychiatry, University of California, San Francisco, and
Training Analyst, C.G. Jung Institute, San Francisco, California; Private Practice,
San Francisco and Corte Madera, California

Edward P. Shafranske, Ph.D., ABPP
Professor and Director of PsyD Program, Pepperdine University, Los Angeles, California; and Lecturer, Department of Psychiatry and Biobehavioral Sciences,
David Geffen School of Medicine, University of California, Los Angeles, Los Angeles, California

Len Sperry, M.D., Ph.D.
Professor, Mental Health Consulting Program, Florida Atlantic University, Boca
Raton, Florida, and Clinical Professor, Department of Psychiatry, Medical College
of Wisconsin, Milwaukee, Wisconsin

Dan J. Stein, M.D., Ph.D.
Professor, Department of Psychiatry and Mental Health, University of Cape
Town, Cape Town, South Africa

Stephen Strack, Ph.D.
Clinical Professor of Psychology, Alliant International University, Los Angeles, and
Fuller Graduate School of Psychology, Pasadena, California

Margaret L. Stuber, M.D.
Jane and Marc Nathanson Professor of Psychiatry, David Geffen School of Medicine, University of California, Los Angeles, California

Samuel B. Thielman, M.D., Ph.D.
Adjunct Assistant Professor of Psychiatry, Department of Psychiatry and Health
Behavior, Duke University School of Medicine, Durham, North Carolina; Re-
gional Medical Officer/Psychiatrist, U.S. Department of State, Embassy of the
United States, London, England

Robert J. Ursano, M.D.
Professor of Psychiatry and Neuroscience; Chair, Department of Psychiatry; and Director, Center for the Study of Traumatic Stress, Uniformed Services University of the Health Sciences, Bethesda, Maryland

George E. Vaillant, M.D.
Senior Psychiatrist, Brigham and Women's Hospital, and Professor of Psychiatry, Harvard Medical School, Boston, Massachusetts

H.M. Van Praag, M.D., Ph.D.
Professor Emeritus, University of Groningen, Utrecht, Maastricht, The Netherlands, and The Albert Einstein College of Medicine, New York, New York

Joseph Westermeyer, M.D., Ph.D.
Professor of Psychiatry and Adjunct Professor of Anthropology, University of Minnesota; Medical Director, Addictive Disorders Service, Minneapolis VA Hospital, Minneapolis, Minnesota

C. Paul Yang, M.D., Ph.D.
Associate Clinical Professor, University of California, San Francisco, and Staff Psychiatrist, San Mateo South County Mental Health Services, Redwood City, California

DISCLOSURE STATEMENT

The research collaboration that produced this monograph was supported with funding from the American Psychiatric Association. This effort preceded the official revision process for *Diagnostic and Statistical Manual of Mental Disorders,* Fifth Edition (DSM-5), and was a component of a separate, rigorous research planning initiative meant to inform the revision of DSM. No private-industry sources provided funding for this research review.

Administrative coordination and oversight of this process was provided by the American Psychiatric Institute for Research and Education, including William E. Narrow, M.D., M.P.H., Emily A. Kuhl, Ph.D., Rocio Salvador, and Darrel A. Regier, M.D., M.P.H. (Executive Director).

The following contributors to this book have indicated financial interests in or other affiliations with a commercial supporter, a manufacturer of a commercial product, a provider of a commercial service, a nongovernmental organization, and/or a government agency, as listed below:

Mary Lynn Dell, M.D., D. Min.—The author has received research support from The Louisville Institute and The Templeton Foundation.

Dan J. Stein, M.D., Ph.D.— The author has received research support and/or consultation support from AstraZeneca, Eli Lilly, GlaxoSmithKline, Jazz Pharmaceuticals, Johnson & Johnson, Lundbeck, Orion, Pfizer, Pharmacia, Roche, Servier, Solvay, Sumitomo, Takeda, Tikvah, and Wyeth.

The following contributors to this book do not have any conflicts of interest to disclose:

Dan G. Blazer, M.D., Ph.D.
Derek Bolton, Ph.D.
C. R. Cloninger, M.D.
Armando R. Favazza, M.D., M.P.H.
Richard J. Frances, M.D.
K. W. M. Fulford, D.Phil., FRCP, FRCPsych
Marc Galanter, M.D.
David M. Gellerman, M.D., Ph.D.

Gerit Glas, M.D. Ph.D.
Linda Glickman, Ph.D.
Philippe Huguelet, M.D.
Allan M. Josephson, M.D.
Paramjit T. Joshi, M.D.
Jocelyn A. Kilgore, M.D.
Harold G. Koenig, M.D.
James W. Lomax, M.D.
Francis G. Lu, M.D.
David Lukoff, Ph.D.
P. Alex Mabe, Ph.D.
William E. Narrow, M.D., M.P.H.
Carol S. North, M.D., M.P.E.
John R. Peteet, M.D.
Philip A. Quanbeck II, Ph.D.
Jennifer Radden, D.Phil.
Teresa A. Rummans, M.D.
John Z Sadler, M.D.
Bruce W. Scotton, M.D.
Edward P. Shafranske, Ph.D., ABPP
Len Sperry, M.D., Ph.D.
Stephen Strack, Ph.D.
Margaret L. Stuber, M.D
Samuel B. Thielman, M.D., Ph.D.
Robert J. Ursano, M.D.
George E. Vaillant, M.D.
H.M. Van Praag, M.D., Ph.D.
Joseph Westermeyer, M.D., Ph.D.
C. Paul Yang, M.D., Ph.D.

INTRODUCTION

John R. Peteet, M.D.
Francis G. Lu, M.D.
William E. Narrow, M.D., M.P.H.

More than 90% of adults in the United States say that they believe in God, and approximately 88% pray (Hoge 1996). For decades following Freud's attacks on religion as immature wish fulfillment, there was little exploration of the territory shared by psychiatry and spirituality. Recently, however, clinical and scholarly interest in the relationship between spirituality, religion, and mental health has grown steadily. Medline contains more than 650 citations to spirituality or religion and psychiatry or mental health in the past 10 years.

In 1994, DSM-IV introduced an "Outline for Cultural Formulation" that encouraged clinicians to consider cultural idioms of distress, explanations of illness, and preferences for care, as well as the role of religion in providing support (American Psychiatric Association 1994). In addition, a V code for Religious or Spiritual Problem was established to help clinicians categorize distressing experiences related to religion or spirituality that were not symptomatic of psychopathology and thereby broaden the differential diagnosis to reduce chances of misdiagnosis.

However, current descriptions of Axis I and II disorders take religious and spiritual considerations into only limited account. As preparations for DSM-V led to the 2002 monograph *A Research Agenda for DSM-V* (Kupfer et al. 2002) and a follow-up volume focused on age and gender issues (Narrow et al. 2007), the Corresponding Committee on Religion, Spirituality, and Psychiatry of the American Psychiatric Association (APA) proposed a review of the innovations in DSM-IV and of relevant recent research with a view to developing an agenda for future research in this area. The APA's Committee on Psychiatric Diagnosis and Assessment and Division of Research provided guidance for this project, which led to a well-attended APA symposium in 2006 that considered the spiritual and religious aspects of major diagnostic categories including psychotic disorders, depression, anxiety and substance use disorders, posttraumatic stress disorder, and disorders of childhood and adolescence.

This volume contains the contributions of the well-known clinicians and researchers who participated in this symposium as well as those of other distinguished scholars. Two expert commentaries follow each of their chapters, to add perspective. The principal charge to authors in addressing major diagnostic categories was to expand the current DSM text on "Age, Gender, and Cultural Considerations" and "Differential Diagnosis" to include the impact of religious/spiritual factors on phenomenology, differential diagnosis, course, outcome, and prognosis. For example, what about the disorder is important to understand in order to distinguish religious/spiritual experiences from psychopathology? What is the prevalence of psychopathological conditions that take a religious/spiritual form? Are these disorders overdiagnosed in people with religious/spiritual commitments? What difference in course or outcome is associated with the presence or absence of religious/spiritual commitments? What changes in the text does evidence support for inclusion in DSM-V?

Each contributor responds to this challenge with a review of existing literature, an analysis of the issues at stake, and suggested wording for a revised DSM. Harold Koenig considers religious issues in schizophrenia and other psychotic disorders. Dan Blazer examines the complex relationship between spirituality and depression. Linda Glickman and Marc Galanter discuss the religious and nonreligious use of substances. Gerrit Glas finds spiritual and existential elements in the phenomenology of anxiety disorders. Robert Cloninger contends that patients with personality disorders can be most clearly understood as having spiritual deficits—that is, deficits in the coherence of their fundamental assumptions and schemas about life. Sam Thielman reviews evidence that an individual's worldview and the moral context of trauma are relevant to coping and the development of posttraumatic stress disorder. Alex Mabe, Mary Lynn Dell, and Allan Josephson consider several ways in which spiritual and religious issues influence disorders of childhood and adolescence.

Three papers address additional ways that religious and spiritual issues have relevance for a revised DSM. Bill Fulford and John Sadler offer a novel approach to the philosophical challenge of distinguishing spiritual phenomena from psychopathology. David Lukoff, Francis Lu, and Paul Yang present evidence for expanding the V code for Religious and Spiritual Problem to include (among others) those presented by New Religious Movements and cults and by life-threatening and terminal illness as well as by mystical, near-death, and spiritual practice–related experiences. Finally, David Gellerman and Francis Lu present a practical framework for incorporating religious and spiritual information into the cultural understanding of the patient.

We recommend changes to the introductory section of the DSM in order to accommodate our consensus that diagnosis should take into account the psychological impact of patients' concerns with meaning, loss, isolation, autonomy, or guilt. Such existential concerns may be found not only in personality, depressive, adjustment, and anxiety disorders but also in nonpathological conditions such as demoralization or subsyndromal anxiety. PubMed now contains 110 references to existential distress. Consider the following proposed revised wording in the introduction to DSM-IV-TR (American Psychiatric Association 2000, p. xxxi):

Each of the mental disorders is conceptualized as a clinically significant behavioral or pathological syndrome or pattern that occurs in an individual and that is associated with present distress (e.g., a painful symptom) or disability (i.e., impairment in one or more important areas of functioning) or with a significantly increased risk of suffering death, pain, disability, or an important loss of freedom. In addition, this syndrome or pattern must not be merely an expectable and culturally sanctioned response to a particular event, for example, the death of a loved one. Whatever its original cause, it must currently be considered a manifestation of a behavioral, psychological or biological dysfunction in the individual. Neither deviant behavior (e.g., political, religious, or sexual) *nor existential distress* nor conflicts that are primarily between an individual and society are mental disorders unless the deviance, *distress,* or conflict is a symptom of dysfunction in the individual as described above.

In applying this definition of mental disorder, clinicians often find the distinction between normal and pathological experience confusing, especially when confronting experiences that human beings have, such as pain, suffering, existential distress, and religious, spiritual, or mystical experiences. Since DSM-III (American Psychiatric Association 1980), the manual has used the "clinical significance criterion" to make the distinction between normative experience and pathological experience. In assessing clinical significance (i.e., distinguishing normal from pathological experience), clinicians must elicit the individual's cultural and individual values and worldviews that crucially frame whether the patient's experiences are "for the worse" and impede the patient's seeking and fulfilling his or her own ideals. By making the patient's values explicit, the clinician can avoid pathologizing normal human experiences or overlooking evidence of psychopathology (American Psychiatric Association 2006; Josephson and Peteet 2004).

Given that pathology can only be clearly defined in relation to health, we further recommend that future research attempt to characterize important domains of normal human functioning that are impaired by psychiatric disorders, such as in the areas of thinking, feeling, and willing as well as in relating effectively to the individual's social, cultural, existential, and spiritual context.

As the commentaries to the chapters make clear, the challenge of incorporating religious and spiritual considerations into an increasingly evidence-based DSM is an iterative process. Yet these thoughtful and provocative contributions demonstrate several important reasons to continue pursuing the task. A DSM that more fully incorporates these ideas could help clinicians recognize their importance to the ways that patients understand and approach their emotional difficulties. It could help them to better appreciate how religious and spiritual concerns may impede—and spiritual resources may promote—recovery and how mental health and religious professionals can collaborate in identifying and achieving healthy goals. Finally, it could locate the diagnostic categories of contemporary Western psychiatry within a larger historical, philosophical, and cultural context.

References

American Psychiatric Association: Diagnostic and Statistical Manual of Mental Disorders, 3rd Edition. Washington, DC, American Psychiatric Association, 1980

American Psychiatric Association: Diagnostic and Statistical Manual of Mental Disorders, 4th Edition. Washington, DC, American Psychiatric Association, 1994

American Psychiatric Association: Diagnostic and Statistical Manual of Mental Disorders, 4th Edition, Text Revision. Washington, DC, American Psychiatric Association, 2000

American Psychiatric Association: Religious/Spiritual Commitments and Psychiatric Practice Resource Document, December 2006. Available at: http://www.psych.org/Departments/Edu/Library/APAofficialDocumentsandRelated/ResourceDocuments/200604.aspx. Accessed March 17, 2010.

Hoge DR: Religion in America: the demographics of belief and affiliation, in Religion and the Clinical Practice of Psychology. Edited by Shafranske EP, Maloney HME. Washington, DC, American Psychological Association, 1996, pp 21–41

Josephson AJ, Peteet JR (eds): Handbook of Spirituality and Worldview in Clinical Practice. Washington, DC, American Psychiatric Publishing, 2004

Kupfer DJ, First MB, Regier DA (eds): A Research Agenda for DSM-V. Washington, DC, American Psychiatric Publishing, 2002

Narrow WE, First MB, Sirovatka PJ, et al: Age and Gender Considerations in Psychiatric Diagnosis: A Research Agenda for DSM-V. Washington, DC, American Psychiatric Publishing, 2007

1

SPIRITUALITY AND DEPRESSION

A Background for the Development of DSM-V

Dan G. Blazer, M.D., Ph.D.

Of all the psychiatric disorders, the depressive disorders have been most closely correlated with ordinary spiritual experience, and the burden of depression may be increasing throughout the world (Kessler et al. 2003; World Health Organization 2001). Although psychotic episodes have often been interpreted as unique spiritual insights and persons with ongoing apparent psychotic experiences have assumed the role of spiritual leaders (such as shamans), the struggle with depression reaches to the very core of the spiritual experience in many faith traditions. For example, even a severe depression has been viewed as an adaptive component, beneficial to the self and others in some religious traditions, such as the "dark night of the soul" described by St. John of the Cross (1959). In other cases, a moderate depressed mood is viewed as a necessary stage in the journey of spiritual growth, found in the mysticism of many faith communities. One reason for the tight intertwining of depression and spirituality is the blurred distinction between clinical

Portions of the chapter were previously published as Blazer DG: "Spirituality, Depression and Suicide: Introduction." *The Southern Medical Journal* 100:733–734, 2007, and Blazer DG: "Spirituality, Depression and Suicide: A Cross-Cultural Perspective." *The Southern Medical Journal* 100:735–736, 2007.

depression and normal problems of living. Major depression, viewed primarily as a biological illness, has especially been challenged as a diagnosis too narrowly conceived (Blazer 2005; Horowitz 2002; Parker 2005).

At the same time, depression is viewed as emotional suffering that is especially open to spiritual interventions. Depression has often been thought to derive from shame and guilt secondary to alienation from a higher being or sin against others. Therefore, only through spiritual exercises, such as repentance and prayer, can these symptoms be alleviated. Although modern psychiatry has done much to temper the view that depression is a spiritual condition rather than an illness, among some of the most conservative religious groups the older view persists. Healing for these people can only occur within the context of the faith community through spiritual counseling (Adams 1970).

In this chapter I concentrate on depression and do not explore bipolar disorder. The rich, complex, and at times paradoxical interactions between depression and spirituality are reviewed. These interactions provide a context for understanding the depressed mood among many of our patients that a sterile diagnostic system cannot capture. The mental health professional, therefore, will not be effective (even though a drug may be efficacious) unless this context is recognized and incorporated into the therapeutic process.

I begin with a review of the historical intertwining of spirituality and depression and follow this with a consideration of cultural factors. Next I explore the interplay between depression and existential issues that are the focus of many faith traditions. A review of depression from a developmental perspective follows. Then I review the current empirical studies, including studies of the phenomenology of presentations of depression as it might be shaped by spirituality; studies of the potential adaptive capacity of depression; studies of religious affiliation and the prevalence of depression; studies of the frequency of religious participation and depression; studies of religious salience and spiritual activities and depression; studies of depression and religious coping; studies of religion/spirituality and the course of depression; and studies of spirituality, depression, and chronic illness. I complete this discussion by suggesting areas that can be addressed in future research of spirituality and depression to inform both our psychiatric nomenclature and clinical practice.

Historical Background

The interrelationship between a depressed mood and spiritual struggle/growth (including the view that the melancholic person may possess unique spiritual gifts) dates to ancient times. Job, in the Hebrew Bible, cries out in the anguish of his depressed mood, "May the day of my birth perish, and the night it was said, 'A man is born'...Why is light given to those in misery, and life to the bitter of soul, to those who long for death that does not come...?" (Job 3:1–20). Nevertheless, he challenged his friends who accused him of some sin that separated him from God or tried to philosophically isolate him because of his severe disturbance of mood: "But I have a mind as well as you; I am not inferior to you...What you know, I also know; I am not inferior to you...you are worthless physicians, all of you! If only you would be altogether silent! For you, that would be wisdom" (Job 12:3; 13:2–5). Although he struggled mightily with God, his struggle was not an extraordinary experience.

The development of the Jewish faith as it approaches suffering has not followed a simple path. A history of persecution through pogroms and culminating in the Holocaust during World War II has shaped Jewish thought appreciably (Bowker 1970). Nevertheless, certain elements of the Jewish response to suffering include a stark realism regarding suffering (the refusal to invoke a supernatural solution to cover or abolish the agonizing realities); intense feelings of family and community; involvement in the suffering of others; and a vision of the Day of Atonement. In other words, suffering brings a more clear view of life.

The relation of depression to a more clear view of life is also observed in Iranian Shi'ism (Good et al. 1985). A core of this variant of Islam embodies a vision whereby tragedy and grief are religiously motivated emotions. Typical religious rituals help the community recollect the struggles and martyrdom of the Shi'a imams. Religious grieving recognizes the suppression of the righteous by the world and the sacrifice of the community in striving toward righteousness. Personal emotional suffering is often interpreted as a reflection of the suffering of the entire community of martyrs. Children first learn to grieve as part of a religious activity. The depressed express their depressed mood in part as one of heightened sensitivity. They view themselves as more sensitive to the social environment, a special vulnerability to the hurtful aspects of social relations or public events. This concept of depression in no way decreases the Iranian concern for the depressed nor the recognition of the personal suffering associated with depressive episodes. The depressed in Iran seek care and condolences, as do the depressed in North America.

The core of the Hindu and Buddhist approach to suffering is detachment, and the struggle is to safeguard detachment from turning into indifference (Bowker 1970). The soul liberated from suffering is a soul unified, and that unity extends horizontally as well as vertically. A soul so liberated leads to a life of submission, gratitude, forgiveness, self-sacrifice, and self-awareness. If one's thoughts are not so liberated—that is, continue to be attached to sinful desires and egoism—the outcome can be emotional states such as anger, resentment, shame, guilt, low self-esteem, confusion, and loss of a sense of self (Juthani 2004). The Hindu and Buddhist patient is rarely self-referred for emotional suffering but usually is brought by the family to the clinician when all other resources are exhausted. Symptoms are therefore often tied to the complex family structure, and the family should be included in therapy.

Among Christians, suffering and melancholy are viewed with ambivalence among those seeking spiritual growth. Religious melancholy has been, through much of Western history, an integral part of spiritual growth yet at the same time a symptom that spiritual growth has stalled. Depression was not merely the self turning inward due to a painful and self-absorbed temperament. The emotional suffering of depression inextricably derived from one's experience with God and the world around. This led to a desire to explain emotional (and physical) suffering, with the result that many Christians were exercised by the problem of theodicy (the difficulty of defending the justice and righteousness of God in the face of suffering) (Bowker 1970).

Stress and fear often lead to depression. One of the ancient interpretations of a depressed mood was weariness in doing good works, *acedia* as described by the ancients. The Apostle Paul encouraged the Thessalonians to "never tire of doing what is right" (2 Thessalonians 3:13), for if they did tire they could slip into acedia. In other words, some depressed withdraw from the world because they are weary of its stresses.

People suffering from acedia might see the world clearly enough, yet lose hope in God; they would fear God. For example, Jonah (in the Hebrew scriptures) was weary; he became angry with the world and with God because the Ninevites repented (Jonah 4). He probably knew their repentance would not last and that they would return to their sin, but he believed they had cheated the wrath of God. "It would be better for me to die than to live," he said while watching and waiting upon the city. The stress of preaching to this sinful nation drained whatever fervor Jonah felt for his godly mission; his anger and depression wearied him. Acedia overtook him and he withdrew from the city. The answer to acedia was the hope found in the events of Jesus's life (including the resurrection).

Yet the hope in Jesus did not abolish suffering and depression. Within the Christian mystic tradition, a period of profound melancholy has been described— the "dark night of the soul" (Underhill 1961, pp. 380–395). This period of desolation and fatigue reflects a disharmony between the self and the world as one grows spiritually. The dark night reflects an exhaustion of the old state and the "growing pain" to the new state of spiritual consciousness. The greatest pain, deriving from the dark night, is the sense of the absence of God (the Divine Absence). This in turn leads to a redoubled desire to unite with God. This sense of God's absence is accompanied by a heightened sense of sin, the loss of old passions for the world, and the recognition that peace and joy cannot be found in the world. Depression serves as a purification of the will and defeat of the person's rebellion against God. To put it more simply, the dark night builds Christian character.

Robert Burton (1577–1640) described a depressive variant called *religious melancholy* (Burton 1621/1948; Jackson 1986). This variant was derived in large part from superstition; it affected the brain, heart, will, understanding, and even the soul itself. Persons so afflicted could experience either religious melancholy in "excess" or in "defect." Melancholy in excess was similar to the enthusiasm described earlier, yet Burton did not view this excess as a gift of the gods but rather of "the first mover... is the Devil." (Burton 1621/1948, p. 879) Others permitted the Devil to lay hold upon them by infecting them with melancholy humor; this led the person to forsake God (and God in turn forsook them). They suffered "a sickness of the soul without any hope or expectation of amendment: which commonly succeed fear; for whilst evil is expected, we fear; but when it is certain, we despair." Such persons "cannot obtain what they would, they become desperate, and many times either yield to the passion by death itself" (p. 936; quoted in Jackson 1986, p. 331). Burton's view has been the predominant view in Western society. Despite the association of depression through our history with keen insight, the experience of a depressed mood by the religious suggests spiritual sickness rather than a spiritual gift.

Later writers viewed religious melancholy as alternating with religious enthusiasm. During periods of enthusiasm, Jonathan Edwards witnessed among his parishioners outcries, faintings, and convulsions. Yet they would then lapse into a sense of the displeasure of God, of being in danger of damnation. They could not sleep at nights, and when they did sleep, they would awaken with fear, heaviness, and distress and become fixated on concerns about their bodies (Rubin 1994).

By the late nineteenth century, depression as a consequence of inward and outward religious activities was seen as a sign of excess (Ribot 1896/1903). During the twentieth century, religious melancholy basically passed away, perhaps having given way to a religion of healthy mindedness. The idea of passing through a dark night of the soul is scarcely heard as a condition of spiritual growth. Depression is now viewed as an illness or faulty thinking largely divorced from one's healthy spiritual growth. Positive religious experiences are viewed by the religious as being a powerful tool to overcome depression (LeHaye 1974). Some exceptions have emerged in fundamentalist religious groups. For example, Jay Adams (1970), in *Competent to Counsel,* cites King David (Psalm 32:4) as evidence that depression is from God and considered merciful punishment of God warning him and leading him to repentance.

Cultural Considerations

No discussion of depression and spirituality can be complete without a discussion of depression and culture, for culture and religion are so intertwined. The recognition of the ongoing negotiation between religion and culture ranges from ongoing discussions by mainline Protestant theologians about the proper stance of religion with culture (Niebuhr 1951) to commentaries on the dramatic revolts against culture by fundamentalist religious groups across many of the world's religions (Lawrence and Denny 1995). Perhaps of most importance for any discussion of depression and spirituality is a discussion of those cultural forces that augment, shape, and perpetuate depression. A culturally shaped depression may be manifested as a spiritual crisis or challenge.

Nussbaum (2001) goes so far as to suggest that emotions are socially constructed. Emotions are not feelings that well up in some natural and untutored way from our natural selves; they are contrivance, social constructs. We learn how to feel. Emotions are taught to us through stories. If they can be learned, they can be unlearned (cognitive therapy). Lutz (1985) proposes a theory and examples of emotion as aspects of cultural meaning systems people use in attempting to understand the situations in which they find themselves (Blazer 2005). Emotions are socially negotiated. The social context surrounding the person gives meaning to feeling and behavior and provides criteria for judging his or her own emotions and the emotions of others.

Margaret Field, in her ethnographic study of Ghana, explored the close connection between culture and religion. She found that women who were depressed around the age of menopause (they had completed their childbearing years) visited a shrine to gain relief from that depression. The depression arose out of the fear of sorcery and evil spirits that made them barren (Field 1960). They felt that they had become useless because they no longer could bear children and therefore had become witches. In many cases the depressed women were not considered mentally ill, for if they believed they had caused harm to others, they were taken at their word. If the woman was restless, agitated, and unable to sleep, a spirit had overtaken her. She would rarely seek help for her illness.

Eaton and Weil (1976; Schwab and Schwab 1978) studied the Hutterites (from 1950 to 1955), a small group of people who isolated themselves for cultural and religious reasons in the northern great plains of the United States and Canada. They prized the simple life and had a reputation for mental health (namely, because the members of the group had similar lifestyles and shared the same sentiments, leading to group cohesion). This sheltered lifestyle was thought to shield them from social risks for mental disorders. Yet the Hutterites' protective social structure was associated with guilt feelings among those who feared that they might not live up to group expectations and a high frequency of symptoms of depression.

Karp (1996), in reflecting upon his own chronic depressive illness, emphasizes the "socially generated meanings of illness." Although the core syndrome of depression may be observed universally across cultures, there are widely varying experiences of depression. All too often the physician leaves out the "illness narrative" (as suggested by Kleinman [1988a]) and is uninterested in hearing the patient's illness experience. The physician listens only to gather the data necessary to make a diagnosis. Although not religious himself, Karp noted that depression at times in our society today may be a "gift" that helps one gain a greater meaning of the mystery of human suffering. He went on to maintain that the social disconnection generated by an ethic of individualism in America is an important element in the proliferation of mood disorders.

In summary, although the biological substrate of depression is universal, cultural factors shape the expression and meaning of the emotions as they emerge. In addition, the social pressure of certain cultures, such as the Hutterite culture, may very well increase the biological vulnerability to depression. Spirituality is so tightly interwoven with many prevailing cultures (such as the cultures in Ghana and among the Hutterites) that no exploration of the frequency and symptoms of depression can be divorced from the context of the prevailing religious orientation of the culture.

Yet these isolated cultures may appear on the surface to have very little influence upon a diverse culture such as found in North America. The psychiatrist must recognize that, despite the multilayered and intersecting cultural influences that virtually everyone encounters daily, unique cultural influences continue to shape thoughts and behaviors. People retreat into their subcultures, often as an escape from the confusion of such a diverse environment. Retreat into a religious subculture may be one of the most common means of retreat.

Existential Issues and Depression

Societal pressures may augment the association of depression with existential concerns. These pressures may emerge in the form of an existential crisis (Yalom 1980), and such crises may lead to spiritual growth or despair. Jeffrey Smith (1997), in his book *Where the Roots Reach for Water: A Personal and Natural History of Melancholia*, chronicles his own prolonged sacred journey through his experience with depression. Depression opened his eyes to a higher being and the world. After years of attempting to cover over, escape, or yield to the desire to end his life through suicide, Smith realized depression was his lot in life, his "thorn in the flesh." His mindset changed as he sought what good could come from his melancholy mood; good did come.

Smith quotes Susan Sontag, "Precisely because the melancholy character is haunted by death, it is melancholics who best know how to read the world" (p. 186). Knowing how to read the world, for Smith, means being rooted in the world and in faith:

> This is what melancholia taught me: wherever this body takes root—in whatever soil would feed it, in whatever water will wash it...if faith be intact it is a oneness, inseparable from the oneness all about it. So now you see the pilgrim walking across the plain, and his striding body, with the legs branched out from the trunk, takes the shape of the root...roots that hold him, and each of us, afoot; you see the roots that hold this landscape...together as one. (p. 274)

Although Smith would never wish depression upon another and would have gladly rid himself of the pain of melancholy, he recognized that the experience of depression was instrumental in his spiritual growth. Thomas Moore (1992), in his popular book *Care of the Soul,* devoted a chapter to the "gifts" of depression:

> Depression grants the gift of experience not as a literal fact but as an attitude toward yourself. You get a sense of having lived through something, of being older and wiser. You know that life is suffering, and that knowledge makes a difference. You can't enjoy the bouncy, carefree innocence of youth any longer....If we pathologize depression, treating it a syndrome in need of cure, then the emotions...have no place to go except into abnormal behavior and acting out. (pp. 139, 147)

Both Smith and Moore speak of a generic spirituality. Loss of hope is also a core symptom of depression and often leads to an existential crisis (Brown and Harris 1978). As Delbanco (1999) notes:

> Human beings need to organize the inchoate sensations amid which we pass our days—pain, desire, pleasure, fear—into a story. When that story leads somewhere and thereby helps us navigate through life to its inevitable terminus in death, it gives us hope....We must imagine some end if we are to keep at bay the...suspicion that one may be adrift in an absurd world. The name for that suspicion—for the absence or diminution of hope—is melancholy...the dark twin of hope. (pp. 1–2)

The swelling prevalence of depression in Western society as we turned the century, coupled with rising rates of suicide, perhaps reflected an increasingly dominant hopelessness within society (Blazer 2005).

Another frequent symptom of depression is a profound sense of *loss of meaning* (Blazer 2005; Lundin 1993). Our society may perpetuate such a loss. A central theme of liberal democracy is the abolishment of authority. All explanations of events, all meta narratives, are equally valid but also equally brought under suspicion. Some would overthrow all entrenched beliefs and attitudes, whatever those beliefs and attitudes might be. Nothing remains sacred. Stephen Carter, in *The Culture of Disbelief,* suggests that beliefs are not so much attacked as restricted and trivialized (Blazer 1998; Carter 1992). For example, an orthodox Jew who enlists in the armed forces wishes to wear his skullcap under his military headgear. He is not permitted to do so in the name of religious freedom and the separation of church and state. Religious beliefs are accepted as long as they are not expressed in words or actions toward others of a different persuasion. What does it "mean" to be an orthodox Jew if one cannot practice one's beliefs? As described by David Lyon, "Like ice-floes on the river during spring break-up, the world of meaning fractures and fragments, making it hard even to speak of meaning as traditionally conceived" (Lyon 1994, p. 11).

Psychiatrists have through most of the twentieth century recognized the importance of meaning to mental health (Blazer 2005; Frankl 1962; Yalom 1980). Victor Frankl, in *Man's Search for Meaning,* described a therapeutic approach to psychotherapy that actually underlies many forms of psychotherapy today—logo (or meaning) therapy (Frankl 1962; Wulff 1991). When depression is considered strictly from the perspective of a medical diagnosis, the psychiatrist is all too quick to answer the question, "Why did I become depressed?" with "You have a chemical imbalance." That answer does not consider the heart and soul of the question (Blazer 1998, p. 136). Thomas Moore (1992), in *Care of the Soul,* wrote: "The great malady of the twentieth century, implicated in all of our troubles and affecting us individually and socially, is 'loss of soul,'…It is impossible to define precisely what the soul is…[yet] we say certain music has soul or a remarkable person is soulful. …Soul is revealed in attachment, love and community, as well as in retreat" (pp. xi–xii).

The theme of existential issues and depression (and other physical and emotional suffering) was explored by the President's Council on Bioethics. This panel posed the question of whether biotechnology (primarily through medications) might lead to a pursuit of pleasure and happiness that extended "beyond therapy" (President's Council on Bioethics 2003). Peter Kramer (1994) originally piqued the public's attention to the idea that medications could lead one to feel "better than normal" and therefore take antidepressant therapy beyond therapy in his book *Listening to Prozac.* The President's Council suggested that as many as 20% of students on elite college campuses now take or have taken prescription "mood brighteners." The suggestion that the new-generation antidepressants, especially the selective serotonin reuptake inhibitors (SSRIs), actually can alter a person's native temperament therefore presents ethical issues that in the past were restricted to the use of recreational drugs. From the perspective that gives primacy to personal freedom and an individual's right to pursue happiness as he or she defines it, the use of mood brighteners would appear to be largely unproblematic. Yet suffering and adaptation to suffering has been in the past largely the province of faith communities (Bowker 1970). One concern expressed among the spiritual is that mood-brightening drugs will estrange us emotionally from life as it really is.

Spirituality and Depression: A Developmental Perspective

Erik Erikson, perhaps more than any other author, focused upon the interaction of spirituality and depression from a developmental perspective (Erikson 1958, 1982; Erikson and Kivnick 1986; Wulff 1991). The developmental task of old age is the achievement of integrity, and failure to do so leads to despair. Integrity is the acceptance of one's one and only life cycle, especially a courageous facing of death. Despair arises when the person fails to accept as ultimate the life cycle drawing to a close. Wisdom, a detached concern with life itself coupled with mature judgment and discernment, arises when integrity gains a victory over despair. For most, however, the essence of wisdom is not an individual achievement but is provided by a living religious or philosophical tradition.

According to Erikson, although individual religious faith is vulnerable to pathological distortion, and religious traditions have at times exploited human weaknesses, faith and tradition, in their more nurturing forms, are vital for the attainment of human maturity (Wulff 1991). Although spanning the life cycle, religion is especially important for the first and last developmental tasks—the lifelong quest for basic trust and developing a sense of cosmic order (integrity). In some extraordinary people, such as Martin Luther (whom Erikson describes as examples of homo religiosus) the quest for integrity becomes a lifelong challenge (Erikson 1958; Wulff 1991). Because these people are unsatisfied with the traditional answers to the most difficult questions about life's meaning, they are burdened by a melancholy world mood (Erikson 1958). Yet this mood is not to be considered pathological, because it may be the most true adaptation to the human condition. For such people, the identity crisis is especially painful, and the search for integrity is enduring. Yet the struggle can lead to an ideological breakthrough not only for the person but for society as a whole.

In a study of adolescents (mostly white), existential well-being (life has meaning), but not religious well-being (I believe God loves and cares for me), was associated with lower frequency of depressive symptoms (Cotton et al. 2005). Many studies of the association of spirituality and the frequency of depressive symptoms or major depression, however, have focused on the elderly. One reason is that late life is intuitively associated with existential issues closely associated with the elderly. Victor Frankl (1962), for example, described a condition in which one's primary or intrinsic religion remains suppressed. In such cases, the striving for meaning is thwarted, leaving an existential vacuum reflected in depression, suicide, drug addiction, and alcoholism. Symptoms include a sense of meaninglessness, emptiness, and futility.

Review of the Literature on the Association of Religion/Spirituality and Depression

PHENOMENOLOGY

There have been virtually no studies of differences in the symptoms of depression resulting from a particular religious orientation, although cultural differences (as discussed earlier) may serve as a proxy in some situations. Robert Burton (1621/1948), in *The Anatomy of Melancholia,* listed sorrow, suspicion, anxiety, horror of conscience, fearful dreams and visions, and the temptation of melancholic individuals to do away with themselves. He believed melancholic individuals to be compelled against their will to harbor impious thoughts and to blaspheme against God.

He believed the cure to be a life of religious moderation, calm reason, and measured fellowship and work (Rubin 1994).

The psychologist Theodule Ribot during the late nineteenth century (Ribot 1896/1903) theorized that at its extreme religious passion could pass over into two general forms: the depressive, wherein the individual became obsessed with feelings of guilt and fear, and the exalted, a transitory and relatively passive state marked by intense feelings of love (Wulff 1991).

The problems associated with previously being involved in a fundamentalist religious group have been described as the "shattered faith syndrome" by the founder of Fundamentalists Anonymous. Symptoms that have been associated with this syndrome include chronic guilt, anxiety, and depression; low self-esteem; loneliness and isolation; distrust of other people or groups; bitterness and anger over lost time; aversion to any structure or authority; lack of basic social skills; and guilt and anxiety about sex (Wulff 1991; Yao 1987).

Today the prevailing view among psychiatrists is that people with depression may express their symptoms in terms of religion (depression is an underlying disease, and religion is merely the idiom or vocabulary in which patients express their symptoms). In a study comparing involutional depressive patients in French Canada and Hungary (Hungary being more secular and Canada being more influenced by Catholic traditions), the Canadians were more likely to be agitated and to link their depression with self-blame based on religious beliefs (Boszormenyi 1979). Guilt is frequently assumed to be a symptom of depression closely connected to depression. Yet some claim that feelings of guilt are much less commonly associated with depression in the non-Western world (Murphy 1982). Guilt has been attributed to the influence of the Judeo-Christian heritage, including its effects on Islam. Other writers do not believe the differences between the expression of guilt across cultures (and religions) are significant (Kleinman 1998b). Hopelessness is one symptom that is frequently associated with the lack of meaning and purpose in life. Sadness might be considered the opposite of religious ecstasy. In addition, certain depressive symptoms may predispose a person to a dramatic spiritual experience.

What symptoms might lead to sudden and dramatic change (such as the conversion experience of the Apostle Paul)? Miller and de Baca (2001) described these changes as "quantum changes." Quantum change is out of the ordinary, and therefore a sense of crisis precedes such changes. Before change, people often were unhappy. They usually felt a deep sense of alienation from their faith communities and society at large, similar to the alienation coined "anomie" by Durkheim (1951) as a predisposition to suicide. The change is characterized by vividness (absolutely clear when it happens—often accompanied by profound emotion), surprise (rarely remembered as willful), benevolence (a life-changing gift), and permanence (no going back).

DEPRESSION AS ADAPTIVE

One theme that must be considered in any discussion of depression and spirituality is the potential adaptive capacity of depression. Depression itself can be viewed as an adaptive response that is not as effective compared with the past (Blazer 2005). Some forms of depression may be protective, whereas other (usually more severe) forms are toxic to the organism. For example, Hybels et al. (2002) found that mild depression was associated with increased longevity among women in a controlled study of older adults.

That major depression is an adaptation gone awry is an idea with a long history. Charles Darwin proposed that pain or suffering of any kind, if persistent, causes depression and lessens the power of action. Depression therefore may be well adapted to assist the organism in withdrawal from unexpected stressors (Darwin 2001). Nesse (2000) asked, "Is depression an adaptation, an adaptation gone awry, or a pathological state unrelated to any function?" The answer is probably all of the above. Investigators of Nesse's question must distinguish severe depression from mild depression because mild depression may be adaptive in some circumstances. If some variants of depression are adaptive, then the association of depression and spirituality becomes even more complex and nuanced.

There is no clear point at which pathological depression can be differentiated from nonpathological depression, just as there is no clear point at which an adaptive fever can be distinguished from a maladaptive fever (Kendler and Gardner 1998). Depressed individuals move from subthreshold to threshold depression and back again easily through time (Judd and Akiskal 1999). Mild depression may initially be adaptive, yet becomes maladaptive if it becomes severe, even though the mechanisms that precipitate the depression may be identical.

A mild depression may help people to disengage from pursuing a goal that is unattainable (Willner et al. 1992). The extant literature supports this idea. The pursuit of large goals requires constructing expensive social enterprises that are difficult to reverse—marriages, friendships, careers, reputation, status, and group membership. Major setbacks in these enterprises precipitate life crises. Depression may enable a person to both decrease investment in the current unsatisfying life enterprise and also to prevent the premature pursuit of alternatives. Failure to disengage can cause depression, and depression can make it harder to disengage (leading to negative feedback loops). In addition, the costs of low mood may be small compared with those of inappropriate high mood (which may not read a situation accurately). Withdrawal into a period of spiritual searching or faith community may be one way in which the depressed recalibrate their expectations.

Yet we must be careful not to glamorize depression, especially the more severe episodes. Peter Kramer (2005) noted:

> As I spoke with audiences about mood disorders, I came to believe that part of what stood between depression and its full status as disease was the tradition of he-

roic melancholy....One medical philosopher asked what it would mean to prescribe Prozac to Sisyphus, condemned to roll his boulder up the hill.

That variant of the *what if* question sent me to Albert Camus's essay on Sisyphus, where I confirmed what I thought I had remembered—that in Camus's reading, Sisyphus, the existential hero, remains upbeat despite the futility of his task. The gods intend for Sisyphus to suffer. His rebellion, his fidelity to self, rests on the refusal to be worn down. Sisyphus exemplifies resilience, in the face of full knowledge of his predicament. Camus says that joy opens our eyes to the absurd— and to our freedom. It is not only in the downhill steps that Sisyphus triumphs over his punishment: "The struggle itself toward the heights is enough to fill a man's heart. One must imagine Sisyphus happy."

SPIRITUALITY AND THE SYMPTOMS OF DEPRESSION

Religious Affiliation and Depression

Early epidemiological studies of the association of depression and spirituality focused upon the association of religious affiliation and depression (Koenig et al. 2001). Although a large body of literature during most of the twentieth century suggested that Jews were at increased risk for developing depression, even when other factors were controlled (Sanua 1992), recent studies have been less consistent. Kennedy et al. (1996) found that being Jewish was a risk factor for both the prevalence and incidence of depression among older adults. In contrast, Idler and Kasl (1992) found that Jews had a lower risk of developing depression than Catholics in a 3-year follow-up of older adults. If Jews are at increased risk for depression, two factors have been suggested to explain the finding. First, Jews of Eastern European descent may be more willing to admit to negative affects, creating a negative response bias. In addition, Jews may express depression more frequently because they experience reduced rates of alcohol abuse and dependence (Koenig et al. 2001).

Findings for Catholics in the United States are equally equivocal. For example, in a secondary analysis of data from the New Haven and Los Angeles Epidemiologic Catchment Area surveys, the prevalence of depressive disorders among Catholics was approximately 50% of that among Jews (Koenig et al. 2001; Levev et al. 1997). In a study exploring the frequency of depressive symptoms, however, investigators found no differences between white Catholics and whites from other faiths (although they found that African American Catholics scored at lower frequency) (Jones-Webb and Snowden 1993).

In a community-based study from North Carolina, investigators found that Pentecostals were three times more likely to experience major depression than non-Pentecostals (Meador et al. 1992). Reasons for this discrepancy may include the aggressive evangelistic outreach of Pentecostals to persons in lower socioeconomic classes and other groups at high risk for mental disorders and the optimistic message that may attract the depressed to Pentecostal congregations (Koenig et al. 2001).

Religious/Spiritual Activities

Measures of religious involvement have often been aggregated into multi-item scales that record both public (e.g., church attendance) and private (e.g., private prayer) activities (Koenig et al. 2001). When these measures are used, they have consistently been negatively associated with measures of depressive symptoms, although the association is decreased in highly controlled studies (Brown and Gary 1994; Fehring et al. 1987; Kendler et al. 1997). In general, measures of participation in organized religion have been more strongly associated with an absence of depression than intrinsic religiosity or participation in a nonorganized religion in older adults (Bosworth et al. 2003; Ellison 1995; Koenig et al. 2001; Parker et al. 2003). In another study, church attendance was "inversely associated with depressive symptoms among whites, but not among blacks" (Ellison 1995). Koenig et al. (1997) found that the rate of depression in subjects who attended religious services once per week or more was only half that of subjects who attended services less than once per week, even after the researchers controlled for physical health, social support, age, sex, and race. In a study of rural, low-income mothers, both religious beliefs and more involvement in a faith community were negatively related to depressive symptoms (Garrison et al. 2004).

Religious/Spiritual Salience and Motivation

The evidence of an association between religious salience/motivation and depression is mixed. In a study of 118 Jewish seniors, spirituality was not correlated with loneliness or depression. On the other hand, having a sense of meaning or purpose in life was inversely correlated with depression and loneliness (Springer et al. 2003). In contrast, investigators of 162 terminally ill patients with cancer and AIDS found that spiritual well-being was associated with lower levels of depression as measured by the Hamiton Rating Scale for Depression, yet religious practices were not (Nelson et al. 2002). In yet another study among elderly hospitalized subjects, religiousness and spirituality were consistently associated with fewer depressive symptoms (Koenig et al. 2004).

Religious/Spiritual Coping and Depression

Loewenthal et al. (2001), in a study of Christians, Hindus, Jews, Muslims, and persons with no religion in the United Kingdom, found in general that religious activity was not seen as particularly helpful for depression. Faith and prayer were seen as the most helpful aspects of religion. Muslims believed more strongly than other groups in the efficacy of religious coping methods to combat depression, were most likely to say they would use religious coping behavior, and were least likely to say they would seek social support or professional help for depression. Christians thought that both prayer and others praying for the sufferer were more effective than did most other groups. The Jewish participants endorsed the effectiveness of maintaining religious practice and consulting a religious leader more strongly than did most other groups. Men saw religious coping as relatively more effective than did women (men may be more reluctant to seek professional help). In general, however, those who valued religious coping were just as likely to seek secular mental health services.

Srinivasan et al. (2003) found that among patients in Canada referred for a depressive disorder, patients strongly rejected attributing depression to spiritual deficits. VanderCreek et al. (2004) studied religious and nonreligious coping methods among persons with positive religious coping (such as seeking religious direction, purification, and forgiveness). They found that these positive coping methods were associated with less depression but that negative religious coping (such as viewing God as punishing them) was associated with more depression. Subjects could make either positive or negative use of religion, and self-reported depression was more frequent among those with negative coping.

In yet another study, overall spirituality among the urban poor, as measured by the Spiritual Involvement and Belief Scale (Hatch et al. 1998), was associated with lower frequency of depressive symptoms. Specific items associated with less depression included belief in a higher power and ideas such as my life has a purpose; I can find meaning in times of hardship; and my spiritual life fulfills me in ways that material possessions do not. In contrast to other studies, church attendance and quantity of prayer were not associated with fewer depressive symptoms (Doolittle and Farrell 2004).

In a large study of the Canadian population, worship attendance was associated with fewer depressive symptoms, but those who stated that values or faith was important or perceived themselves to be spiritual/religious had higher levels of depressive symptoms (Batez et al. 2004).

Does the association between religious involvement and depression change as a function of the amount and/or type of life stress encountered? There is partial support of the stress buffering hypothesis. In a study of female twins, the negative association between personal religious devotion and depressive symptoms became stronger as stressful life circumstances increased (Kendler et al. 1997; Koenig et al. 2001). On the other hand, some cross-sectional studies have suggested that certain life stressors may make highly religious people more vulnerable to depression. In one study, for people who had encountered family stressors (such as marital problems), organizational and non-organizational religious involvement were associated with a greater likelihood of depression (Strawbridge et al. 1998). In the same study, for people who reported having encountered nonfamily stressors, such as financial problems and health problems, both organizational and non-organizational religious involvement were associated with lower frequency of depression.

RELIGION/SPIRITUALITY AND THE COURSE OF DEPRESSION

Park et al. (1990) found that greater religiousness predicted less depression over time and buffered the negative effects of life stress (particularly uncontrollable life stress) among college students. This association was true for Protestants but not for Catholics. Koenig et al. (1998) followed depressed older adults who were hospitalized for medical problems. Intrinsic religious motivation was associated with more rapid remission of the depression. In a study of 62 subjects with a diagnosis of major depression followed for 3 months, higher perceived emotional support from family and friends at baseline was a predictor of positive outcome. In contrast, spiritual well-being had a minimal effect on outcome (Nasser and Overholser 2005).

SPIRITUALITY, DEPRESSION, AND CHRONIC ILLNESS

There is evidence that religion can buffer depression and support the healing process (Koenig and Larson 1998). In a study of female breast cancer patients from Croatia, high religiosity was associated with lower frequency of depression but not with the intensity of pain perception. The type of operation and tumor stage were not associated with depression or religiosity, but mastectomized patients who belonged to the high-religiosity group were less depressed (Aukst-Margetic et al. 2005). A group from the United Kingdom found, among cancer patients treated in a hospice facility, a negative correlation between overall spiritual well-being (especially the existential effect) and depression. However, no correlation was found between religious well-being (such as strength of religious belief) and depression (McCourbie and Davies 2006). In another study of patients with rheumatoid arthritis, spirituality was found to facilitate emotional adjustment and resilience, even in the midst of significant depressive symptoms (Bartlett et al. 2003).

Future Research

- Epidemiological and clinical databases subject to latent class analysis of the symptoms of depression and other symptoms often associated with depression (such as somatic symptoms and anxiety symptoms) should be analyzed to compare both the cross-sectional patterns and longitudinal trajectories of symptom clusters by religious affiliation and reported religious involvement.
- Among people who are strongly socialized into religious communities, it is critical to

  1. Better understand which symptoms are clear intermediate phenotypes of those psychobiological abnormalities that lead to depressive symptoms and which symptoms are socially constructed.

2. Consider depressive symptoms within the context of a person's faith community. Guidelines to better understand the unique characteristics of faith communities and how these faith communities view and shape depressive symptoms can derive from qualitative research of these communities.
3. Consider depressive symptoms within the context of biopsychosocial development (Engel 1980) but complement the biopsychosocial model with a spiritual developmental model, one that includes both generic aspects of spiritual growth and particular aspects within different faith communities.
4. Distinguish between those symptoms of depression, given the context from which they arise, that are appropriate targets for therapeutic intervention and those that are "beyond therapy"—that is, symptoms that may be adaptive and appropriate within the context from which they arise (Blazer 2005; President's Council on Bioethics 2003).
5. Determine what (if any) symptoms of depression uniquely predispose a person to seek spiritual solace or to experience a profound change in their lives (such as a conversion experience).

Summary

- Not all religious groups are protected from depression by religion or spirituality, but the evidence is generally positive regarding the association.
- Public religious activities appear more protective than private religious activities and attitudes against depression.
- Religious involvement may be a moderator of risk factors for depression, such as stressful life events.
- Religious involvement may protect against depression associated with severe and chronic illnesses such as cancer, but not against the direct symptoms of the diseases (such as pain).

Proposed Statement for the Text of DSM-V

Of all the psychiatric disorders, the depressive disorders have been most closely correlated with ordinary spiritual experience. Depressive symptoms and spiritual experience are closely intertwined across the spectrum from mild to severe. Mild symptoms are frequently signs of spiritual development in most faith traditions and severe symptoms have at times been associated with the development and resolution of spiritual crises. In addition, spirituality has been thought to be a key to the amelioration of depressive symptoms in many faith traditions. Therefore, the clinician should carefully explore the spiritual context from which depressive symptoms emerge, the meaning of the symptoms to the patient, and the complex interplay of traditional psychiatric therapies with the potentially aggravating or nurturing characteristics of the spirituality of the patient.

References

Adams J: Competent to Counsel. Grand Rapids, MI, Baker Book House, 1970

Aukst-Margetic B, Jakovljevic M, Margetic B, et al: Religiosity, depression and pain in patients with breast cancer. Gen Hosp Psychiatry 27:250–255, 2005

Bartlett S, Piedmont R, Bilderback A, et al: Spirituality, well-being, and quality of life in people with rheumatoid arthritis. Arthritis Rheum 49:778–783, 2003

Batez M, Griffin R, Bowen R, et al: The association between spiritual and religious involvement and depressive symptoms in a Canadian population. J Nerv Ment Dis 192:818–822, 2004

Blazer D: Freud vs. God: How Psychiatry Lost its Soul and Christianity Lost its Mind. Downers Grove, IL, InterVarsity Press, 1998

Blazer D: The Age of Melancholy: Major Depression and Its Social Origins. New York, Routledge, 2005

Bosworth H, Park KS, McQuoid D, et al: The impact of religious practice and religious coping on geriatric depression. Int J Geriatr Psychiatry 18:905–914, 2003

Boszormenyi Z: A comparative study of involutional depressive patients in French Canada and in Hungary. Psychiatric Clin (Basal) 13:156–163, 1979

Bowker J: Problems of Suffering in the Religious World. Cambridge, United Kingdom, Cambridge University Press, 1970

Brown D, Gary L: Religious involvement and health status among African-American males. J Natl Med Assoc 86:825–831, 1994

Brown G, Harris T: Social Origins of Depression: A Study of Psychiatric Disorder in Women. New York, Free Press, 1978

Burton R: The Anatomy of Melancholy (1621). Edited by Dell F, Jordan-Smith P. New York, Tudor, 1948

Carter S: The Culture of Disbelief. New York, Basic Books, 1992

Cotton S, Larkin E, Hoopes A, et al: The impact of adolescent spirituality on depressive symptoms and health risk behaviors. J Adolesc Health 36:529–535, 2005

Darwin F (ed): The Life and Letters of Charles Darwin. Honolulu, HI, University Press of the Pacific, 2001

Delbanco A: The Real American Dream: A Meditation on Hope. Cambridge, MA, Harvard University Press, 1999

Doolittle B, Farrell M: The association between spirituality and depression in an urban clinic. Prim Care Companion J Clin Psychiatry 6:114–118, 2004

Durkheim E: Suicide: A Study in Sociology. Translated by Spaulding JA, Simpson G. New York, Free Press, 1951

Eaton J, Weil R: Culture and Mental Disorders. New York, Free Press, 1976

Ellison C: Race, religious involvement and depressive symptomology in a southeastern US community. Soc Sci Med 40:1561–1572, 1995

Engel G: The clinical application of the biopsychosocial model. Am J Psychiatry 137:535–544, 1980

Erikson E: Young Man Luther: A Study in Psychoanalysis and History. New York, WW Norton, 1958

Erikson E: The Life Cycle Completed: A Review. New York, WW Norton, 1982

Erikson E, Kivnick H: Vital Involvement in Old Age: The Experience of Old Age in Our Time. London, WW Norton, 1986

Fehring R, Brennan P, Keller ML: Psychological and spiritual well-being in college students. Res Nursing Health 10:391–398, 1987

Field M: Search for Security: An Ethnographic Study of Rural Ghana. New York, WW Norton, 1960

Frankl V: Man's Search for Meaning: An Introduction to Logotherapy. Translated by Lasch I. Boston, MA, Beacon Press, 1962

Garrison M, Marks L, Lawrence F, et al: Religious beliefs, faith community involvement and depression: a study of rural, low-income mothers. Womens Health 40:51–62, 2004

Good B, Good M, Moradi R: The interpretation of depressive illness and dysphoric affect, in Culture and Depression. Edited by Kleinman A, Good B. Berkeley, University of California Press, 1985, pp 369–428

Hatch R, Burg M, Maberhaus D: The Spiritual Involvement and Beliefs Scale: developing and testing of a new instrument. J Fam Pract 46:476–486, 1998

Horowitz A: Creating Mental Illness. Chicago, IL, University of Chicago Press, 2002

Hybels C, Pieper C, Blazer D: Gender differences in the relationship between subthreshold depression and mortality in a community sample of older adults. Am J Geriatr Psychiatry 10:283–291, 2002

Idler E, Kasl S: Religion, disability, depression, and the timing of death. Am J Soc 97:1052–1079, 1992

Jackson SW: Melancholia and Depression: From Hippocratic Times to Modern Times. New Haven, CT, Yale University Press, 1986

Jones-Webb R, Snowden L: Symptoms of depression among blacks and whites. Am J Pub Health 83:240–244, 1993

Judd L, Akiskal H: Delineating the longitudinal structure of depressive illness: beyond thresholds and subtypes (Presentation). Nuremberg, Germany, German College of Neuropsychopharmacology, 1999

Juthani N: Hindus and Buddhists, in Handbook of Spirituality and Worldview in Clinical Practice. Edited by Josephson A, Peteet J. Washington, DC, American Psychiatric Publishing, 2004, pp 125–138

Karp D: Speaking of Sadness. New York, Oxford University Press, 1996

Kendler K, Gardner C: Boundaries of major depression: an evaluation of DSM-IV criteria. Am J Psychiatry 155:172–177, 1998

Kendler K, Gardner C, Prescott C: Religion, psychopathology, and substance use and abuse: a multimeasure, genetic-epidemiologic study. Am J Psychiatry 154:322–329, 1997

Kennedy G, Kelman H, Thomas C, et al: The relation of religious preference and practice to depressive symptoms among 1,855 older adults. J Gerontol 51B:301–308, 1996

Kessler R, Berglund P, Demler E, et al: The epidemiology of major depressive disorder: results from the National Comorbidity Survey Replication (NCS-R). JAMA 289:3095–3105, 2003

Kleinman A: The Illness Narratives: Suffering, Healing, and the Human Condition. New York, Basic Books, 1998a

Kleinman A: Rethinking Psychiatry: From Cultural Category to Personal Experience. New York, The Free Press, 1998b

Koenig H, Larson D: Use of hospital services, religious attendance and religious affiliation. Southern Med J 91:925–932, 1998

Koenig H, Cohen H, George L, et al: Attendance at religious services, interleukin-6 and other biological indicators of immune function in older adults. Int J Psychiatry Med 27:233–250, 1997

Koenig H, George L, Peterson B: Religiosity and remission from depression in medically ill older patients. Am J Psychiatry 155:536–542, 1998

Koenig H, McCullough M, Larson D: Handbook of Religion and Health. New York, Oxford University Press, 2001

Koenig H, George L, Titus P: Religion, spirituality, and health in medically ill hospitalized older patients. J Am Geriatr Soc 52:554–562, 2004

Kramer P: Listening to Prozac: A Psychiatrist Explores the Antidepressant Drugs and the Remaking of the Self. New York, Viking Penguin, 1994

Kramer P: There's nothing deep about depression. New York Times Magazine, April 17, 2005. Available at: http://www.nytimes.com/2005/04/17/magazine/17DEPRESSION.html?scp=1&sq=Kramer&st=nyt.

Lawrence B, Denny F: Defenders of God: The Fundamentalist Revolt Against the Modern Age. Columbia, University of South Carolina Press, 1995

LeHaye T: How to Win Over Depression. Grand Rapids, MI, Zondervan, 1974

Levev I, Kohn R, Golding J, et al: Vulnerability of Jews to affective disorders. Am J Psychiatry 154:941–947, 1997

Loewenthal K, Cinnirella M, Evdoka G, et al: Faith conquers all? Beliefs about the role of religious factors in coping with depression among different cultural-religious groups in the UK. Br J Med Psychol 74:293–303, 2001

Lundin R: The Culture of Interpretation: Christian Faith and the Postmodern World. Grand Rapids, MI, William B. Eerdmans, 1993

Lutz C: Depression and the translation of emotional worlds, in Culture and Depression: Studies in the Anthropology and Cross-Cultural Psychiatry of Affect and Disorder. Edited by Kleinman A, Good B. Berkeley, University of California Press, 1985

Lyon D: Postmodernity. Minneapolis, MN, University of Minnesota Press, 1994

McCourbie R, Davies A: Is there a correlation between spirituality and anxiety and depression in patients with advanced cancer. Support Care Cancer 14:379–385, 2006

Meador K, Koenig H, Turnbull J, et al: Religious affiliation and major depression. Hosp Community Psychiatry 43:1204–1208, 1992

Miller W, de Baca J: Quantum Change: When Epiphanies and Sudden Insights Transform Ordinary Lives. New York, Guilford, 2001

Moore T: Care of the Soul. New York, HarperCollins, 1992

Murphy H: Comparative Psychiatry: the International and Intercultural Distribution of Mental Illness. New York, Springer-Verlag, 1982

Nasser E, Overholser J: Recovery from major depression: the role of support from family, friends, and spiritual beliefs. Acta Psychiatr Scand 111:125–132, 2005

Nelson C, Rosenfeld B, Breitbart W, et al: Spirituality, religion, and depression in the terminally ill. Psychosomatics 43:213–220, 2002

Nesse R: Is depression an adaptation? Arch Gen Psychiatry 57:14–20, 2000

Niebuhr H: Christ and Culture. New York, Harper & Row, 1951

Nussbaum M: Upheavals of Thought: The Intelligence of Emotions. New York, Cambridge University Press, 2001

Park C, Cohen L, Herb L: Intrinsic religiousness and religious coping as life stress moderators for Catholics and Protestants. J Person Soc Psychol 59:562–574, 1990

Parker G: Beyond major depression. Psychol Med 35:467–474, 2005

Parker M, Roff L, Klemmack D, et al: Religiosity and mental health in Southern, community-dwelling older adults. Aging Ment Health 7:390–397, 2003

President's Council on Bioethics: Beyond Therapy: Biotechnology and the Pursuit of Happiness. New York, Regan Books/Harper Collins, 2003

Ribot T: The Psychology of Emotions. New York, Charles Scribner's Sons (Original French Edition, 1896), 1903

Rubin J: Religious Melancholy and the Protestant Experience in America. New York, Oxford University Press, 1994

Sanua V: Mental illness and other forms of psychiatric deviance among contemporary Jewry. Transcultural Psychiatric Research Review 29:197–233, 1992

Schwab JJ, Schwab ME: Sociocultural Roots of Mental Illness: An Epidemiologic Survey. New York, Plenum Medical Book Company, 1978

Smith J: Where the Roots Reach for Water: A Personal and Natural History of Melancholia. New York, North Point Press, 1997

Springer M, Newman A, Weaver A, et al: Spirituality, depression, and loneliness among Jewish seniors residing in New York City. J Pastoral Care Counsel 57:305–318, 2003

Srinivasan J, Cohen N, Parikh S: Patient attitudes regarding causes of depression: implications for psychoeducation. Can J Psychiatry 48:493–495, 2003

St. John of the Cross: Dark Night of the Soul. Translated by Peers E. New York, Image Books, 1959

Strawbridge W, Shema S, Cohen R, et al: Religiosity buffers effects of some stressors on depression but exacerbates others. J Gerontology Soc Sci 53:S118–S126, 1998

Underhill E: Mysticism. New York, Dutton, 1961

VanderCreek L, Paget S, Horton R, et al: Religious and nonreligious coping methods among persons with rheumatoid arthritis. Arthritis Rheum 51:49–55, 2004

Willner P, Muscat R, Papp M: Chronic mild stress-induced anhedonia: a realistic animal model of depression. Neurosci Biobehav Rev 16:525–534, 1992

World Health Organization: World Health Report 2001: Mental Health, New Understanding, New Hope. Geneva, Switzerland, World Health Organization, 2001

Wulff D: Psychology of Religion: Classic and Contemporary Views. New York, Wiley, 1991

Yalom I: Existential Psychotherapy. New York, Basic Books, 1980

Yao R: An Introduction to Fundamentalists Anonymous. New York, Fundamentalists Anonymous, 1987

Commentary 1A

COMMENTARY ON "SPIRITUALITY AND DEPRESSION"

James W. Lomax, M.D.

Dr. Blazer's chapter on spirituality and depression is an exhaustive literature review by a distinguished psychiatric epidemiologist. It contains several carefully and modestly stated core concepts of everyday clinical importance to practitioners.

One such concept is that *mild* depression can be either "adaptive" or a response to what is "wrong" in the social environment. Religious-based ordering of experiences in the social environment is healthily adaptive when the results are prosocial—the formation of communities with shared values, aims, and goals. Such community qualities also characterize other health-promoting groups such as Alcoholics Anonymous (Vaillant 1995). Stressed or insecure humans tend to read "different" as "dangerous" and to construct "different" groups as "evil." Aggression channeled by such ordering may lead to self-hatred/depression when internalized or aggressive action toward others seen as containing externalized, disavowed aspects of the self. What Blazer adds to these familiar constructs is that mild depression may be a signal of something wrong in the social environment, not the depressed person.

Living in complex communities is inherently stressful and produces fear or anxiety that "often leads to depression." The ancient interpretation of a depressed mode is described as "weariness in doing good works" or acedia. Potential religious solace may therefore reside in "the hope found in the events of Jesus's life" and the associated promise of an afterlife where good people and deeds are predictably rewarded and bad people or deeds are predictably punished.

The section on cultural considerations includes content underrepresented in the education of most mental health professionals. A specific example is that "cultural factors shape the expression and meaning of the emotions as they emerge." Blazer notes that "the social pressure of certain cultures, such as the Hutterite culture, may very well increase the biological vulnerability of depression." Pursuing such questions requires overcoming a research confound not specifically mentioned in this chapter: the effect of the cultural setting on world religions. Islamics or Catholics in different communities construct very different goods to be pursued and behaviors to be rewarded. It is extremely difficult to identify *the* definitive research population to determine how a particular religious faith tradition, separate from its cultural context, influences the incidence and severity of depression.

Blazer observes that people "retreat into their subcultures" as an escape from the confusion of diversity. Retreat into religious subcommunity *can* be an important solace. However, such solace comes at an enormous price if the retreat is a final destiny to be defended (or from which to create wars) as opposed to a respite for periodic renewal. Unfortunately, the "defensive" function of such religious "ties that bind" can also become problematic when homogeneity (instead of unity) or rules (instead of principles) become criteria by which the group members measure all things. Religious organizations formed out of a "spiritual" seeking of connectedness also create religious disputes and wars.

Blazer wonders if the increasing prevalence of depression in Western society reflects a "dominant hopelessness." Many humans have trouble finding solace in living with ambiguity. Accepting inevitable ambiguity or multiple "truths" may therefore be experienced as a "profound loss of meaning." The possibility does exist to experience diversity and ambiguity with what Blazer defines as wisdom: a "detached concern with [the specific details of] life itself coupled with mature judgment and discernment, [which] arises when integrity gains victory over despair" (Erikson 1982).

Depression is indeed not a unitary phenomenon, even though the neurobiology of any depressed mood state may have fundamental similarities in terms of the spectrum of neurotransmitters and the neurocircuitry involved. Mild depression *may* be adaptive as a retreat from unexpected stressors providing a moratorium after major losses of relationships, role, or status. Depressive withdrawal to engage in spiritual searching, engagement in a faith community, or reflective thinking may be a key step allowing reattachment to new people, aims, or goals. A critical determinant for the outcome of such a withdrawal is whether such spiritual searching occurs in an attachment relationship in which relearning takes place (Vaillant 1988, 2002).

Blazer advocates discerning the specific type of cognitive religious coping employed by the individual and notes the difference in health outcomes between positive religious coping and negative religious coping (Pargament 2004). The "idea" or image that one has of God is also a source of either help or harm (Rizzuto 2001).

Future research recommendations include using contemporary neuroimaging technology to clarify the neurobiology of specific personality temperaments and brain circuitry involved in different types of spiritual or religious participation. We should identify characterological adaptations (utilizing psychometric measures of defense mechanisms, self, object relationships) associated with different religious constructs and prioritizations. We should differentiate religious from cultural determinants of health outcomes. Finally, we should determine whether nonreligious social interaction in groups like Alcoholics Anonymous has a similar moderating effect on symptom severity in depression.

References

Erikson E: The Life Cycle Completed: A Review. New York, WW Norton, 1982

Pargament KI, Koenig HG, Tarakeshwar N, et al: Religious coping methods as predictors of psychological, physical and spiritual outcomes among medically ill elderly patients: a two-year longitudinal study. J Health Psychol 9:713–730, 2004

Rizzuto AM: Does God help? What God? Helping whom? The convolutions of divine help, in Does God Help?: Developmental and Clinical Aspects of Religious Belief. Edited by Akhtar S, Parens H. New York, Jason Aronson, 2001, pp 19–51

Vaillant GE: Attachment, loss and rediscovery. Hillside J Clin Psychiatry 2:148–164, 1988

Vaillant GE: Hope, alcoholism and Alcoholics Anonymous. Presentation at the Psychotherapy and Faith Conference, Houston, TX, October 1995

Vaillant GE: The past and how much it matters, in Aging Well. Boston, MA, Little, Brown, 2002, pp 83–113

Commentary 1B

COMMENTARY ON "SPIRITUALITY AND DEPRESSION"

Teresa A. Rummans, M.D.
Philip A. Quanbeck II, Ph.D.

Dr. Blazer's discussion of spirituality and depression highlights the complex nature of the interaction between the two. Only in mankind's recent history have spirituality and depression been separated to this extent. Blazer traces the history of this phenomenon, explores the cultural and religious factors contributing to this division, and brings us back to the reality that the two are more closely related than not. The importance of this unifying, rather than dividing, approach is profound because it sets the stage for advancing our understanding of the treatment of depression in the larger context, which maximizes the spiritual benefits and minimizes the medical morbidity.

Dr. Blazer begins his discussion with a reference to the concept of the "dark night of the soul," which is a term associated with traditions of mysticism—and, in particular, St. John of the Cross. This notion of spiritual crisis is not particular to one religious tradition, nor is it unique to spirituality. "Depression has often been thought to derive from shame and guilt secondary to alienation from a higher being or sin against others" writes Dr. Blazer; however, "modern psychiatry has done much to temper the view that depression is a spiritual condition rather than an illness."

Neither guilt nor shame can be confined to a theological or psychological view. In religious traditions that emphasize correct religious practice, failure to observe the boundaries of religious law or tradition does mean that guilt is incurred. This is not necessarily a subjective situation but an objective reality. In contrast, guilty feelings are subjective and may be present even when objective guilt is not involved. In some religious traditions and some psychological treatments, there are practices for alleviating "guilt" and "feelings of guilt."

Similarly, shame has an objective and subjective character. Subjectively, shame can be understood as embarrassment or the desire to hide or cover oneself. Objectively, shame can refer to social rejection or the public display of misplaced hopes or values. In religious contexts one might be considered as shamed before divine holiness. If depression derives from shame and guilt associated with one's alienation from a higher being, guilt or infractions against others can be remedied by actions. However, as Blazer suggests, shame implies some insurmountable flaw that the person cannot overcome. In this case, religious shame can be connected to the experience of depression and understood as a spiritual condition.

Blazer describes a person's spiritual struggle, one that is often viewed as depression in the Judeo-Christian culture, through the Biblical description of Job's suffering. This struggle is ascribed to not examining one's inner motives fully. Although on the surface, depression may appear as the source of his struggle, Job's response to his condition suggests not depression but shame, as symbolized by his covering of himself with ashes and his move to silence before the divine.

From the Western tradition of thought, the "conversion" of St. Paul the Apostle has been explained by "interior" reasons or "introspective consciousness" as noted by Stendahl (1963). Blazer himself describes this phenomenon as a dramatic religious conversion by Paul that had its origin in prior internal psychological struggles that might be understood as "depression." Stendahl argued that this is not always the case. In the instance of the Apostle Paul, Stendahl noted that he did not exhibit internal doubt, discord, or depression prior to his conversion but instead exhibited a robust conscience. The implication then is that Paul's "conversion" was not a psychological break or a way of resolving a problem of internally felt guilt. Stendahl proposed instead that the conversion cannot be understood in psychological terms but rather as arising from actions outside of the person of Paul. Spiritual struggles then cannot be understood as psychological struggles alone.

In the process of outlining the historical view of spirituality and depression, Blazer makes a worthy attempt to be inclusive of, and pay respect to, the experience of world religions such as Islam and Buddhism and to some degree a generic animism. This approach shows us that there is an intermingling of cultural considerations with both spiritual beliefs and depressive symptoms.

Blazer makes an argument for acknowledging a kind of religious experience that, although it might appear to present itself in ways that mimic depression, may in fact express authentic religious experience, struggle, and journey. In such cases, the goal is not the quick amelioration of the symptoms but the respectful engagement of the person and the experience. In many ways contemporary practitioners of pastoral care and counseling have become more psychologically sophisticated. They too share in the risk of medicalizing or psychologizing experiences. Blazer is boldly trying to carve out a third way.

Similar to theologians, scientists have demonstrated that most empirical research ultimately brings spirituality and depression together, and the review of the current data by Dr. Blazer confirms this. It is interesting that no studies of differences in symptoms of depression resulting from a particular religious orientation exist. Although cultural and religious differences may impact the rate of depression and the way in which symptoms present, most depressive symptoms, including dysphoria, withdrawal, feelings of guilt, and hopelessness, are universal. Like spirituality, which is on a continuum from healthy to pathologic, depression, as Dr. Blazer points out, can actually be adaptive as well as incapacitating and life threatening. With milder forms of depression, individuals may avoid pursuing goals that are unattainable and recalibrate their expectations. However, in more severe forms one's ability to function in any way is impaired. Inward expressions of spirituality have been associated with a sense of purpose and meaning in life and a better chance of maintaining a sense of well-being even in the face of deteriorating physical health. Outward expressions of spirituality manifested as solely religious activities have generally been shown to be negatively associated with depressive symptoms. Coping with chronic and even terminal illness is more effective with religious and spiritual coping skills such as prayer and involvement in supportive religious communities (Bostwick and Rummans 2007). Individuals using these skills are less likely to consider suicide and are more accepting of death when faced with it (Bostwick and Rummans 2007). Treatments that have combined traditional psychological treatments such as cognitive-behavioral therapy with religious content and pastoral care were found to be better in improving and maintaining that improvement in depression than those using psychological therapy alone (Mueller et al. 2001). In addition to Dr. Blazer's recommendations for future research to focus on presentation and etiology, we must also explore ways in which the positive aspects of spirituality can be incorporated into our treatment armamentarium to help those with depressive symptoms.

References

Bostwick JM, Rummans TA: Spirituality, depression and suicide in middle age. Southern Med J 100:746–747, 2007

Mueller PS, Plevak DJ, Rummans TA: Religious involvement, spirituality, and medicine: implications for clinical practice. Mayo Clin Proc 76:1125–1235, 2001

Stendahl K: Paul and the introspective conscience of the West. Harv Theol Rev 56:199–215, 1963

2

SCHIZOPHRENIA AND OTHER PSYCHOTIC DISORDERS

Harold G. Koenig, M.D.

This chapter examines the role of religion and spirituality in the diagnostic process that is basic to effective treatment of persons with schizophrenia and other psychotic disorders. This includes conditions associated with delusions, hallucinations, and disordered thought processes. In DSM-IV-TR (American Psychiatric Association 2000), this category includes schizophrenia, schizophreniform disorder, schizoaffective disorder, delusional disorder, brief psychotic disorder, shared psychotic disorder, psychotic disorder due to a general medical condition or substance abuse, and psychotic disorder not otherwise specified. Patients with major depression and bipolar disorder can also present with psychotic symptoms, although such presentations are considered in the chapter on mood disorders.

In this chapter I explore how religious beliefs, practices, and experiences influence the clinical presentation, assessment, course and outcome of schizophrenia and other psychotic disorders. The chapter is divided into five sections that cover

1. Background information on how religious communities have historically viewed persons with schizophrenia and other psychotic disorders and how mental health professionals have viewed devoutly religious persons;
2. Phenomenology related to the presentation and prevalence of psychotic and nonpsychotic religious beliefs, experiences, and practices in persons with and without psychoses;
3. Diagnostic issues related to distinguishing culturally normative religious belief and experiences from religious delusions and hallucinations;

31

4. Religious or spiritual resources that may impact the course and outcome of schizophrenia and other psychotic disorders; and

5. Future research needed to help clarify the impact of religious beliefs, practices, and experiences on the assessment, diagnosis, and course of these disorders.

Historical Background

Although some cultures have viewed persons with psychotic disorders as possessing special spiritual powers or insights, many religions throughout history and up to the present have understood psychosis in terms of possession by spirits or demons (Koenig 2005). In order to rid the person of demons, believers have often turned to exorcism. This treatment not only has been widespread in certain fundamentalist Christian groups but also has been present at one time or another in almost every major religion (Numbers and Amundsen 1998; Sullivan 1989). One can understand how such interpretations of psychosis could have developed, given that one-third of psychotic persons (in Western countries) have delusions or hallucinations with religious content (Cothran and Harvey 1986; Siddle et al. 2002a). Members of religious communities today seldom have difficulty distinguishing normative, culturally sanctioned religious belief, experience, and practice from psychotic symptoms with religious content, which are usually viewed as abnormal and due to sickness or demonic influences.

Sigmund Freud did not believe that mental illness was the result of demonic possession or the work of spirits. Instead, he believed that religion itself was evidence for (or produced) neurosis and suggested that religious beliefs were illusions bordering on the psychotic (Freud 1927/1962). Although Freud never directly attributed psychosis to religion, he understood religious beliefs as rooted in fantasy and illusion. His negative view of religion has pervaded the mental health field over the years, as evidenced in modern writings (Ellis 1988; Watters 1992) and in the personal religious involvement of psychiatrists (Curlin et al. 2005; Neeleman and King 1993). Eventually, religion would be used to illustrate psychopathology in the psychiatric nomenclature (Larson et al. 1993). Given mental health professionals' negative views toward religion, it is not surprising that religious communities have developed antagonism toward psychiatrists, whom they see as unsympathetic to their deeply held personal beliefs and values.

Phenomenology

In this section I describe the prevalence of psychotic and nonpsychotic religious beliefs and practices in persons with and without mental illness. In psychotic patients, how common are religious delusions, how common is nonpsychotic religious involvement, and is there a relationship between the two? Is there an association between religious involvement and proneness to psychosis in persons without mental disorder? Does religious involvement precede or follow the development of psychosis, and what does this tell us about religion's role in the etiology or exacerbation of psychosis?

RELIGIOUS DELUSIONS

Delusional ideas exist on a continuum with normal beliefs, and religious beliefs lie on a continuum from normal beliefs to overvalued ideas to religious delusions (Siddle et al. 2002a). One study has suggested that religious delusions result from a combination of overactivity of the left temporal lobe and underactivity of the left occipital lobe (Puri et al. 2001).

The prevalence of religious delusions in psychotic persons varies depending on geographical location (7% in Japan and 80% in Afro-Caribbean populations), type of psychotic disorder, and how religious delusions are defined.

United States

A small study of 41 patients with schizophrenia or mania admitted to a state psychiatric facility in New York reported that 13 had religious delusions—39% with schizophrenia (9 of 23 patients) and 22% (4 of 18 patients) with mania (Cothran and Harvey 1986). In a study of 1,136 psychiatric inpatients in Kansas City, Missouri; Pittsburgh, Pennsylvania; and Worcester, Massachusetts, Appelbaum et al. (1999) identified 328 patients who were possibly or definitely delusional: 93 had religious delusions (28% of those with delusions, 8% of all patients). Religious delusions were most common in patients with schizophrenia: 36% of those with delusions and 25% of all patients with schizophrenia. Religious delusions were next most common in bipolar disorder: 33% of those with delusions and 15% of all patients with bipolar disorder. Of all delusion types, religious delusions were the most pervasive and held with the greatest conviction.

Great Britain

In the largest and most detailed study to date in Great Britain, researchers examined the prevalence of religious delusions among 193 inpatients with schizophrenia (Siddle et al. 2002a). A total of 45 patients (24%) had religious delusions using strict criteria (Sims 1995). Examples of delusions (in order of frequency) were hearing a voice or other hallucination attributed to God or the devil; believing oneself to be God, Jesus, or an angel; and believing that one was possessed by the devil or demons. Subjects with religious delusions had more severe symptoms, especially hallucinations and bizarre delusions, poorer functioning, longer duration of illness, and were on more antipsychotic medication compared with patients with nonreligious delusions.

Western Versus Non-Western Countries

Are religious delusions in Western countries more common than in non-Western ones, and does the content of religious delusions reflect the local religion? One small study of four Chinese patients with schizophrenia in Hong Kong found that the content of delusions and hallucinations reflected Chinese religious beliefs involving Buddhist gods, Taoist gods, historical heroic gods, and ancestor worship (Yip 2003).

In a larger and more systematic study that compared delusions in 126 Austrian versus 108 Pakistani patients with schizophrenia, researchers found significantly more grandiose, religious, and guilt delusions in Austrian patients (largely Christian) than in Pakistani patients (largely Muslim) (Stompe et al. 1999). In the largest study to date outside the United States, investigators compared the delusions of 324 inpatients with schizophrenia in Japan with those of 101 similar patients in Austria and 150 in Germany (Tateyama et al. 1998). Themes of persecution and religious themes of guilt/sin were more common among patients in Austria and Germany than in Japan (21% vs. 7%, respectively), whereas delusions of reference such as "being slandered" were more common in Japan, where shame plays a more dominant role in the culture than religion. These results were confirmed in a study of 429 hospitalized patients with schizophrenia in Japan that involved 95 psychiatric hospitals in a nationwide multicenter field trial (Kitamura et al. 1998). Religious delusions were present in 11% of patients; this tied tactile hallucinations for the *lowest prevalence* among 26 positive symptoms. Delusions of reference (such as being slandered), however, were present in 74% of patients.

Summary

In the United States religious delusions are present in about 25%–39% of patients with schizophrenia and about 15%–22% of those with mania/bipolar disorder. In Great Britain and Europe, about 21%–24% of patients with schizophrenia have religious delusions, and in Japan the rate is 7%–11%. The content of religious delusions appears to reflect the local religious/cultural environment. Research in the United States has found that religious delusions are pervasive and held with great conviction. In the United Kingdom, schizophrenic persons with religious delusions have more positive symptoms, poorer functioning, and require more antipsychotic medication (based on one study). In Japan, religious delusions are much less common and cluster together with grandiose delusions.

NONPSYCHOTIC RELIGIOUS ACTIVITY

How common are nonpsychotic religious beliefs, activities, and experiences among those with schizophrenia and other psychotic disorders compared with those without mental disorder? In their study of 41 psychotic patients with schizophrenia or mania in New York, Cothran and Harvey (1986) found that those with religious delusions reported higher overall religiosity but had fewer fundamentalist beliefs and were less involved in religious communities compared with nondelusional patients or normal control subjects. At least one other study in the United States (Ohio) has also reported a positive association between religious activity and severity of religious delusions (Getz et al. 2001).

Studies in Great Britain have consistently found a cross-sectional association between religious involvement and psychotic symptoms. For example, in a small case-control study of 21 psychotic outpatients with schizophrenia, 52 depressed or suicidal psychiatric outpatients, and 26 orthopedic control subjects in London, investigators found that patients with schizophrenia reported more religious experiences compared with depressed or orthopedic patients (48% and 38% vs. 17%, respectively) (Neeleman and Lewis 1994). These findings were consistent with the results of an earlier study in London that found a positive relationship between religiousness and schizotypal thinking in a sample of 67 patients with schizophrenia (Feldman and Rust 1989). Finally, in the most detailed religious evaluation to date, Siddle et al. (2002a) found a positive correlation between religious delusions and religious activity on cross-sectional analysis of 193 schizophrenic inpatients in Great Britain.

Despite these positive correlations between psychotic patients and religious activity, investigators may have had a hard time distinguishing psychotic from nonpsychotic religious beliefs, activities, and experiences. Interestingly, during a 1-month course of hospitalization and treatment, Siddle et al. (2002b) reported that patients' need for religion, faith, and God and their concern about religion for the benefit of others declined slightly (differences were small but statistically significant).

PERSONS WITHOUT MENTAL ILLNESS

Is religious involvement associated with more or fewer psychotic-like symptoms in persons without diagnosed mental illness? Studies of nonclinical samples of teenagers and adults in Great Britain shed further light on the relationship between religiousness and psychosis. One such study examined the association between religiosity and schizotypal thinking in 492 British teenagers (Joseph and Diduca 2001). In the overall sample, scores on a Christian attitude scale were correlated with higher scores on a perceptual aberration scale but with lower scores on magical ideation and impulsive nonconformity (other schizotypal symptoms). The results differed by gender. Among boys, there was a significant positive association between Christian attitudes and magical ideation, but among girls there was a significant negative association between Christian attitudes and impulsive nonconformity. Researchers concluded that religiosity was associated with greater psychosis-proneness in boys, but less psychosis-proneness in girls.

These findings replicated an earlier British study of the relationship between religious orientation and psychosis-proneness among 195 university students ages

18–49 years (Maltby et al. 2000). In that study, intrinsic religiosity was associated with more borderline personality traits in men but not women. In the most recent study by these investigators of 308 English people aged 20–59 years, intrinsic religiosity was found to be related to *lower* (not higher) levels of schizotypal thinking in the overall sample, but this inverse relationship was stronger in women than in men (Maltby and Day 2002). Finally, Feldman and Rust (1989) reported significantly less schizotypal thinking among those who were more religious when studying a sample of 140 British adults without mental health problems (but as reported earlier, more schizotypal thinking in religious patients with schizophrenia). Again, however, all of these studies were cross-sectional, precluding any causal inferences.

CAUSAL DIRECTION

What is the causal direction of the relationship between religious activity and psychosis? Do psychotic symptoms precede or follow an increase in religiousness? As noted above, most studies are cross-sectional and thus tell us little about the order of causation. Whether or not religion causes psychosis may also depend on the type of religion and the suddenness or speed at which religious convictions develop.

Type of Religion

There is some evidence from case reports that manic episodes may be induced by religious practices such as Eastern meditation (Yorston 2001). Systematic research studies provide further information. Investigators compared the strength of religious belief between 121 nonpsychotic and 88 psychotic inpatients at a psychiatric facility in Illinois (Armstrong et al. 1962). Religious beliefs were stronger in nonpsychotic patients versus psychotic patients among Catholics and Protestants, but stronger in psychotic than nonpsychotic patients among Unitarians. Ullman (1988) reported similar findings in a small sample that compared Jewish and Catholic converts to Baha'i and Hare Krishna converts. Examining 10 converts each to Judaism, Catholicism, Baha'i, and the Hare Krishna faith, Ullman found that Baha'i and Hare Krishna converts were significantly more likely to report a history of a psychotic episode requiring hospitalization (25% vs. 5%) and to report a chaotic lifestyle prior to conversion (75% vs. 40%).

A third systematic study compared delusional thinking in 142 Hare Krishnas, Druids, Christians, nonreligious people, and psychotic inpatients. Hare Krishnas and Druids scored higher in delusional thinking than either Christians or nonreligious persons and could not be distinguished from psychotic inpatients. Finally, a study of patients with first-onset schizophrenia from four ethnic groups in Great Britain (Trinidadian, London white, London Asian, and London African-Caribbean) found that these patients were likely to have recently converted to a new religious faith in order to regain self-control as their self-concept began to change with the onset of their illness (Bhugra 2002). Rather than indicating that involvement in a particular religion may lead to psychosis, this suggests that psychosis itself may precipitate a change in affiliation to a less traditional religious group.

Religious Conversion

Information on the causal relationship between religion and psychosis may be obtained by studying the psychiatric symptoms surrounding religious conversion. Besides conversion to nontraditional religious groups as discussed earlier, the intense psychological experience associated with religious conversion in some well-established traditions may play a role in precipitating psychosis in vulnerable individuals (Sedman and Hopkinson 1966). For example, John Cuidad (considered the patron saint of psychiatric nurses) and Anton Boisen (founder of Clinical Pastoral Education) experienced episodes of psychosis requiring hospitalization immediately following their dramatic religious conversions (Koenig 2005).

More important than the fact of religious conversion may be the speed at which conversion takes place. There is some evidence that sudden religious conversion increases the risk of a psychotic episode (Wootton and Allen 1983). Over a century ago, William James (1902) wrote that sudden conversion was more often seen in the "sick soul" than in the "healthy minded." An individual's intrinsic vulnerability to psychotic illness, then, may predispose to sudden religious conversion, rather than sudden conversion leading to psychosis. James' ideas were based almost entirely on clinical experience or case reports rather than systematic research.

Religious conversion does not always occur during a time of emotional stress or psychological vulnerability, and often may be precipitated by much more mundane social events. In perhaps the largest systematic study to date, Heirich (1977) studied the factors associated with religious conversion in a sample of 152 recently converted Catholic Pentecostals in Ann Arbor, Michigan, compared with 158 control subjects. Life stress and emotional problems among converts were not significantly different from that in nonconverted control subjects. Instead, most relevant in bringing about conversion were discussions with friends, relatives, or religious professionals. Bear in mind that Heirich's sample consisted of healthy persons without mental illness.

Other Research

Early reports in the clinical literature, based largely on individual case studies, suggested that religious beliefs were particularly common prior to the onset of schizophrenia (Margolis and Elifson 1983; Spero 1983). However, systematic research reveals otherwise. Wilson et al. (1983) compared the religious histories of 72 inpatients with schizophrenia at two psychiatric hospitals in North Carolina with those of 109 healthy control subjects. Patients with schizophrenia were actually less likely to have a history of religious conversion experiences than healthy control subjects. In another study of 63 persons without psychiatric illness, Wilson (1972) reported that religious conversion was associated with personality integration, increased ability to communicate with others, decreased use of alcohol, and decreased symptoms of depression, anxiety, confusion, and anger, but not psychiatric decompensation.

Other studies of persons with schizophrenia suggest an increase in religious activity *following* a first psychotic breakdown. Unfortunately, the methodology used in these studies seldom allows detailed pinpointing of when an increase in religiousness occurred in relationship to the onset of psychotic illness. In one Austrian study of 639 first-time admissions for patients with delusions (Gutierrez-Lobos et al. 2001), the investigators reported that delusions with religious content were more common among patients with schizophrenia than in those with delusions resulting from other psychiatric disorders (as other researchers have documented—see "Religious Delusions" earlier in this chapter). In research conducted in India, a quarter of patients with schizophrenia (22%–27%) reported an increase in religious activity following diagnosis (Bhugra et al. 1999; Indian Council of Medical Research 1988). Does this indicate an increased turning to religion to cope with the stress of schizophrenic symptoms in a highly religious population (India)? Do areas of the brain responsible for religious or spiritual activities become more active as a physiological response to brain changes that occur with the onset of schizophrenia? Can religious activity stimulate brain activity that leads to psychosis in vulnerable persons? The answers to such questions remain largely unknown and will depend on future research.

Summary

Cross-sectional studies of patients with schizophrenia, especially those in Great Britain, suggest a positive association between religious activity and psychotic symptoms in persons with psychiatric illness. When studying community populations without diagnosed mental illness, most investigators do not find an association between psychosis-proneness and religion, although the findings are influenced by gender in some studies, with religiousness being associated with more psychosis-proneness in men but less among women. Involvement in nontraditional religious groups appears to be associated with a greater likelihood of psychosis than involvement in traditional religious groups, although psychosis may stimulate a switching of affiliation. Finally, religious conversion—especially when sudden and dramatic—has been associated with the onset of psychotic illness, and an increase in religious activity has been noted around the time of first psychotic break, especially in patients with schizophrenia. Carefully done studies that pinpoint the time relationship between the onset of psychotic symptoms and increase in religious activity are needed.

Diagnostic Issues: Distinguishing Religion From Psychosis

Not only are religious delusions common in persons with psychosis, they can also be associated with poor outcomes and risk of self-harm. Cases have been reported of psychotic persons who, carrying out Matthew 5:29–30, gouged out both eyes, castrated themselves, or amputated a limb (Erol and Kaptanoglu 2000; Favazza 1989; Kushner 1967; Moselhy et al. 1995). A particularly disturbing case recently involved a mother from McKinney, Texas, who killed her baby daughter by cutting off both arms, impelled by psychotic delusions and hallucinations to follow this scripture (Whitley 2006). There is little doubt that religious delusions can have terrible consequences—at least in selected cases. Cothran and Harvey (1986) commented that the religiosity of patients with religious delusions was of a different nature than the religiousness of normal control subjects.

In highly religious areas of the world, such as the United States, the ability to distinguish religious beliefs that are normal for a person's culture and social group from those that suggest a mental disorder in need of treatment is of considerable clinical importance. The border between fantasy and reality is often elusive, especially when one is dealing with individual beliefs whose truth cannot be objectively verified.

The following study illustrates how difficult it may be to separate religious delusions and hallucinations from normal religious experiences. Stifler et al. (1993) compared 30 psychiatric inpatients with psychotic disorders and religious delusions with 30 senior members of contemplative/mystical groups and 30 hospital staff members in Danville, Virginia, based on scores obtained on the Hood Mysticism Scale. Although staff subjects could be distinguished from mystics and patients with psychosis, mystics could not be distinguished from those with psychosis based on their scores alone. Although mystical experiences may be similar between patients with psychosis and deeply spiritual normal subjects, other differences exist that distinguish these individuals.

Pierre (2001) provided several suggestions to differentiate religious delusions and hallucinations from normal religious experiences. First, he pointed out that entire delusional subcultures exist and that this must be taken into consideration when evaluating a patient's beliefs. Second, he emphasized that religious delusions, like other psychotic symptoms, can be a consequence of neurological lesions (often temporal lobe) that should always be ruled out. Third, he noted that it is helpful to have input from religious professionals who are more familiar with the patient's religious beliefs than the clinician, and that members of the patient's religious community usually have no difficulty distinguishing those with religious delusions from normal persons in the congregation (except in delusional subcultures). Finally, he pointed out that for religious delusions to be pathological, they must have an impact on the patient's social or occupational functioning; if functioning is un-impaired, then the religious belief—no matter how bizarre—is not pathological. Of relevance in terms of diagnostic classification, Pierre noted that although DSM-III-R (American Psychiatric Association 1987) and earlier versions tended to make normal religious beliefs pathological, DSM-IV (American Psychiatric Association 1994) perhaps went too far the other way, overrestricting the requirements necessary to make a diagnosis of religious delusions.

In addition, Lukoff (1985) noted that the person with psychosis does not usually have insight into the incredible nature of his or her claims and may even embellish the account in a self-promoting way. This contrasts with the nonpsychotic person who often readily admits the extraordinary or unbelievable nature of the things that he or she is claiming. Lukoff also emphasized the consequences of the psy-chotic person's experiences: loss of the ability to hold down a job, legal problems with police or due to failure to fulfill obligations, homicidal or suicidal threats and behaviors, and problems with thinking clearly (with conceptual disorganization). Summarizing the important distinctions, Lukoff stated: "When persons show widespread deficiencies in handling the everyday commonsense tasks involved in independent living combined with severe inability to establish 'intersubjective re-ality' with others in their psychosocial environment, they meet the criteria for a psychotic state" (pp. 165–166). In contrast, a person having spiritual or mystical experiences usually over time has a positive outcome in terms of psychological and social growth and maturity. However, Lukoff readily acknowledged that there may be times when mystical and psychotic states overlap so extensively that they may be hard to tease apart without extensive follow-up.

SUMMARY

There appears to be a convergence of opinion by experts in the field that there are specific criteria that can be used to separate persons with religious, spiritual, or mystical experiences from those with psychotic experiences symptomatic of un-derlying severe mental illness. The religious/spiritual person without severe mental illness usually recognizes the extraordinary or unbelievable nature of their experi-ences (insight), shares their experiences or ideas with another group of people (in-tersubjective reality), has no disturbances in thought processes (conceptual disorganization, looseness of associations, thought blocking), is able to handle ev-ery day commonsense tasks (maintain a job, stay out of legal problems), is not dan-gerous to others or self (low risk), and usually has a positive outcome over time. Bear in mind, however, that persons with psychotic disorders may have *healthy* re-ligious/spiritual ideas and experiences that can be enriching for them and their lives.

Impact of Religion on Course and Outcome

Although religious delusions may be correlated with degree of religious involvement, whether a psychotic patient either 1) is actively religious or 2) has religious delusions may influence prognosis in different ways.

RELIGIOUS DELUSIONS

A number of studies have reported worse long-term prognosis for patients with schizophrenia with religious delusions (Doering et al. 1998; Thara and Eaton 1996), although this is not always the case (McCabe et al. 1972; Siddle et al. 2004). For example, the most detailed study of religious activity and religious delusions in schizophrenia to date ($N = 155$) did not find that either patients with religious delusions ($n = 40$) or patients who described themselves as religious ($n = 106$) responded less well to 4 weeks of treatment than other patients (Siddle et al. 2004). However, as noted before, patients with religious delusions had more severe illness and greater functional disability than other patients. Thus, further long-term studies are needed to determine whether patients with religious delusions respond less well to treatment than other psychotic patients.

NONPSYCHOTIC RELIGIOUS ACTIVITY AS A RESOURCE

At least four longitudinal studies in patients with schizophrenia suggest that certain types of religious activity predict a *better* prognosis over time. First, in their follow-up study of 210 patients with schizophrenia, Schofield et al. (1954) identified 13 factors associated with a good prognosis, one of which was regular church attendance. In a second study, 128 African-American patients with schizophrenia consecutively admitted to seven hospitals and mental health centers in Missouri were assessed on admission, discharge, and 12 months later or on rehospitalization (whichever came first). Religious involvement at baseline was examined in relationship to frequency of rehospitalization during follow-up (Chu and Klein 1985). Patients from urban areas ($n = 65$) were less likely to be rehospitalized if their families encouraged religious worship during the hospital stay. Both urban and rural patients were also less likely to be hospitalized if their family was Catholic and were more likely to be hospitalized if they had no religious affiliation.

In a third study, conducted in India, researchers followed 386 outpatients with schizophrenia for 2 years, examining factors predicting readmission for psychotic exacerbations (Verghese et al. 1989). This is the largest study to date of religious influences on the course of schizophrenia. Investigators found that patients who reported a decrease in religious activities at baseline experienced a more rapid deterioration over time, prompting researchers to conclude that "Religiosity is important in Indian culture and the increase in religiosity that was related to better outcomes in the present study could be a means of effectively handling the anxiety of the patient" (p. 502).

Finally, Jarbin and von Knorring (2004) followed 88 patients in Sweden with adolescent-onset psychotic disorders (the majority with schizophrenia or schizo-affective disorder) for 10.6 years; 25% made suicide attempts during follow-up. Factors *inversely* associated with attempted suicide on follow-up were satisfaction with safety, family relations, health, and religion. When concurrent symptoms of anxiety and depression were controlled for, only satisfaction with religious belief remained a significant inverse predictor. How might religious belief/involvement serve as a resource to impact the course of schizophrenia and other psychotic disorders in a positive way?

RELIGION AS A COPING BEHAVIOR

The person with schizophrenia or other psychotic disorder has a lot to cope with, and it is not surprising that many end up committing suicide. It is also easy to see why some turn to religion for comfort and hope, when few other options exist.

In a small study of 28 patients with schizophrenia and other psychotic disorders (mostly schizophrenia) living in Maryland, Lindgren and Coursey (1995) found that 47% indicated that spirituality/religion helped "a great deal," 57% prayed every day, and 76% thought about God or spiritual/religious matters daily. In another study of 406 patients with schizophrenia and other psychotic disorders at a Los Angeles County mental health facility, more than 80% indicated they used religion to cope (Tepper et al. 2001). In this study, the majority of patients spent nearly half of their total coping time in religious activities such as prayer. These findings prompted investigators to conclude that religion serves as a "pervasive and potentially effective method of coping for persons with mental illness, thus warranting its integration into psychiatric and psychological practice" (p. 660).

Other studies support this conclusion. Sullivan (1993) interviewed 40 psychiatric patients in Springfield, Missouri, finding that nearly half (48%) indicated that spiritual beliefs and practices were essential to their coping with mental illness. Likewise, in an Internet survey of persons with severe mental illness, Russinova et al. (2002) found spiritual practices common among alternative health practices used. Of the 157 individuals who responded, 40 had schizophrenia, 70 had bipolar disorder, and 39 had major depression. The majority of patients with schizophrenia (58%) and major depression (56%) indicated that the most common alternative health practice that helped them to cope was religious/spiritual activity. Even among those with bipolar disorder, "meditation" was the only other alternative practice that was more common than religious/spiritual activity (54% vs. 41%).

A study in Great Britain assessed importance of religious faith and religious coping in 52 consecutively admitted psychotic patients (Kirov et al. 1998). The majority (70%) indicated they were religious and 22% reported that religion was the *most important* aspect of their lives. Two-thirds of these patients (61%) said they used religion to cope with their mental illness, and 30% said that their religiousness had increased since the onset of their illness. Researchers reported that those who indicated they used religion to cope had better insight into their illness and, interestingly, were more compliant with antipsychotic medication.

The research findings, however, are not always positive. In a small qualitative study conducted in Sioux Center, Iowa, researchers did not find that the faith community played much of a role in the coping of 17 people with severe and persistent mental illness (Bussema and Bussema 2000). Many indicated that they felt estranged from their religious communities, whom they did not view as supportive. Even in this study, however, the majority indicated that their personal religious beliefs were important in providing a sense of meaning and hope.

There is also evidence that the way in which people use religion to cope may influence its helpfulness. Yangarber-Hicks (2003) examined relationships between religious coping styles, adaptive functioning, and recovery activities in persons with severe and persistent mental illness living in Cincinnati, Ohio. On the one hand, those who coped using a "collaborative/deferring" approach (i.e., problem solving through a partnership with God and at times deferring to God) reported higher quality of life and more frequent involvement in recovery-enhancing rehabilitation activities. On the other hand, a coping style that was self-directed without God's help or one that involved pleading to God for direct intervention was associated with worse outcomes.

The type of psychotic disorder may also influence the use of religion to cope. In a study of 356 persons with severe and persistent mental illness, Reger and Rogers (2002) examined the differences in religious coping between individuals with schizophrenia, schizoaffective, bipolar, and depressive disorders. They reported that patients with chronic schizophrenia or schizoaffective disorder were more likely to report that religion helped them to cope. Note from an earlier section in this chapter that religious delusions were also reported to be more common in patients with schizophrenia.

Degree of religious coping may depend on what part of the world a person lives in. Wahass and Kent (1997) interviewed small samples of Western ($n=33$) and non-Western ($n=37$) patients with schizophrenia to find out about how they coped with auditory hallucinations. Investigators found that non-Western patients (from Saudi Arabia) were more likely than Western patients (from Great Britain) to use religion to cope (43% vs. 3%, respectively). Whereas Saudi patients prayed, read the Koran, or listened to religious cassettes to help, British patients depended more on distraction and other nonreligious coping behaviors.

Even in areas of the world where religious beliefs are less common, religion may still be an important source of coping for those with schizophrenia and other psychotic disorders. A study of 79 psychiatric patients in New South Wales found that 79% rated spirituality as very important, 82% thought their therapist should be aware of their spiritual beliefs, and 67% reported that spirituality helped them to cope (D'Souza 2002).

Thus, it appears that religious coping is common among persons with psychotic disorders in the United States, the Middle East, and Wales but is less common in Great Britain and Europe, although not less helpful (Kirov et al. 1998). Because all of these studies are cross-sectional, we do not know whether religion is more common in persons with schizophrenia and other psychotic disorders because it helps them to cope with their distressing symptoms, whether religion somehow contributes to the development of psychotic disorder (whether due to parental influences during childhood, destabilizing religious influences during early adulthood, or religious conversion experiences [Watters 1992]), or whether psychotic illness leads to an increase in religious activity.

In summary, although there is relatively little systematic research on the relationship between religion and psychotic disorders, the limited evidence thus far suggests that religious beliefs do not usually "cause" or worsen these disorders, but that psychosis is not uncommonly expressed in religious terms (especially in cultures where religion is widely prevalent). Religious beliefs, in fact, may help the persons with schizophrenia and other psychotic disorders to cope better, and may affect compliance, thus reducing the frequency of relapse and hospitalization. Further studies, however, are clearly needed.

Future Research

The lack of carefully designed and executed research on religion, spirituality, and psychotic disorders (phenomenology, diagnosis, impact on course and outcome) is a major barrier to diagnostic assessment and clinical applications. There is almost no research question in this area that has been adequately examined, so the possibilities in terms of future studies are almost endless and present a unique opportunity for investigators.

In order to better understand diagnostic issues related to religion and psychotic disorders, further systematic research is critical. Although a more comprehensive research agenda has been outlined elsewhere (Koenig 2005), areas in need of study can be divided into three groups: 1) presentation, 2) assessment/diagnosis, and 3) impact on course and outcome.

PRESENTATION

More information is needed on how religious delusions or hallucinations differ from the beliefs and experiences that are considered normative in a particular religious tradition and culture. A more careful description of the phenomenology (e.g., religious delusions, hallucinations) in different religious environments in the United States and around the world is needed. Specific research questions include

- How do people with schizophrenia and other psychotic disorders from different religious traditions present in terms of symptoms or experiences with religious content?
- What distinct features separate these persons demonstrating psychopathology from healthy persons in their religious tradition?
- In persons with schizophrenia and other psychotic disorders, how can one distinguish religious beliefs, practices, and experiences that have a positive impact on coping and disease course from those that negatively impact prognosis (and are part of their psychopathology)?
- How is the expression of religiousness different in persons actively symptomatic with psychotic disorders from those with psychotic disorders whose symptoms are controlled?
- What effect does treatment with antipsychotic medication have on religious beliefs, behaviors, and experiences (both "normal" and pathological ones) in persons with schizophrenia and other psychotic disorders?
- What is the relationship between religious conversion experiences and the onset of psychotic disorders? What kinds of religious conversions are linked with the precipitation of psychosis (i.e., those that are slow and gradual vs. sudden; conversion to one religious tradition vs. another; etc.)? Does a predisposition to schizophrenia and other psychotic disorders make one more likely to experience certain types of religious conversion?
- What effects do age, gender, ethnicity, and education/socioeconomic status have on the answers to these questions?
- What effects do the presence of various medical and neurological conditions have on the answers to these questions (including HIV/AIDS with and without nervous system involvement)?
- Are there specific biological and/or psychodynamic causes for religious delusions or hallucinations? (Or are these entirely culturally determined?)

ASSESSMENT AND DIAGNOSIS

Clinical measures are needed to help guide clinicians on how to assess persons with strong religious beliefs, practices, and experiences and to differentiate them from persons expressing their psychopathology in religious terms. Such tools, based on established diagnostic criteria, need to be able to separate healthy religious expressions from pathological ones when these may coexist in persons with schizophrenia and other psychotic disorders. Specific research questions are:

- Can a simple set of diagnostic criteria be identified that differentiate healthy from pathological expressions of religion, based upon long-term effects on course and outcome?
- Can a brief spiritual history be developed that operationalizes these criteria in a user-friendly format that can sort out healthy expressions of religion that can be supported and encouraged from pathological expressions that require treatment?
- Are different versions of this spiritual history needed for persons from different religious traditions (or will "one size fits all" be sufficient)?

DISEASE COURSE AND OUTCOME

Information is needed on how both pathological and nonpathological religious beliefs, practices, and experiences impact the course of schizophrenia and other psychotic disorders. Specific research questions are

- Do persons with religious delusions or hallucinations have a worse prognosis or response to treatment? How is compliance affected?
- Are there specific types of religious delusions or hallucinations that portend a particularly poor prognosis?
- What impact do "healthy" religious beliefs, practices, and experiences have on disease course/outcome for persons with schizophrenia and other psychotic disorders? Are there certain practices that are healthier than others (i.e., involvement in religious community vs. private religious activities)? Are certain religious practices synergistic with biological treatments in terms of efficacy?
- Is the impact of religious delusions or healthy religious beliefs on disease course stronger for certain psychotic disorders more than for others (e.g., schizophrenia vs. bipolar mania vs. delusional disorder)?
- How does religious involvement affect the risk of comorbid substance abuse in persons with schizophrenia and other psychotic disorders? How does it affect the course of illness in this population?
- Can sensitive and sensible spiritual interventions be developed (specific for each religious tradition) and tested for efficacy (improvement) and side effects (worsening psychosis)?
- Does removal of any religious influences or symbols during the acute treatment phase facilitate or hinder recovery of the religious patients with schizophrenia and other psychotic disorders?

Although much further research is needed to help clarify how religion affects the presentation, diagnosis, course, and outcome of schizophrenia and other psychotic disorders, we already know quite a bit about this area, enough to at least make some preliminary first steps.

Summary and Conclusions

Religious content is present in the psychotic symptoms of a significant minority of patients with psychotic disorders. Religious beliefs and experiences of actively psychotic persons are different in nature from those of nonpsychotic persons, and there are ways to identify when religious expressions become pathological. There may be an increase in religiousness near the time of illness onset, and religious conversion, particularly if sudden, may increase the risk of psychotic decompensation in vulnerable persons. However, it is known that persons with schizophrenia and other psychotic disorders commonly use religion to cope with the stress of their illness, which may confuse the picture. This is especially true in religious areas of the world and for members of certain religious groups. There is some evidence that religious beliefs and activity may reduce frequency of hospital admission, improve compliance with medication, and reduce suicide rates.

Research on religion and mental health in persons with severe mental illness has lagged far behind that in nonpsychiatric or medical populations. This represents a serious gap that interferes with our ability to differentiate psychotic symptoms from normal religious beliefs and experiences and clouds our understanding of how religion can be a resource or a risk factor in this population.

Proposed Statement for DSM-V Section on Schizophrenia and Other Psychotic Disorders: Religious/Spiritual Considerations

Religious/spiritual ideas that appear delusional in one setting (e.g., sorcery and witchcraft) may be considered normal or even encouraged in another. Likewise, visual or auditory hallucinations with a religious content may be a normal part of religious experience (e.g., seeing the Virgin Mary or hearing God's voice). The diagnosis of schizophrenia or other psychotic disorders should never be made in the absence of other symptoms and signs of the diagnosis. The religious/spiritual person without schizophrenia usually recognizes the extraordinary or unbelievable nature of their experiences (insight), shares their experiences or ideas with another group of people (intersubjective reality), has no disturbances in thought processes (conceptual disorganization, looseness of associations, thought blocking), is able to handle everyday commonsense tasks (maintain a job, stay out of legal problems), is not dangerous to others or self (low risk), and usually has a positive outcome over time. Persons with schizophrenia, however, may have healthy religious/spiritual ideas and experiences. Prospective studies suggest that religious/spiritual activities (religious affiliation, worship, regular church attendance, satisfaction with religious belief) predict fewer admissions for psychotic exacerbations, less rapid deterioration over time, and reduce the risk of suicide in persons with schizophrenia. In contrast, religious delusions (held by 25%–39% of psychotic patients with schizophrenia) may portend a worse prognosis, although further research is needed.

References

American Psychiatric Association; Diagnostic and Statistical Manual of Mental Disorders, 3rd Edition Revised. Washington, DC, American Psychiatric Association, 1987

American Psychiatric Association: Diagnostic and Statistical Manual of Mental Disorders, 4th Edition. Washington, DC, American Psychiatric Association, 1994

American Psychiatric Association: Diagnostic and Statistical Manual of Mental Disorders, 4th Edition, Text Revision. Washington, DC, American Psychiatric Association, 2000

Appelbaum PS, Robbins PC, Roth LH: Dimensional approach to delusions: comparison across types and diagnoses. Am J Psychiatry 156:1938–1943, 1999

Armstrong RG, Larsen GL, Mourer SA: Religious attitudes and emotional adjustment. J Psychol Stud 13:35–47, 1962

Bhugra D: Self-concept: Psychosis and attraction of new religious movements. Mental Health, Religion and Culture 5:239–252, 2002

Bhugra D, Corridan B, Rudge S, et al: Early manifestations, personality traits and pathways into care for Asian and white first-onset cases of schizophrenia. Soc Psychiatry Psychiatr Epidemiol 34:595–599, 1999

Bussema KE, Bussema EF: Is there a balm in Gilead? The implications of faith in coping with a psychiatric disability. Psychiatr Rehab J 24:117–124, 2000

Chu CC, Klein HE: Psychosocial and environmental variables in outcome of black schizophrenics. J Natl Med Assn 77:793–796, 1985

Cothran MM, Harvey PD: Delusional thinking in psychotics: correlates of religious content. Psychol Rep 58:191–199, 1986

Curlin FA, Lantos JD, Roach CJ, et al: Religious characteristics of U.S. physicians: a national survey. J Gen Intern Med 20:629–634, 2005

D'Souza R: Do patients expect psychiatrists to be interested in spiritual issues? Australas Psychiatry 10:44–47, 2002

Doering S, Muller E, Kopcke W, et al: Predictors of relapse and rehospitalisation in schizophrenia and schizoaffective disorder. Schizophr Bull 24:87–98, 1998

Ellis A: Is religiosity pathological? Free Inq 18:27–32, 1988

Erol S, Kaptanoglu C: Self-inflicted bilateral eye injury by a schizophrenic patient. Gen Hosp Psychiatry 22:215–216, 2000

Favazza AR: Why patients mutilate themselves. Hosp Community Psychiatry 40:137–145, 1989

Feldman J, Rust J: Religiosity, schizotypal thinking, and schizophrenia. Psychol Rep 65:587–593, 1989

Freud S: Future of an Illusion (1927), in Standard Edition of the Complete Psychological Works of Sigmund Freud. Translated by Strachey J. London, England, Hogarth, 1962, p 43

Getz GE, Fleck D, Strakowski SM: Frequency and severity of religious delusions in Christian patients with psychosis. Psychiatry Res 103:87–91, 2001

Gutierrez-Lobos K, Schmid-Siegel B, Bankier B, et al: Delusions in first-admitted patients: gender, themes and diagnoses. Psychopathology 34:1–7, 2001

Heirich M: Change of heart: a test of some widely held theories about religious conversion. Am J Sociol 83:653–680, 1977

Indian Council of Medical Research: Multicentre Collaborative Study of Factors Associated With the Course and Outcome of Schizophrenia. New Delhi, Indian Council of Medical Research, 1988

James W: The Varieties of Religious Experience. New York, The New American Library, 1902

Jarbin H, von Knorring AL: Suicide and suicide attempts in adolescent-onset psychotic disorders. Nord J Psychiatry 58:115–123, 2004

Joseph S, Diduca D: Schizotypy and religiosity in 13–18 year old school pupils. Mental Health, Religion and Culture 4:63–69, 2001

Kirov G, Kemp R, Kirov K, et al: Religious faith after psychotic illness. Psychopathology 31:234–245, 1998

Kitamura T, Okazaki Y, Funinawa A, et al: Dimensions of schizophrenic positive symptoms: an exploratory factor analysis. Eur Arch Psychiatry Clin Neurosci 248:130–135, 1998

Koenig HG: Faith and Mental Health. Philadelphia, PA, Templeton Foundation Press, 2005

Kushner AW: Two cases of auto-castration due to religious delusions. Br J Med Psychol 40:293–298, 1967

Larson DB, Thielman SB, Greenwold MA, et al: Religious content in the DSM-III-R glossary of technical terms. Am J Psychiatry 150:1884–1885, 1993

Lindgren KN, Coursey RD: Spirituality and serious mental illness: a two-part study. Psychosocial Rehabilitation Journal 18:93–111, 1995

Lukoff D: The diagnosis of mystical experiences with psychotic features. Journal of Transpersonal Psychology 17:155–181, 1985

Maltby J, Day L: Religious experience, religious orientation and schizotypy. Mental Health, Religion and Culture 5:163–174, 2002

Maltby J, Garner I, Lewis CA, et al: Religious orientation and schizotypal traits. Pers Individ Dif 28:143–151, 2000

Margolis RD, Elifson KW: Validation of a typology of religious experience and its relation to the psychotic experience. J Psychol Theol 11:135–141, 1983

McCabe MS, Fowler RC, Cadoret RJ, et al: Symptom differences in schizophrenia with good and poor prognosis. Am J Psychiatry 128:49–63, 1972

Moselhy HF, McKnight A, MacMillan J: The challenge of self-mutilation: a case report and review of literature. Eur J Psychiatry 9:161–165, 1995

Neeleman J, King MB: Psychiatrists' religious attitudes in relation to their clinical practice: a survey of 231 psychiatrists. Acta Psychiatr Scand 88:420–424, 1993

Neeleman J, Lewis G: Religious identity and comfort beliefs in three groups of psychiatric patients and a group of medical controls. Int J Soc Psychiatry 40:124–134, 1994

Numbers RL, Amundsen DW: Caring and Curing: Health and Medicine in the Western Religious Traditions. Baltimore, MD, Johns Hopkins University Press, 1998

Pierre JM: Faith or delusion: at the crossroads of religion and psychosis. J Psychiatr Pract 7:163–172, 2001

Puri BK, Lekh SK, Nijran KS, et al: SPECT neuroimaging in schizophrenia with religious delusions. Int J Psychophysiol 40:143–148, 2001

Reger GM, Rogers SA: Diagnostic differences in religious coping among individuals with persistent mental illness. Journal of Psychology and Christianity 21:341–348, 2002

Russinova Z, Wewiorski NJ, Cash D: Use of alternative health care practices by persons with serious mental illness: perceived benefits. Am J Publ Health 92:1600–1603, 2002

Schofield W, Hathaway SR, Hastings DW, et al: Prognostic factors in schizophrenia. Journal of Consultation Psychology 18:155–166, 1954

Sedman G, Hopkinson G: The psychopathology of mystical and religious conversion experiences in psychiatric patients. Confin Psychiatr 9:1–19, 1966

Siddle R, Haddock G, Tarrier N, et al: Religious delusions in patients admitted to hospital with schizophrenia. Soc Psychiatry Psychiatr Epidemiol 37:130–138, 2002a

Siddle R, Haddock G, Tarrier N, et al: The validation of a religiosity measure for individuals with schizophrenia. Mental Health, Religion and Culture 5:267–284, 2002b

Siddle R, Haddock G, Tarrier N, et al: Religious beliefs and religious delusions: response to treatment in schizophrenia. Mental Health, Religion and Culture 7:211–223, 2004

Sims A: Symptoms in the Mind: an Introduction to Descriptive Psychopathology, 3rd Edition. London, England, WB Saunders, 1995

Spero MH: Religious patients in psychotherapy. Br J Med Psychol 56:287–291, 1983

Stifler KR, Greer J, Sneck W, et al: An empirical investigation of the discriminability of reported mystical experiences among religious contemplatives, psychotic inpatients, and normal adults. J Sci Study Relig 32:366–372, 1993

Stompe T, Friedman A, Ortwein G, et al: Comparison of delusions among schizophrenics in Austria and in Pakistan. Psychopathology 32:225–234, 1999

Sullivan LE: Healing and Restoring: Health and Medicine in the World's Religious Traditions. New York, Macmillan, 1989

Sullivan WP: "It helps me to be a whole person": the role of spirituality among the mentally challenged. Psychosocial Rehabilitation Journal 16:125–134, 1993

Tateyama M, Asai M, Hashimoto M, et al: Transcultural study of schizophrenic delusions: Tokyo versus Vienna versus Tubingen (Germany). Psychopathology 31:59–68, 1998

Tepper L, Rogers SA, Coleman EM, et al: The prevalence of religious coping among persons with persistent mental illness. Psychiatr Serv 52:660–665, 2001

Thara R, Eaton WW: Outcome of schizophrenia: the Madras longitudinal study. Aust N Z J Psychiatry 30:516–522, 1996

Ullman C: Psychological well-being among converts in traditional and nontraditional religious groups. Psychiatry 51:312–322, 1988

Verghese A, John JK, Rajkumar S, et al: Factors associated with the course and outcome of schizophrenia in India: results of a two-year multicentre follow-up study. Br J Psychiatry 154:499–503, 1989

Wahass S, Kent G: Coping with auditory hallucinations: a cross-cultural comparison between Western (British) and non-Western (Saudi Arabian) patients. J Nerv Ment Dis 185:664–668, 1997

Watters W: Deadly Doctrine: Health, Illness, and Christian God-Talk. Buffalo, NY, Prometheus Books, 1992

Whitley G: The Devil and Doyle Davidson: did a preacher's obsessions push Dena Schlosser over the edge? Dallas Observer, May 18, 2006. Available online http://www.dallasobserver.com/Issues/2006-05-18/news/feature_full.html. Accessed July 9, 2006

Wilson WP: Mental health benefits of religious salvation. Dis Nerv Syst 36:382–386, 1972

Wilson WP, Larson DB, Meier PD: Religious life of schizophrenics. Southern Med J 76:1096–1100, 1983

Wootton RJ, Allen DF: Dramatic religious conversion and schizophrenic decompensation. J Relig Health 22:212–220, 1983

Yangarber-Hicks NI: Religious coping styles and recovery from serious mental illness. Dissertation Abstracts International: Section B: the Sciences and Engineering 63:3487, 2003

Yip K: Traditional Chinese religious beliefs and superstitions in delusions and hallucinations of Chinese schizophrenic patients. Int J Soc Psychiatry 49:97–111, 2003

Yorston GA: Mania precipitated by meditation: a case report and literature review. Mental Health, Religion and Culture 4:209–213, 2001

Commentary 2A

COMMENTARY ON "SCHIZOPHRENIA AND OTHER PSYCHOTIC DISORDERS"

Armando R. Favazza, M.D., M.P.H.

Dr. Koenig's chapter takes on the daunting task of discerning the relationship between religious beliefs, practices, and experience and the clinical presentation, assessment, course, and outcome of persons with schizophrenia and other psychotic disorders. I use the word *daunting* because the literature is relatively sparse and inconclusive. Koenig clearly writes on multiple occasions about "weak evidence," "some evidence," cross-sectional studies that "tell us little about the order of causation," individual case studies, findings that "suggest" some conclusion, unfortunate methodology, how "further studies…are clearly needed," and that "there is almost no research question in this area that has been adequately examined."

Koenig makes too much of geography, for example, "Degree of religious coping may depend on what part of the world a person lives in," although at other times he more appropriately refers to cultural differences. Also, I had hoped that Koenig would help us make some sense of a study involving 492 British teenagers in which "In the overall sample, scores on a Christian attitude scale were correlated with higher scores on a perceptual aberration scale but with lower scores on magical ideation and impulsive nonconformity." Perceptual aberration? What exactly does this mean? There was a gender difference so that "religiosity was associated with greater psychosis-proneness in boys." Is "psychosis-proneness" a concept with proven clinical significance?

There are some unexplained concepts mentioned in the chapter. What counts as "religious activities"? The United States may be a "religious nation" from certain points of view, but from another perspective religious institutions are in trouble—for example, animosity among rival Baptist churches is at an all-time high, Presbyterians are splintering into different camps, the Catholic and Episcopalian Churches are importing priests from Africa, and half of American Jews have married outside their faith and only one-third of their children are being reared Jewish. Religion and spirituality are mentioned in many of the studies, but spirituality is a fuzzy concept that nowadays can connote anything from fervent Pentecostal worship to participating in ecological causes to tapping into vibrations that supposedly emanate from outer space or from the rocks of Sedona, Arizona.

Koenig writes of the antagonism between psychiatry and religion, but physicians, perhaps because they see so many children die and good persons suffer, have long been skeptical about religion. "Three physicians, two atheists" was a medieval aphorism. Freud's description of religion as fostering neurosis certainly has influenced psychiatric thinking, but times have changed. Nowadays psychiatrists are paid mainly to make a diagnosis, to dispense medications, and to leave therapy to other mental health professionals. In such a climate, it has been my experience that agnostic and even atheistic psychiatrists are more than willing to seek out the clergy as allies in providing care to patients and to regard church congregations as potentially healing resources. In fact, the pendulum has swung so far that many psychiatrists now regard churches as types of mental health centers. Although religious organizations may promote mental health through such activities as caring human contacts, forums for the discussion of values and behaviors, material help, praying, and moral support in times of crisis, the ultimate purposes of religion are not mental health and euthymia but rather salvation and the quest for holiness.

In my view, the most solidly established findings in Koenig's review are the following:

1. Some religious phenomena, such as seeing a vision of the Virgin Mary or hearing God call one's name, may be normal in certain cultural contexts and do not necessarily signify psychosis.
2. As opposed to psychotic persons, people who have unusual religious, spiritual, or mystical experiences have insight into the extraordinary nature of their experiences, talk about them with others, have no symptoms of a thought disorder (such as loose associations or thought blocking), are able to handle everyday tasks (hold a job, avoid legal problems), and pose no danger to themselves or others.
3. When the clinician is unsure about whether a patient is psychotic because of religious claims, the patient's peers—such as church members—should be consulted. They commonly will be able to identify the patient's behaviors as either abnormal or within the group's concept of normality.

4. Rapid conversion from a traditional religion to a cultic or somewhat "exotic" religion (such as Hare Krishna or Druidism) is usually associated with emotional turmoil and may either be caused by or result in psychosis.

5. Psychotic persons demonstrating high religiosity and concrete thinking may interpret certain biblical passages literally and may harm themselves (eye enucleation, self-castration) or others (sacrifice children).

6. Persons with schizophrenia and other psychotic disorders may have healthy religious/spiritual ideas and experiences.

Since the writing of Koenig's chapter, two articles of interest have been published based on what appears to be the same sample of 100 Swiss outpatients with psychotic disorders. In one study (Mohr et al. 2006), some subjects reported that religion instilled hope, purpose, and meaning in their lives (71%), whereas it induced spiritual despair in others (14%). Subjects also reported that religion lessened (54%) or increased (10%) psychotic symptoms, increased social integration (28%) or social isolation (3%), reduced (33%) or increased (10%) the risk of suicide attempts , reduced (14%) or increased (3%) substance abuse, and fostered adherence to (16%) or opposition to (15%) psychiatric treatment. The other study (Huguelet et al. 2006) found that psychiatrists were often unaware of their patients' religious involvements and that patients usually were reluctant to talk about religion with their psychiatrists, often for fear of being hospitalized.

References

Huguelet P, Mohr S, Borras L, et al: Spirituality and religious practices among outpatients with schizophrenia and their clinicians. Psychiatr Serv 57:366–372, 2006

Mohr S, Brandt P-Y, Borras L, et al: Toward an integration of spirituality and religiousness into the psychosocial dimension of schizophrenia. Am J Psychiatry 163:1952–1959, 2006

Commentary 2B

COMMENTARY ON "SCHIZOPHRENIA AND OTHER PSYCHOTIC DISORDERS"

Philippe Huguelet, M.D.

Commenting on a chapter written by Harold Koenig is not an easy task. Indeed, this author's comprehensive knowledge is accompanied by an outstanding capacity for clearly describing complex phenomena.

Koenig describes the phenomenology related to religious beliefs in individuals with and without psychosis. His description calls attention to the challenges clinicians face when caring for individuals with psychosis who report religious, spiritual, or mystical experiences. Koenig provides detailed descriptions of the characteristics and outcomes associated with religious delusions, as well as the role of nonpsychotic religious activities as a resource for individuals with psychosis. For all these issues, the author underscores the need for more research.

The two comments in this review, one about delusions with religious content and the other about religious/spiritual coping, lead to a common conclusion.

First, Koenig shows that religious delusions may be associated with a worse prognosis. Yet what makes delusions with religious content appear in certain individuals? Are they due to biological factors (i.e., specific neurobiological alterations), psychological factors (e.g., as an attempt to cope with unusual psychological experiences), or social factors (perhaps supported by the fact that the prevalence of delusions with religious content varies across countries and cultures) (Siddle et al. 2002)? Delusions with religious content can be observed in different disorders (e.g., manic episodes, depressive disorders) but also in various types of delusions. Recent research on medication-free individuals with schizophrenia has indicated that delusions can be separated into three distinct categories: delusions of influence (e.g., delusions of being controlled, thought withdrawal, thought insertion, mind reading), self-significance delusions (delusions of grandeur, reference, religious delusions of guilt/sin), and persecutory delusions (Kimhi et al. 2005). In fact, religious content can be found in *each* of these categories. Patients may have the conviction that they are being controlled by God or that their thoughts come from God; they may think that they *are* God; or they may be convinced that they are being persecuted by the Devil or some other religious figure. This observation provides some evidence that delusions with religious content are unlikely to reflect a unitary phenomenon with a common neurocognitive or neurobiological underpinning. Thus, they should not be considered as a special kind of delusion. Rather, delusions with religious content may be related to former personal and social experiences and thus understood in the context of a person's life and culture (Drinnan and Lavender 2006). Rhodes and Jakes (2004) suggested that religious experience represents patients' attempts to interpret their anomalous experiences—that is, a way to cope with distressing events such as hallucinations. Consequently, research on delusions with religious content should consider these different forms of delusion.

My second comment concerns Koenig's examination of whether religion helps individuals with psychosis. Religious conversion has been associated with the first psychotic breakdown in certain cases. Research on this topic does not lead to any firm conclusions as to how these events may interact, but some hypotheses can be formulated. First, as described by Koenig, it is possible that, at least in the case of some brief psychotic conditions, conversion could be such an intense and disorienting experience that it may destabilize predisposed individuals, serving as a precipitant. Second, the conversion of individuals with recent psychotic onset may be due to a neurocognitive alteration related to their disorder. Third, the need to find coping strategies to deal with the appalling consequences of the appearance of a psychotic condition may lead to religious conversion. Koenig cites literature supporting this last hypothesis, and recent studies provide further evidence (Fallot 2007; Mohr et al. 2006). The latter study concluded that religious coping was important among persons with psychotic disorders. Even if most of the patients in this study had long-term psychotic conditions, qualitative analyses showed that positive coping was also present among patients with a short duration of illness. Thus, religion may play a strong supportive role in the recovery from serious disorders such as schizophrenia.

At this time, no firm evidence exists showing religion to be more harmful than beneficial to individuals with psychosis. Rather, it may constitute a coping mechanism, used to deal with both psychological (or neuropsychological) issues and existential difficulties. This could explain why delusions with religious content are more prevalent among patients with less favorable outcomes, because these individuals may have more problems and symptoms to cope with. Clinicians are often reluctant to broach religious topics with their patients with psychosis (Huguelet et al. 2006). According to recent literature (Andreasen 2007), we think that a phenomenological approach is needed (in terms of understanding subjective experience) in order to understand the very specific role religion plays for each patient and thus avoid stigmatizing individuals whose delusions feature religious content. In this way, it might be possible to begin disentangling the pathological aspects from the useful coping mechanisms religion provides.

References

Andreasen NC: DSM and the death of phenomenology in America: an example of unintended consequences. Schizophr Bull 33:108–112, 2007

Drinnan A, Lavender T: Deconstructing delusions: a qualitative study examining the relationship between religious beliefs and religious delusions. Mental Health, Religion and Culture 9:317–331, 2006

Fallot RD: Spirituality and religion in recovery: some current issues. Psychiatric Rehabilitation Journal 30:261–270, 2007

Huguelet P, Mohr S, Borras L, et al: Spirituality and religious practices among outpatients with schizophrenia and their clinicians. Psychiatr Serv 57:366–372, 2006

Kimhi D, Goetz R, Yale S, et al: Delusions in individuals with schizophrenia: factor structure, clinical correlates, and putative neurobiology. Psychopathology 38:338–344, 2005

Mohr S, Brandt PY, Gillieron C, et al: Toward an integration of religiousness and spirituality into the psychosocial dimension of schizophrenia. Am J Psychiatry 163:1952–1959, 2006

Rhodes JE, Jakes S: The contribution of metaphor and metonymy to delusions. Psychology and Psychotherapy: Theory, Research and Practice 77:1–17, 2004

Siddle R, Haddock G, Tarrier N, et al: Religious delusions in patients admitted to hospital with schizophrenia. Soc Psychiatry Psychiatr Epidemiol 37:130–138, 2002

3

SUBSTANCE USE DISORDERS AND SPIRITUALITY

Marc Galanter, M.D.
Linda Glickman, Ph.D.

The United States today provides fertile ground for the growth in diverse combinations of psychoactive substances and spiritual practices. Because drug-influenced religious behavior and ideation might easily take a form similar to elements of a DSM diagnosis, it is important to know the specific religious and social context within which it occurs. In this chapter, therefore, we focus on an area that is of importance in developing accurate clinical categories and diagnoses.

Knowledge of the spiritual contexts of substance use may be important both in determining an accurate diagnosis and in understanding how the social context influences a patient's behavior. Psychoactive substances can produce a variety of different behaviors that might lead to an erroneous diagnosis of psychosis, and other diatheses that may be mistakenly ascribed to general psychiatric disorders (Brown et al. 2001; Shaner et al. 1993). Similarly, knowing a patient's controlled involvement with a psychoactive sacrament within an organized religious context might prevent a mistaken diagnosis of substance abuse or dependence. Because diverse presentations continue to develop at the intersection of the absorption with both spirituality and psychoactive substances of all kinds, in both the United States and other countries, clinicians' need for information on this phenomenon is likely to grow.

Social Trends Related to Use of Psychoactive Substances in Spiritual Practices

Many current activities ensure there will be experiences with drugs and spirituality in this and other countries rich in psychoactive substances, religious experimentation, and a fascination with all manner of drugs. Such experimentation is moving from its traditional locations in bohemian circles, cults, and among Native Americans into the mainstream. Numerous social trends come together to create an environment in which novel and extensive combinations of psychoactive substances and spiritual practices can develop. A number of such trends are important: 1) the continuing influence of the 1960s counterculture, 2) the search for intense spiritual experiences in industrialized countries, 3) the constant creation of religious and quasireligious cults, 4) the growth and growing interest in the Native American Church with its peyote sacrament, 5) active and widespread legal and illicit drug cultures, 6) easy access to information and substances through the Internet, 7) widespread foreign travel, including drug tourism and fascination with exotic foreign drug cultures, 8) a network of producers and sellers of illicit synthetic drugs, 9) the large variety of psychoactive substances naturally occurring in the United States, 10) large new immigrant communities from regions where the use of psychoactive substances for spiritual uses is common, 11) the growth in the use and legitimacy of hallucinogens among young people, and 12) the association of many such substances with natural healing. In the following subsections, we provide examples of how these issues have come to relate to the process of psychiatric diagnosis.

RELIGIOUS REVIVAL IN THE WEST

The 1960s' music and alternative lifestyles celebrated the links between psychoactive substances and spiritual seeking, and counterculture influences remain strong, with some moving into the cultural mainstream. The counterculture notion of life as a personal spiritual quest, pursued in and out of organized religion and facilitated through the use of psychoactive substances, has wide currency. A similar emphasis is seen in the growth of evangelical Christianity with its emphasis on an intensely intimate relationship with God, often involving trance states (Luhrmann 2004). It appears that the search for ecstatic states has moved farther into the mainstream, beyond established religious circles (Bourguignon 2003). Widespread interest and use of mood-altering natural substances in the world of alternative medicine moves people closer to an interest, and possible acceptance, of stronger, perhaps illicit, natural substances (Barnes and Powell-Griner 2004).

PEYOTE RITUALS

Psychedelic substances may be at the center of informal groups or, as in the case of the Native American Church, the central sacrament of a full-fledged church. This widely studied and publicized religious denomination, with 300,000, largely Native American, members from many Indian nations, is considered the leading edge in America for the contention that use of a psychedelic sacrament in a religion, in this case peyote, is protected by the First Amendment (Calabrese 2001; Garrity 2000; Lewton 2000). A substantial body of literature supports the notion that peyote is used safely in this practice with considerable spiritual and therapeutic effects, including as a treatment for alcoholism and mental illness, without leading to dependency (Albaugh and Anderson 1974; Calabrese 1997).

Mescaline, the principal psychoactive alkaloid compound among more than 60 found in peyote, produces a strong intoxication peaking within 2–4 hours, ending within 6 hours. As with other hallucinogens, mescaline produces changes in perception, thought, and mood. Bergman, a psychiatrist on the Navajo reservation, reported only one adverse reaction per 70,000 peyote ingestions (Bergman 1971). There is no strong evidence of long-term cognitive or psychological deficits among Native Americans using peyote regularly in the Native American Church (Halpern and Sewell 2005). However, there still is reason to suspect that frequent long-term users of mescaline and other hallucinogens might experience neuropsychological deficits, because these substances bind to some of the same neuroreceptors involved in psychotic disorders, and there is evidence that hallucinogens may damage the central serotonergic systems (Halpern and Pope 1999; Halpern et al. 2005; Pechnick and Ungerleider 2004). Mescaline use is likely to become more widespread as the Internet drug culture expands. Cacti other than peyote, such as the San Pedro and Peruvian torch, also contain mescaline and can be purchased online or from garden shops (Halpern and Sewell 2005).

HALLUCINOGENS AND RAVES

Many psychoactive substances grow naturally in North America (Halpern and Sewell 2005). Information about how to find and prepare them, about the large variety of psychoactive substances, and on ways to obtain them is readily available on the Internet as a magnet for young people (Boyer et al. 2005; Morris and Avorn 2003). After a decline from the mid-1970s to the late 1980s, hallucinogen use among young people rose through the 1990s. In 2004, 6.2% of high school seniors reported using a hallucinogen within the past year, whereas 9.7% had used one at least once in their lifetime (Hunt 1997; Office of National Drug Control Policy 2006). Helping to fuel the new legitimacy and extensive use among young people is the rave culture, in which large numbers of young people dance into the early hours of the morning to electronically synthesized music. Rave participants often are involved with polydrug use, most notably MDMA (3,4-methylenedioxymeth-amphetamine, or ecstasy) (Check 2004; Hutson 2000). Rave culture may, in certain cases, be construed to have the strong spiritual components characteristic of other social settings, producing feelings of connectedness centered on collective trance experiences. A Canadian study found that 42% of respondents interpreted their experience with raves in spiritual terms (Takahashi and Olaveson 2003). It remains to be seen whether the current use of psychedelic substances will lead to a lifetime of experimentation, as occurred among many in the 1960s counterculture.

Part of the 1960s' new age seekers' culture, and widely used in the 1970s as an adjunct to psychotherapy, MDMA became illegal in 1985. MDMA, a synthetic amphetamine analog, is typically inhaled or taken orally in tablets or capsules. Onset of a sudden amphetamine-like rush begins after 30 minutes; a plateau is reached within 3–4 hours, with acute effects lasting 6–8 hours. Acute negative effects include depersonalization, accelerated thinking, impaired decision making, anxiety, panic, and depression (Freese et al. 2002; McDowell 2004). Hangover effects of 24 hours or longer include lethargy, anorexia, and depressed mood. MDMA use may be accompanied by comorbid psychiatric disorders that typically began before the use of the substance (Gouzoulis-Mayfrank and Daumann 2006).

MDMA works by increasing the release of serotonin and inhibiting its reuptake. Resulting increases in blood pressure and temperature appear to be implicated in deaths from a condition resembling heat stroke. As the user continues to take MDMA the adverse effects increase, leading to a reduction of usage. Some users take large amounts regularly during the week, not only for weekend parties. Although abstinence appears to result in a diminishment of long-term effects, evidence is accumulating that heavy MDMA use can lead to long-term memory impairment (Medina et al. 2005; Rodgers 2000).

AYAHUASCA AND IBOGAINE

Ease of foreign travel, glowing claims of the virtues of psychoactive substances, and fascination with exotic locales and cultures, combined with numerous people (often with considerable experience with psychoactive substances) in search of new spiritual experiences, have produced the new phenomenon of *drug tourism* (Dobkin de Rios 1994). Travelers to the Amazon region in search of an authentic setting for an ayahuasca retreat with a shaman (Winkelman 2005), or on a similar journey to West Africa for an encounter with ibogaine, often speak in glowing terms about this experience in their search for spiritual growth or therapeutic results. Ibogaine and ayahuasca have similar trajectories in their introduction in the United States. Heavily promoted, they are likely to increase in importance here.

Ayahuasca, a tea preparation made from a combination of plants in the Amazon basin, is widely used for spiritual and healing purposes in rural and urban areas of Brazil, Peru, and elsewhere (Dobkin de Rios 1996). Urban healers deal with a wide variety of DSM disorders, including drug abuse, diagnosed and treated as either natural or supernatural in origin (Grob et al. 1996). As with ibogaine and peyote in the Native American Church, its current use is not of long traditional standing; instead, as with the others, it is a product of a movement responding to colonialism, particularly massive depopulation from disease and forced labor, taking a form combining Christianity and modern spiritualist traditions (Fernandez and Fernandez 2001). Ayahuasca, the most widely used hallucinogen in Amazonia, is used by more than 70 different ethnic groups there and officially sanctioned in Brazil for use by 22 religious groups (Dobkin de Rios 1996; Winkelman 2005). Most prominent are Santo Daime, the largest Brazilian sect, and the Uniao do Vegetal church. The acute effects of ayahuasca, lasting 3–4 hours, peak within the first hour of ingestion; the accompanying vomiting is seen as a form of spiritual purging (Halpern and Sewell 2005). Subjective effects include visual hallucinations, dream-like reveries, and a heightened feeling of alertness (McKenna et al. 1998). The sparse literature on frequent, long-term users of ayahuasca in a controlled religious context indicates there is little association with current psychiatric disorders among them, but a stronger association with remitted past diagnoses, including alcohol abuse (McKenna et al. 1998).

Similarly, ibogaine became the central sacrament of numerous sects of the Bwiti religion, the fastest growing indigenous religion in Africa. Bwiti, which considers itself a form of Christianity, is open to all groups and was a unifying force in Gabon's liberation struggle (Samorini 1995). Centered in former French colonies in Equatorial Africa, Bwiti initiates undergo an intense 3-day vision quest facilitated by high doses of ibogaine in a communal ritual setting (Fernandez 1982; Samorini 1995). Ibogaine, an alkaloid found in the root bark of a shrub, appears to produce its effects through complex interactions between multiple neurotransmitter systems (Alper 2001). Psychotropic effects appear within 1–3 hours after ingestion, with a duration of from 4–8 hours. Informants report a waking dream in which the person enters a visual landscape, often involving contact with transcendent beings. Alper (2001) argued that these reports appear more consistent with dreams rather than with hallucinations. A further "evaluative" phase follows in which the subject processes the experience of the acute phase. French chemist Robert Goutarel hypothesized that ibogaine produces a state similar to rapid eye movement sleep, heightening reprocessing of previously learned ideas. Little is known about its long-term psychological effects (Alper 2001). Ibogaine may become particularly attractive to some African immigrants and to African Americans because of its African origins (Shine et al. 1995).

Both ibogaine and ayahuasca are widely touted for their therapeutic properties. As with the Native American Church, ibogaine- and ayahuasca-involved religious groups appear to help initiates deal with problems of substance abuse. Much is made of the healing power of ayahuasca in its ritual context as an effective enhancer of a process akin to Western psychotherapy (Andritzky 1989; Grob et al. 1996). Such explorations, similar to the highly touted therapeutic promise of earlier fashionable hallucinogens such as lysergic acid diethylamide (LSD; Strassman 1995), have helped to create a demand for research to incorporate them into mainstream medicine. This process is particularly apparent in the longstanding controversy about the possible benefits of ibogaine in drug treatment. Although in 1993 the U.S. Food and Drug Administration approved a clinical trial for ibogaine, the National Institute on Drug Abuse did not fund it, citing safety concerns (Vastag 2002, 2005). An active advocacy movement with strong ties to 1960s pro-psychedelic activism, AIDS activism, and scientists has grown up around ibogaine (Alper 2001). Moreover, an estimated 30–40 clinics in Europe and the Caribbean have treated more than 5,000 addicted patients with the drug. Privately funded early-phase trials are anticipated (Vastag 2005). Along with contributing to the favorable view of hallucinogens in the counterculture, youth culture, and beyond, the ibogaine drug treatment advocacy milieu has produced a growing number of Americans exposed to the substance. Following the example of the Native American Church, religious denominations claiming the First Amendment right to legally use ayahuasca or ibogaine as a sacrament have been started (Dobkin de Rios and Grob 2005).

CANNABIS

New immigrant groups bring their distinctive local combinations of psychoactive drugs and spirituality. *Ganja,* the Hindu word for cannabis, is widely used and accepted throughout Jamaica for its medicinal and spiritual properties (Broad and Feinberg 1995). Used as a sacrament by groups professing the Rastafari religion, a Jamaican variant of Orthodox Christianity, ganja and its spiritual properties are likely to be embraced not only by West Indians in the United States but by American young people attracted to the peace, love, music, and drugs image of the Rastafarian culture (Hickling and Griffith 1994; Redington 2006). Cannabis preparations, often in the form of a drink similar to a milk shake, are widely used in India to celebrate special occasions in a manner similar to the way alcohol is used in the United States. Grown in profusion throughout India, cannabis is deeply embedded in numerous spiritual traditions (Morningstar 1985). Such use may be part of the experience of U.S. immigrants from the subcontinent, even in the face of severe penalties from the immigration authorities for drug convictions (Mautino 2002). When smoked, marijuana typically produces a euphoric reaction lasting 3–4 hours; however, the response may be dysphoric instead. Taken at a high dosage, marijuana may produce paranoid ideation similar to that associated with LSD and other hallucinogens. It may also serve as a trigger for panic attacks, paranoia, and psychosis for individuals predisposed to psychiatric illnesses (Gold et al. 2004). Among the approximately 1 million Americans receiving treatment for marijuana abuse annually, most come to the attention of clinicians through referrals after positive results on a drug test or for evaluation for persistent social, academic, or health problems.

BETEL NUTS

Preparations containing the areca nut, the seed of the areca palm, are used extensively throughout Asia and the Pacific Islands and are legally available to immigrant groups in the United States (Changrani and Gany 2005; Gupta and Warnakulasuriya 2002). Such preparations, often termed *betel nut,* taking numerous local forms, often combined with tobacco, are deeply embedded in these cultures. Producing an energizing feeling of well-being, and associated with social events, healing, suppression of hunger, artistic inspiration, spirituality, or helping people cope with the stresses of everyday life, among a myriad of such cultural meanings, areca nut is commonly made available to young children (Strickland 2002; Williams et al. 2002). There are some findings that support the claim that areca nut produces euphoria and has antidepressant, analgesic, and sedative properties (Strickland 2002). Concern for its spread among young people in New York City led to legislative efforts to ban areca nut sales to minors (Changrani and Gany 2005).

CREATIVITY

Psychoactive substances may be part of the complex relationship between artistic creation, bohemian lifestyles, mood disorders, and spirituality. Such a relationship appears to have occurred among the abstract expressionist artists of the New York School, where alcohol abuse, depressive disorders, and a spiritual form of painting combined to create a major movement in modern art (Schildkraut et al. 1994). Psychoactive substances may become part of a spiritually infused artistic career that parallels the more direct spiritual seeking of other users. Within an artistic or religious milieu, the lure of psychoactive substances as a shortcut to desired results can lead to experimentation with the possibility of developing formal or informal groups of users.

This review demonstrates the complexity of the fast-changing forms the relationship between psychoactive substances and spiritual practices takes in our society. New cultural forms are likely to arise often and quickly. For some persons the substance is a sacrament in a well-organized ritual ceremony in a religion (Baker 2005). For others, a cult, a small group of like-minded friends, a "scene" (such as raves), individualized inspiration gained from the Internet or elsewhere, a lifelong search for spiritual experience or a related search for healing (sometimes from drug abuse), a set of practices adapted from an immigrant's homeland, or any number of varied social contexts may provide support and motivation for an individual's involvement. Often the distinction between spiritual and therapeutic involvement may not be easy to make, evoking ancient and contemporary traditions of spiritual healing. New hybrid cultural forms are likely to arise, as they have in the past, because of our complex culture with many strands conducive to combining substance use and spirituality.

Much remains to be learned about this phenomenon. Psychiatrists' awareness of the contours of this growing, large-scale connection is important to help understand the social context of patients' drug involvement and symptoms as well as to develop accurate diagnoses and effective treatment. This review highlights the protean connections between psychoactive substances and spiritual practices, and some of the reasons for them, as a contribution to that end.

Options for DSM-V

DIAGNOSTIC CATEGORIES

Substance use may be normative within a religiously grounded subculture and may be confused with a pattern of abuse by a diagnostician. Such patterns of use may result in conflict with close relations or authorities because of cultural differences. The text of the DSM-V can make this distinction clear so it is not considered a sign of pathology.

The following paragraphs refer to DSM-IV-TR diagnostic categories (American Psychiatric Association 2000). Phrases in italics illustrate options to addressing the intersection between substance use and abuse and spirituality.

- **297.3 Shared Psychotic Disorder** *(Folie à Deux)*: The following diagnostic criterion for shared psychotic disorder is given: "is not due to the direct physiological effects of a substance (e.g., a drug of abuse, a medication, or a general medical condition)." The following could be added: *but could result from a consensual belief system of a religious movement.*
- **Substance Abuse:** The following material is included in the narrative preceding the diagnostic criteria for substance abuse: "The person may continue to use the substance despite a history of undesirable, persistent, or recurrent social or interpersonal consequences (e.g., marital difficulties or divorce, verbal or physical fights)." The following could be added: *This aspect of substance abuse should be distinguished from difficulties encountered by individuals who are members of a religious group whose practice of ritualized substance use may lead to conflict with nonmembers or legal authorities (e.g., culture-bound use of agents such as khat or peyote).*
- **Substance Dependence:** With regard to remission of substance dependence: "The following specifiers apply if the individual is on agonist therapy or in a controlled environment" *or in ongoing attendance at a mutual support program.*

In a mutual support group: This specifier is used if the individual is in voluntary regular attendance in an abstinence-oriented mutual support program or religious sect, and no criteria for dependence or abuse have been met for at least the past month. Examples of this are spiritually oriented 12-Step groups such as Alcoholics Anonymous and abstinence-oriented religious groups.

RELIGIOUS/CULTIC EXPERIENCES ASSOCIATED WITH SUBSTANCE USE

Some behaviors included as diagnostic criteria within the DSM structure may emerge in response to experiences associated with membership in an intensely affiliative religious or cultic group. These behaviors may appropriately qualify a person for a pathologic diagnosis. Others, on the other hand, may be incorrectly construed as pathologic as they may be normative in such groups. Descriptions of a number of the diagnoses in the DSM-V can therefore be qualified accordingly. For example:

- **300.15 Dissociative Disorders Not Otherwise Specified:** "Example 3. States of dissociation that occur in individuals who have been subjected to periods of prolonged and intense coercive persuasion (e.g., brainwashing, thought reform, or indoctrination while captive)." This could be added: *Such states, which remit, may take place during induction into a cultic group or the experience of an intense religious experience (possibly substance-induced), and should not be termed pathologic.*
- **309 Adjustment Disorder:** In the context of the description of this syndrome, the following is included in the DSM-IV-TR: "Individuals from disadvantaged life circumstances experience a high rate of stressors and may be at increased rate for the disorder." This could be added: *Persons leaving religious movements with intense affiliative ties (which may be related to spiritually oriented substance use) under adverse circumstances are also at increased risk.*

Summary

Each substance has its own mixture of spiritual uses, cultural and social contexts, psychological effects, and potential involvement in the process of making a DSM-based diagnosis. The possibility that such usage may be therapeutic to the individual, although little understood, should be considered as well. How clinicians explore such patients' related substance use and spiritual involvement, and how such information, or its absence, impacts on their diagnoses and treatments, remains unstudied. Well-controlled substance usage within an individual or group spiritual context should not be considered dependence. A diagnosis of dependence should depend more on disturbance of patterns of substance use and of important elements of the person's life, rather than on the amount and persistence of usage (Gold et al. 2004). Determining whether a strongly held drug-related spiritual belief is delusional should be seen in the same contextual light.

According to Pierre (2001), the content of a delusion is less salient than the way it is maintained, as in the case of excessive preoccupation. Just as novel mixtures of new and old substances, spiritual subcultures, and the varieties of spiritual experience continue to proliferate in our increasingly global society, so does psychiatric diagnosis need to more fully engage this domain. It is likely that new manifestations of the connections between spirituality, social settings, psychoactive substances, and their clinical effects will occupy the careful attention of clinicians for some time to come.

References

Albaugh BJ, Anderson PO: Peyote in the treatment of alcoholism among American Indians. Am J Psychiatry 131:1247–1250, 1974

Alper KR: Ibogaine: a review. Alkaloids Chem Biol 56:1–38, 2001

American Psychiatric Association: Diagnostic and Statistical Manual of Mental Disorders, 4th Edition, Text Revision. Washington, DC, American Psychiatric Association, 2000

Andritzky W: Sociopsychotherapeutic functions of Ayahuasca healing in Amazonia. J Psychoactive Drugs 21:77–89, 1989

Baker JR: Psychedelic sacraments. J Psychoactive Drugs 37:179–187, 2005

Barnes PM, Powell-Griner E: Contemporary and alternative medicine use among adults: United States, 2002. Adv Data 27:1–19, 2004

Bergman RL: Navajo peyote use: its apparent safety. Am J Psychiatry 128:695–699, 1971

Bourguignon E: Faith, healing and "ecstasy deprivation": secular society in a new age of anxiety. Anthropology of Consciousness 14:1–19, 2003

Boyer EW, Shannon M, Hibberd PL: The internet and psychoactive substance use among innovative drug users. Pediatrics 115:302–305, 2005

Broad K, Feinberg B: Perceptions of ganja and cocaine in urban Jamaica. J Psychoactive Drugs 27:261–276, 1995

Brown ES, Suppes T, Adinoff B, et al: Drug abuse and bipolar disorder: comorbidity or misdiagnosis? J Affect Disord 65:105–115, 2001

Calabrese JD: Spiritual healing and human development in the Native American Church: toward a cultural psychiatry of peyote. Psychoanal Rev 84:237–253, 1997

Calabrese JD: The Supreme Court versus peyote: consciousness alteration, cultural psychiatry and the dilemma of contemporary subcultures. Anthropology of Consciousness 12:4–19, 2001

Changrani J, Gany F: Paan and gutka in the United States: an emerging trend. J Immigr Health 7:103–108, 2005

Check E: The ups and downs of ecstasy. Nature 429:126–128, 2004

Dobkin de Rios M: Drug tourism in the Amazon. Anthropology of Consciousness 5:16–19, 1994

Dobkin de Rios M: On human pharmacology of hoasca: a medical anthropology perspective. J Nerv Ment Dis 184:95–98, 1996

Dobkin de Rios M, Grob CS: Interview with Jeffrey Bronfman, representative Mestre for the União do Vegetal church in the United States. J Psychoactive Drugs 37:189–191, 2005

Fernandez JW: Equatorial excursions: the quest for revitalizing dreams and visions, in Bwiti: An Ethnography of the Religious Imagination. Princeton, NJ, Princeton University Press, 1982, pp 470–493

Fernandez JW, Fernandez RL: "Returning to the path": The use of Iboga[ine] in an equatorial African ritual context and the binding of time, space, and social relationships, in Ibogaine: Proceedings of the First International Conference (The Alkaloids, series ed Cordell GA). Edited by Alper KR, Glick SD. San Diego, CA, Academic Press, 2001

Freese TE, Miotto K, Reback CJ: The effects and consequences of selected club drugs. J Subst Abuse Treat 23:151–156, 2002

Garrity JF: Jesus, peyote, and the holy people: alcohol abuse and the ethos of power in Navajo healing. Med Anthropol Q 14:521–542, 2000

Gold MS, Frost-Pineda K, Jacobs WS: Cannabis, in Textbook of Substance Abuse Treatment, 3rd Edition. Edited by Galanter M, Kleber HD. Washington, DC, American Psychiatric Publishing, 2004, pp 167–188

Gouzoulis-Mayfrank E, Daumann J: Neurotoxicity of methylenedioxyamphetamines (MDMA; ecstasy) in humans: how strong is the evidence for persistent brain damage? Addiction 101:348–361, 2006

Grob CS, McKenna D, Galloway G, et al: Human psychopharmacology of hoasca, a plant hallucinogen used in ritual context in Brazil. J Nerv Ment Dis 184:86–94, 1996

Gupta PC, Warnakulasuriya S: Global epidemiology of areca nut usage. Addict Biol 7:77–83, 2002

Halpern JH, Pope HG: Do hallucinogens cause residual neuropsychological toxicity? Drug Alcohol Depend 53:247–256, 1999

Halpern JH, Sewell RA: Hallucinogenic botanicals of America: a growing need for focused drug education and research. Life Sci 78:519–526, 2005

Halpern JH, Sherwood AR, Hudson JI, et al: Psychological and cognitive effects of long-term peyote use among Native Americans. Biol Psychiatry 58:624–631, 2005

Hickling FW, Griffith EEH: Clinical perspectives on the Rastafari movement. Hosp Community Psychiatry 45:49–53, 1994

Hunt D: Rise of hallucinogen use. National Institute of Justice: Research in Brief, October 1997, pp 1–11

Hutson SR: The rave: spiritual healing in modern western subcultures. Anthropol Q 73:35–49, 2000

Lewton EL: Identity and healing in three Navajo religious traditions: Sa'ah Naaghài Bik'eh Hózhó. Med Anthropol Q 14:476–498, 2000

Luhrmann TM: Metakinesis: how God becomes intimate in contemporary U.S. Christianity. Am Anthropol 106:518–528, 2004

Mautino KS: Immigrants, immigration, and substance use and abuse. J Immigr Health 4:1–3, 2002

McDowell DM: MDMA, ketamine, GHB, and the "club drug" scene, in Textbook of Substance Abuse Treatment, 3rd Edition. Edited by Galanter M, Kleber HD. Washington, DC, American Psychiatric Publishing, 2004, pp 321–333

McKenna DJ, Callaway JC, Grob CS: The scientific investigation of Ayahuasca: a review of past and current research. The Heffter Review of Psychedelic Research 1:65–76, 1998

Medina KL, Shear PK, Corcoran K: Ecstasy (MDMA) exposure and neuropsychological functioning: a polydrug perspective. J Int Neuropsychol Soc 11:753–765, 2005

Morningstar PJ: Thandai and chilam: traditional Hindu beliefs about the proper uses of cannabis. J Psychoactive Drugs 17:141–165, 1985

Morris CA, Avorn J: Internet marketing of herbal products. JAMA 290:1505–1509, 2003

Office of National Drug Control Policy: Facts and figures: hallucinogens. Available at: http://whitehousedrugpolicy.gov/drugfact/hallucinogens/index.html. Accessed April 24, 2006.

Pechnick RN, Ungerleider JT: Hallucinogens, in Textbook of Substance Abuse Treatment, 3rd Edition. Edited by Galanter M, Kleber HD. Washington, DC, American Psychiatric Publishing, 2004, pp 199–209

Pierre JM: Faith or delusion? At the crossroads of religion and psychosis. J Psychiatr Pract 7:163–172, 2001

Redington NH: A sketch of Rastafari history. Available at: http://www.nomadfx.com/old/rasta1.html. Accessed April 15, 2006.

Rodgers J: Cognitive performance amongst recreational users of "ecstasy." Psychopharmacology 151:19–24, 2000

Samorini G: The Bwiti religion and the psychoactive plant Tabernanthe iboga (Equatorial Africa). Integration 5:105–114, 1995. Available at: http://www.ibogaine.org/samorini.html. Accessed April 15, 2006.

Schildkraut JJ, Hirshfeld AJ, Murphy JM: Mind and mood in modern art, II: depressive disorders, spirituality, and early deaths in the abstract expressionist artists of the New York School. Am J Psychiatry 151:482–488, 1994

Shaner A, Khalsa ME, Roberts L, et al: Unrecognized cocaine use among schizophrenic patients. Am J Psychiatry 150:758–762, 1993

Shine BR, Washington R, Rogers RS: Sacred African plant found effective in treating addiction. The City Sun, October 4–10, 1995. Available at: http://www.ibogaine.desk.nl/citysun.html. Accessed April 15, 2006.

Strassman RJ: Hallucinogenic drugs in psychiatric research and treatment. J Nerv Ment Dis 183:127–138, 1995

Strickland SS: Anthropological perspectives on use of the areca nut. Addict Biol 7:85–97, 2002

Takahashi M, Olaveson T: Music, dance and raving bodies: raving spirituality in the central Canadian rave scene. Journal of Ritual Studies 17:72–96, 2003

Vastag B: Addiction treatment strives for legitimacy. JAMA 288:3096, 3099–3101, 2002

Vastag B: Ibogaine therapy: a "vast uncontrolled experiment." Science 308:345–346, 2005

Williams S, Malik A, Chowdhury S, et al: Sociocultural aspects of areca nut use. Addict Biol 7:147–154, 2002

Winkelman M: Drug tourism or spiritual healing? Ayahuasca seekers in Amazonia. J Psychoactive Drugs 37:209–218, 2005

Commentary 3A

COMMENTARY ON "SUBSTANCE USE DISORDERS AND SPIRITUALITY"

Richard J. Frances, M.D.

Galanter and Glickman provide important descriptions and insights into the relationship of specific religious and cultural contexts of substance use that can be valuable in sharpening the cultural relevance of the DSM-V. The danger of over-diagnosing problems with substances and/or of dual diagnosis (especially delusions and psychosis), when substance use is part of a religious rite, has been discussed widely in the literature, is worthy of more study, and is a major reason cultural competence needs to be a key part of medical school and residency curricula. However, there is also a danger that a religious justification for legalization of use can be excessive. For example, I have had patients who like reggae music and marijuana but who do not have a deep reverence for Haile Selassie or other aspects of the religion and embrace Rastafarianism simply as a plea to get out of charges of marijuana possession or dealing, claiming they were just practicing their faith and have First Amendment rights to worship in their own way.

Because DSM-V will be referred to in forensic contexts and public policy debate relating to legalization of drugs, caution in DSM-V wording regarding religious and cultural context of use will be important so as not to inject a bias favoring use of religion as a factor for diminished personal responsibility of use or negative consequences of use. Having said this, the authors provide many helpful suggestions that can be useful in crafting DSM-V text that takes into account the relationship between spirituality, cultural context, and the effects of intoxication, withdrawal, and chronic use of substances and comorbid psychiatric disorders.

Throughout his career, Dr. Galanter, as a leader in the addiction psychiatry field, has increased physicians' awareness of the importance of spirituality and social affiliation in all of our patients' lives and, perhaps especially, in those who use and abuse substances. An understanding of our patients' beliefs and cultural values needs to be taken into account in the assessment and treatment of every patient, which is why any revision of the DSM needs to heed these suggestions.

Commentary 3B

COMMENTARY ON "SUBSTANCE USE DISORDERS AND SPIRITUALITY"

Joseph Westermeyer, M.D., Ph.D.

Drs. Galanter and Glickman have provided us with an informed, thoughtful document that should prove valuable to those framing DSM-V. They have accomplished this contribution by explicating the following topics:

- The spiritual context and goals of much substance use
- Potential drug epidemics related to drug-using rituals from Africa and Latin America
- Potential influences of immigrants, refugees, and illegal migrants who have arrived in the United States in the several tens of millions over the past few decades

Acculturation

Acculturation involves a two-way process in which members of the receiving society, or "natives," influence immigrants, and immigrants affect and modify the receiving society (Markides 1988). Because acculturation does not end with the "first," or migrating, generation, this process continues at least into the native-born, or "second," generation. Many immigrants are exposed to new substances or patterns of use, for which they have no premigration traditions to guide them. Stressors inherent in acculturation itself—including religious and spiritual changes—can foster substance use and abuse (Westermeyer et al. 1984). This process may especially affect young migrants and second-generation migrants who know little about the culture-of-emigration and consequently cathect to indigenous substance use in the United States as a false symbol of cultural identity and successful acculturation. Examples include youth from abstaining Hindu, Moslem, or Christian sects that do not ensocialize their offspring to safe alcohol use. Youth from these families who choose to drink often adapt the patterns taught to them by peers—sometimes not a model conducive to safe use.

Although some immigrants come from societies with substance use comparable with that found in the United States, secular contexts of drinking or drug use may replace the spiritual, religious, and ceremonial constraints that staved off abuse and ensuing problems. An example consists of first- and second-generation Mexican Americans whose drinking exceeds that of Mexicans who remain at home as well as that of the general American population (Caetano 1987). Factors associated with this change-for-the-worse include stressors associated with migration, waning of traditional influences that may constrain amounts or frequency of use, and increased disposable income that can permit expression of celebratory drinking, a valued behavioral expression. Conversion to abstinence-oriented religion has been an effective means for stemming widespread alcohol abuse in some immigrant communities (Porter 2002). Support groups for teenaged second-generation immigrants have also proven effective in fostering traditional spiritual values against alcohol and drug abuse (Weine et al. 2004).

The huge numbers of first- and second-generation immigrants can have momentous effects on local culture in localized areas where they may choose to concentrate. In concentrated settings, the traditions of the culture-of-emigration may persist and even influence the surrounding native community. To appreciate the extent of these influences, consider that more than 15% of the current population in the United States consists of foreign-born immigrants, refugees, and illegal migrants. Because these populations reproduce at a rate generally exceeding the native population, it is likely that their second generation exceeds even this percentage. Close to 100 million of the 300 million inhabitants of the United States may (or will) be first- and second-generation immigrants and refugees (Lim 2006).

Some "cultural migrants" have been in the United States for many generations. Nevertheless, their departure from their traditional home communities into the mainstream society can involve a major cultural relocation (Little Soldier 1995). These migrations share many characteristics of foreign immigration.

Mercantile Motivations May Replace Spiritual Practices

Acculturation often proceeds in an unpredictable fashion, as exemplified by the following illustration. American mercantilism sometimes overwhelms traditional folk or spiritual practices. In many countries, psychoactive substances are produced as a local cottage industry, and their use is controlled by local cultural, spiritual, and religious traditions—influences that may no longer hold sway following migration. Some immigrants have access to sources of drug production in their countries of origin, including khat from the Middle East, cocaine from Latin America, and opiates from Asia and Latin America. In addition, smuggling in many countries comprises a traditional occupation pursued by residents of frontier communities. As traditional influences weaken, and the mercantile or secular values of the United States wax, a small but effective number of foreign-born nationals have chosen to play major roles in the smuggling and sale of illicit drugs (Westermeyer 1982).

V Codes Related to Culture and Spirituality

V codes may be useful in tracing drug use lying at this interface between the old and the new cultures. One V code might consist of the consumption of an illegal substance in a culturally syntonic fashion, such as khat use in the United States by some East Africans (Griffiths et al. 1997). Another V code might describe immigrant youth using locally available but illegal substances as a means of "fitting in" with native-born American adolescents, or as a symbol of cultural alienation.

References

Caetano R: Acculturation and drinking patterns among U.S. Hispanics. Br J Addict 82:789–799, 1987

Griffiths P, Gossop M, Wickenden S: A transcultural pattern of drug use: Qat (khat) in the U.K. Br J Psychiatry 170:281–284, 1997

Lim RF: Clinical Manual of Cultural Psychiatry. Washington, DC, American Psychiatric Publishing, 2006

Little Soldier L: To soar with the eagles: enculturation and acculturation of Indian children. Child Educ 61:185–191, 1995

Markides KS: Acculturation and alcohol consumption among Mexican Americans: a three-generation study. Am J Public Health 78:1178–1181, 1988

Porter E: Protestant faiths appeal to Hispanics and win many over. Wall Street Journal, July 2, 2002, A:1–6

Weine SM, Ware N, Klebic A: Converting cultural capital among teen refugees and their families from Bosnia-Herzegovina. Psychiatr Serv 55:923–927, 2004

Westermeyer J: Poppies, Pipes and People: Opium and Its Use in Laos. Berkeley, University of California Press, 1982

Westermeyer J, Neider J, Vang TF: Acculturation and mental health: a study of Hmong refugees at 1.5 and 3.5 years postmigration. Soc Sci Med 18:87–93, 1984

4

RELIGIOUS AND SPIRITUAL ISSUES IN ANXIETY AND ADJUSTMENT DISORDERS

Gerrit Glas, M.D., Ph.D.

When laypeople are asked to describe a situation in which anxiety is related to some religious or spiritual theme or concern, they usually have little problem doing so. They will refer, for instance, to conditions in which persons fear being punished by God or possessed by some supernatural power. They describe moments of uncertainty, doubt, and anxiety in which people seek divine assistance. Some mention religious interpretations of life events that are accompanied by worry and feelings of apprehension. Still others refer to the existential dimension of anxiety, by saying that anxiety is inherent in human existence and that it is our destiny— as beings endowed with freedom—to face finitude, death, and other uncertainties of the human condition.

References to these religious, spiritual, and existential aspects of anxiety are virtually absent in current classifications of anxiety disorders. This is not very surprising. The history of the concept of anxiety can be read as the history of the gradual peeling off of layers of the broad and encompassing concept of melancholia, which included references to religious matters (Glas 2003). During this process of taxonomic differentiation, spiritual connotations of anxiety and depression were slowly excluded from clinical descriptions of anxiety disorders.

Several interpretations are possible of this state of affairs. Pathological forms of anxiety may in fact be immune from religious and spiritual influences, both *qua* form and *qua* content. This interpretation suggests that religious and spiritual issues only concern the periphery of the disorder and leave its core unaffected, both at the level of symptoms and at the level of the underlying causal mechanisms. According to another hypothesis, religious and spiritual matters are not distinctive in a diagnostic sense. The absence of references to spiritual and religious aspects is simply a reflection of the need for criteria that distinguish the normal from the abnormal. Religious and spiritual phenomena are part of the behavior of both patients and nonpatients and inclusion of these phenomena in the sets of criteria for anxiety and adjustment disorder would not add to the distinctness of diagnostic classes. According to a third interpretation, however, the current lack of attention to spiritual and religious dimensions of anxiety and adjustment disorders should be considered as artificial and in need of reconsideration. This view entails that religious and spiritual issues are intertwined in a much more intrinsic way with the psychopathology of anxiety and other emotional disorders.

In this chapter I review evidence in favor of each of these three interpretations. After a brief conceptual history of anxiety, I discuss empirical research on the interface between anxiety and adjustment disorders and religion/spirituality. I conclude with some suggestions and a research agenda for DSM-V, based on a conceptual framework for the understanding of relationship between psychopathology and religious and spiritual issues.

Conceptual History

Anxiety is a disquieting emotion with an enormous range of behavioral and subjective expressions, all indicating that one is in a state of being threatened. Anxiety can vary from complete paralysis to states of frenzy; from anxious surprise to the most incapacitating forms of terror; from sudden panic to a constant state of worry and concern. Like other emotions, anxiety has physiological, behavioral, and subjective manifestations.

The word *anxiety* is derived from the Indo-German root *Angh,* a term that refers to constriction of the throat and upper chest and that has been associated with feelings of suffocation and strangulation. Throughout history these physical feelings have metaphorically been associated with existential and spiritual experiences of "narrowness" and existential suffocation and of wrestling with disarming and oppressing supernatural powers—be it God, a demon, or fate. When overcome, these experiences may turn out to be part of a process of inner change and growth. Instead of leading to inhibition and paralysis, anxiety then helps to instill virtues such as courage, humility, and commitment to some greater good. The term *anxiety,* accordingly, refers to a condition with a double spiritual and existential meaning. On the one hand it expresses the paralyzing experience of being thrown back on oneself. On the other hand it refers to a crucial phase in the process of transformation in which the person—by an act of self-transcendence—gives up egocentric wish-fulfillment and devotes his or her life to a greater cause. This double meaning of the concept of anxiety can be detected in both mystical traditions and

Protestantism. Mystics and Calvinist Protestants concur that sooner or later in the process of conversion there are moments of existential darkness and oppression preceding the moment of illumination and liberating self-surrender, respectively.

These two meanings of anxiety were preserved in the existentialist tradition that began with the intriguing analysis of anxiety by the Danish philosopher Søren Kierkegaard. Kierkegaard (1844/1980) saw anxiety on the one hand as the counterpart of human freedom and at the other hand as "pedagogical" for the deepening of faith. Anxiety brings us into the "realm of possibility," he said. Those who can face the uncertainty and openness it brings will undergo a process of inner change. Anxiety acquires at least five different existential meanings in Kierkegaard's *The Concept of Anxiety:* anxious surprise, dizziness for the openness of human existence, anxiety intermingled with guilt, demonic anxiety, and pedagogical anxiety. The experience of anxiety is often mingled with those of other moods.

In the existentialist tradition these views returned in secularized form. Kurt Goldstein, a German psychopathologist influenced by Kierkegaard and the early existentialist philosophers, characterized anxiety as an inhibition of the urge for self-realization (Goldstein 1929). Arthur Kronfeld held a similar view (Kronfeld 1935). The element of transformation was preserved in the emphasis on courage as the necessary counterpart of anxiety. It is not without significance that it was a theologian—Paul Tillich—who brought this up (Tillich 1952). Anxiety asks for the "courage to be," according to Tillich. This idea became prominent in existential psychotherapies such as those of Rollo May (1950, 1983) and Irvin Yalom (1980).

Debates about the classification of anxiety have followed a typical course. For centuries anxiety was understood as being part of the much broader concept of melancholia. This lasted until 1850 or so, when the first medical descriptions of anxiety as a syndrome began to appear (Berrios 1996). These descriptions were partly influenced by nonmedical factors such as war and changing societal conditions. Classificatory boundaries became important in discussions of the "war neuroses" and the legitimacy of providing pensions to those with these anxiety syndromes. Anxiety (and later, stress) became associated with the hectic modern lifestyle, for which George Beard (1890) coined the term "American nervousness." In work of both Kraepelin and Freud, one can find descriptions that come close to contemporary distinctions such as those between panic, agoraphobia, other phobias, obsessive-compulsive disorder (OCD), generalized anxiety, and traumatic anxiety (Freud 1926; Kraepelin 1899; Kraepelin and Lange 1927). However, it is no exaggeration to say that the further demarcation of the spectrum of anxiety syndromes was delayed for almost half a century by psychoanalytic thinking about anxiety. Freud invented the—at that time—new and revolutionary idea of anxiety as an inner threat. His theory of anxiety as a signal indicating some underlying neurotic conflict transformed anxiety into a nonspecific emotion not needing any further specification. Attention should be focused on the underlying neurotic problem, not on the phenomenon of anxiety itself.

The reopening of the classification debate on anxiety disorder in the late 1950s and early 1960s was marked by concentration on overt behavior and a search for objective standards. Old psychopathological distinctions were reinvented. Panic disorder became a disorder on its own. References to the existential and psychodynamic vocabularies disappeared. Confronted with the endless variety of fleeting and overlapping manifestations of anxiety, depression, somatic complaints, and personality dysfunction, the psychiatric community concentrated on the identification of at least some more or less fixed and outspoken behavioral categories. This attempt was extremely successful, but at the cost of the existential and psychodynamic components of anxiety.

Why do we need this conceptual history? There are several reasons why such delving into historical detail may be important, but one reason stands above all. Our brief overview shows why it will be difficult to identify *specific* relations between the anxiety disorders and religious and spiritual issues. *Religion* and *spirituality* refer to dimensions of existence that were excluded from DSM and other classifications in order to attain at least some stability of diagnostic concepts. They concern a person's broad outlook on life and suggest a holistic perspective, emerging from one's basic and most fundamental attitudes. They, in short, refer to a different conceptual level than that of symptoms and signs. Our definitions of anxiety disorders, on the other hand, denote specific behavioral and psychological conditions that are conceptualized at a more superficial and tangible level. If religious and spiritual issues are to have an impact on anxiety disorders, one would expect this influence to occur at a global level—that is, in classificatory terms, at subthreshold and subsyndromal levels of anxiety. On closer scrutiny, then, such relations between these issues and religiosity/spirituality could appear to be in fact very complex and mediated by a whole range of intermediate factors.

Scholars agree today that the concepts of religiosity and spirituality are multidimensional. The same holds for anxiety. There is a wide variety of anxiety phenomena. Each form of anxiety has its own place on a conceptual map that is characterized by distinctions such as those between the subjective, behavioral, motor, and physiological aspects of anxiety; between state and trait; and between object/situation-bound and objectless forms of anxiety. The multidimensionality of the constructs of anxiety and religiosity/spirituality implies that in-depth investigation of the relations between different dimensions of these phenomena would in the long run reveal a richer and more complex picture of (causal) relations. What we may expect to emerge, then, is a multifaceted tapestry consisting of numerous threads of reciprocal dependencies and causal relations at different levels. Therefore, in terms of the research agenda at which we are aiming, it seems plausible 1) to search for relationships between religion/spirituality and these nonspecific, more diffuse forms of anxiety and 2) to elucidate the (probably many) causal pathways mediating the effects of religious and spiritual issues on anxiety disorders.

One might argue that the type of research mentioned under item (1) in the previous paragraph does not seem to be helpful for the development and refinement of a classification system. Nonspecific and more diffuse forms of anxiety, however, may be clinically relevant because they may predispose to anxiety disorders and other Axis I disorders.

Religious and Spiritual Issues and Anxiety in the General Population

Given the ubiquity of religiosity/spirituality and anxiety, it is surprising how little research has been done with respect to the relationship between the two. With respect to religious and spiritual issues and anxiety in a medical context there are some studies on religion and OCD as well as on religion and anxiety in somatic disease and on death anxiety. Hardly any study could be found on religion and panic disorder, agoraphobia, social phobia, simple phobia, generalized anxiety disorder, and/or adjustment disorder. We first describe some reviews of the relationship between religion and anxiety in the general population.

In a recent overview, Shreve-Neiger and Edelstein (2004) highlighted a number of studies in which religion is associated with decreased anxiety. Having some type of religious affiliation appears to be related to lower anxiety levels in some studies. Other studies show that contemplative prayer is associated with increased security and less distress, and intrinsic religiosity with less worry and anxiety. *Intrinsic religiosity*, a concept formulated by Allport and Ross (Allport 1950; Allport and Ross 1967), refers to a lifestyle in which religion is personally appropriated and "lived" from within, whereas *extrinsic religiosity* refers to a lifestyle in which religion is related to social convention. Schreve-Neiger and Edelstein then reviewed studies with a relationship between religion and increased anxiety. Some of these appeared to be focused on extrinsic forms of religiosity. Finally, they mentioned a number of studies with no relationship at all between religion and anxiety. The authors concluded that "no study in this review escaped methodological and/or conceptual criticism" (p. 393). Psychometric properties of religiosity measures were unsound (e.g., unpublished measures, unknown reliability and validity), sample sizes were often small, and sampling procedures were poor. Typically, multidimensional measures of religiosity were lacking. Older populations seem to tap into the "more positive and healthful aspects of religion," the authors said. Nevertheless, there may be a relationship between religion and subsyndromal and subthreshold types of anxiety. They concluded that these forms of anxiety should be assessed with general measures of anxiety instead of with the standard diagnostic instruments.

In a comprehensive review of the relationship between religion and medicine, Koenig (2001) found 76 studies examining the relationship between religion and anxiety (7 clinical trials, 69 observational studies). Thirty-five studies found lower levels of anxiety or less fear among more religious people; 17 studies reported no association; 7 reported mixed or complex results; and 10 reported greater anxiety among the more religious. In a study by Koenig et al. (1993), religion and anxiety were only related in the young age group. Church attendees, mainline Protestants, and those considering themselves "born again" showed fewer anxiety disorders, whereas young fundamentalist Pentecostals, persons with no religious affiliation, and frequent religious-television viewers had more anxiety disorders. No specific associations could be found in the middle-aged and old age groups. This study was conducted among participants of the Piedmont Epidemiological Catchment Area survey (1,025 young, 645 middle aged, and 1,299 elderly persons).

Schapman and Inderbitzen-Nolan (2002) specifically investigated a group of 261 adolescents. They found partial support for a positive relationship between religiosity and mental health in general, but no association between more frequent religious involvement and anxiety.

Tapanya et al. (1997) conducted a study on religiosity and worry, comparing elderly (nonpsychiatric) Buddhist Thais and Christian Canadians (N=104; all subjects were between ages 65 and 90 years). They found for both Buddhists and Christians that intrinsic religiosity was associated with less worry. It was furthermore revealed that extrinsic orientation among Buddhists, in contrast to Christians, was linked to greater worry. The authors hypothesized that this might be a result of Buddhists' realization that their extrinsic religious behavior does not help in alleviating individual responsibility or guilt. Belief in the law of the karma implies, they suggested, that there is no escape from the consequences of one's actions through redemption (as in Christianity). Only individual perseverance toward enlightenment will bring forth liberation from the cycle of death and reincarnation. This study is mentioned because it is one of the very few comparing Christian and non-Christian subjects.

Kendler et al. (2003) investigated 2,616 twins with respect to a possible differential relationship between aspects of religion and internalizing and externalizing disorders. This study is relevant for our purposes because anxiety disorder could be related to an internalizing emotional and cognitive style. The authors, moreover, looked for relationships between religious and spiritual issues and psychopathology at a more general level by using the broad and encompassing concepts of internalizing and externalizing disorder. One out of seven religiosity factors could indeed be associated with internalizing disorders (unvengefulness, i.e., "an attitude toward the world emphasizing personal retaliation rather than forgiveness"; the factor was called unvengefulness because the items were scored in the positive direction); four factors with externalizing disorders (general religiosity, involved God, forgiveness, God as judge); and two factors with both internalizing and externalizing disorders (social religiosity, thankfulness). This study is one of the first large epidemiological studies that meets the requirement of a multidimensional measure of religion.

Religious and Spiritual Issues in Obsessive-Compulsive Disorder

All studies reviewed thus far do not distinguish among different anxiety disorder categories. When we look for associations between religion/spirituality and specific anxiety disorders, OCD is obviously the category in which we would expect such relationships to be present. Not only do religious obsessions frequently occur (42% of all obsessions; Tek and Ulug 2001), but one might also hypothesize that there is some relation between particular clinical features of OCD such as thought-action fusion (i.e., the belief that thinking is equal to doing, magical thinking), perfectionism, rituals, and doubt on the one hand and religious practices, thought patterns, and moral concerns on the other hand. Research so far has shown inconsistent results. Abramowitz et al. (2004) indeed found partial support for a relation between high religiosity and obsessional symptoms, compulsive washing/cleaning, and beliefs about the importance of thoughts among Protestant undergraduates. There was strong support for a relation between high religiosity and higher levels of OCD-related cognitions, such as the importance of or a need to control and responsibility for one's thoughts. Highly religious persons also showed lack of tolerance of uncertainty and doubt. Abramowitz et al. (2002) also reported on the development of the Penn Inventory of Scrupulosity, a 19-item self-report scale measuring religious obsessive-compulsive symptoms. Factor analysis showed a two-factor solution with one subscale measuring fears about having committed sin and the other subscale measuring fears concerning punishment from God.

Zohar et al. (2005) could establish a relationship "to some degree" between religiosity on the one hand and perfectionism and parental attitudes to upbringing on the other, but not to obsessive-compulsive behavior. In a second study on OCD and religious change, obsessive-compulsive traits were more prevalent among those who had become more religious than their parents than among those who were less religious than their parents, but the causality of this relationship was unclear. Rassin and Koster (2003) found a relationship between Protestant belief and increased scores on the morality part of the thought-action fusion measure. The thought-action fusion measure distinguishes between a morality and a probability (or likelihood) dimension of thought-action fusion; the *morality dimension* refers to the inclination to believe that thinking something wrong is morally equal to doing something wrong; the *probability (likelihood) dimension* refers to the inclination to think that one's thoughts are the cause of some evil (or good) (Berle and Starcevic 2005). Protestants, in other words, were more inclined to feel excessively responsible for what they were thinking. The authors also found a relationship between Catholic belief and moderate scores on both the morality and the probability parts of the thought-action fusion measure (to think is to cause). Tek and Ulug (2001), however, could not establish any conclusive relationship between religiosity and any clinical feature of OCD, including the presence of religious obsessions. Nor did Greenberg and Shefler (2002) find differences in the experience of religious and nonreligious symptoms of OCD in a group of ultra-orthodox Jewish psychiatric referrals with OCD. In another Israeli sample Hermesh et al. (2003) also could not establish relationships between OCD and percentage of religious patients, intensity of OCD symptoms and degree of religiosity, and percentage of religious obsessions related to religious background.

Religious and Spiritual Issues in Other Anxiety Disorders and Adjustment Disorder

With respect to other anxiety disorders there are very few studies investigating the relationship between religious and spiritual issues and the occurrence of specific anxiety disorders other than OCD. Trenholm et al. (1998) showed in their study that there is a relationship between religious conflict and catastrophic thinking in the genesis of panic disorder. The group consisted of 20 women with panic disorder and/or agoraphobia, 20 women in therapy for other reasons than panic, and a control group of 20 recruited from the general population. The authors used the Religious Conflict subscale of the Survey of Attitudes Towards Religion and Philosophy of Life Scale. The Religious Conflict scale could be subdivided into two subscales: one measuring "positive" religious conflict (questioning and discussing certain teachings of one's church, for example) and one addressing "negative" religious conflict (for instance, wavering faith in one's religion or guilt). The panic group scored significantly higher on negative religious conflict, suggesting that negative religious conflict might be related to catastrophic thinking in panic disorder. Hybels et al. (2000) sought a relationship between social and personal resources and the prevalence of the phobic disorder in a community population (the Duke University Epidemiologic Catchment Area Study). There were no relationships between religiosity (operationalized by church attendance, time spent in religious activities, and perceived importance of religion) and simple phobia, agoraphobia, and social phobia.

Loewenthal et al. (1997) investigated the social circumstances under which anxiety occurred among orthodox Jews in London. Danger and early adversity bore only a weak relationship with anxiety in this sample. Women were more likely to have borderline anxiety than were men. Women had more "eventful lives" than men. The authors concluded that unlike in the general population, danger comes not so much from one menacing or disruptive event but from general overburdening. They speculated that in this traditional religious subculture burden is related to danger of failing to maintain normative standards. Women might be more vulnerable to such overburdening because of their "greater responsibilities for maintaining religious standards and boundaries." The "events" the women were talking about were associated with "rites of passage and religious festivals, which depend on tremendous culinary activity by women" (p. 93).

Kroll et al. (2004) conducted an interesting study on the concept of worry in 225 psychiatric outpatients. Worry about moral issues emerged as a domain distinct from worry about practical matters. Moral worries appeared not to decline with age (in contrast to practical worries) and to be negatively correlated with intrinsic religiosity and positively with neuroticism. From their study these authors drew a line to the study of moral emotions such as remorse, guilt, and shame. They suggested that moral worries are part of the lives of our patients and thus should not be minimized as mere symptoms of depression.

There are at present no quantitative studies on the relationship between religious and spiritual issues and adjustment disorder.

Religious and Spiritual Issues and Anxiety in Medical Illness

There has been a plethora of research on spirituality and psychological well-being in medically ill patients. The relationship between religiosity/spirituality and anxiety in these patients has been studied much less, however. In a review on depression and anxiety in heart failure, Konstam et al. (2005) reported that people with higher levels of religiosity/spirituality responded to illness with better coping or improved adjustment and health-related quality of life compared with individuals who reported lower levels of religiosity/spirituality. McCoubrie and Davies (2006) found a negative correlation between spirituality, in particular the existential aspect, and anxiety (and depression) in patients with advanced cancer (*N*=85). Remarkably enough, religious well-being, and strength of belief had no impact on psychological well-being in their study. Spirituality was measured with the Spiritual Well-Being Scale and the Royal Free Interview for Spiritual and Religious Beliefs, and anxiety was measured with the Hospital Anxiety and Depression Scale. The Spiritual Well-Being Scale has 20 items, 10 measuring one's sense of meaning and purpose (Existential Well-Being) and 10 measuring one's relationship to a higher being, "God" (Religious Well-Being). The results suggest that making sense of one's circumstances and finding meaning and purpose when faced with life-threatening illness "has far more impact on psychological well-being than does religious faith" (McCoubrie and Davies 2006, p. 383). This study was preceded by a similar study by Kaczorowski (1989) in which spiritual well-being (with the Spiritual Well-Being Scale) and anxiety (Spielberger's State-Trait Anxiety Inventory) appeared to be negatively correlated in adults diagnosed with cancer (*N*=114). This relationship was consistent even after correction for gender, age, marital status, diagnosis, group participation, and length of time since diagnosis. Kaczorowski did not make a distinction between the existential and the religious part of the Spiritual Well-Being Scale. Boscaglia et al. (2005) investigated the contribution of spirituality and spiritual coping to anxiety and depression in women with a recent diagnosis of gynecological cancer (*N*=100). Use of negative spiritual coping was found to be associated with higher anxiety scores. People with lower levels of spirituality tended to be more depressed, but this finding did not reach statistical significance.

Religious and Spiritual Issues and Death Anxiety

Studies on death anxiety have also focused on religious and spiritual issues. In a longitudinal study of a community-based sample of the San Francisco East Bay Area, using data of people born in the 1920s, Wink and Scott (2005) investigated the relationship between religiousness and fear of death and dying (the terms were used interchangeably) in old age (*N*=155). They compared two hypotheses, one predicting the presence of a linear relationship between death anxiety and religiousness, the other predicting a more complex relationship. The authors built on earlier findings of a curvilinear relationship between religiosity and death anxiety (death anxiety being highest among people with moderate religiosity; see for instance Nelson and Cantrell 1980) and on studies showing that death anxiety is mediated by the perception that life is meaningful and is related to "inconsistency" between beliefs and practices and to ambivalence (contradictory beliefs)—more inconsistency and/or ambivalence being linked to more death anxiety. The authors found support for the more complex relationship and for the "inconsistency" hypothesis (i.e., lack of congruence between belief in afterlife and religious practices was associated with more death anxiety). Religiosity in middle adulthood predicted death anxiety in late adulthood (a time interval of 25 years!) in the same curvilinear fashion, even after controlling for sociodemographic variables, life satisfaction, social support, and stressors. The authors concluded that firmness and consistency of beliefs and practices, rather than religiousness per se, buffers against death anxiety in old age.

Results of the study of Ardelt and Koenig (2006) in hospice patients and relatively healthy older adults (*N*=103) point in the same direction. Path analyses showed that a sense of purpose in life rather than religiosity had a direct positive effect on subjective well-being and a direct negative effect on fear of dying. Intrinsic religiosity had an indirect positive effect on subjective well-being when mediated by shared spiritual activities. Frequency of prayer did not add much to subjective well-being. Intrinsic religiosity also had a strong direct positive effect on approach acceptance of death. *Approach acceptance of death* refers to longing for afterlife and its expected rewards. Extrinsic religiosity, finally, had an indirect negative effect on purpose in life and was positively related to fear of death. The results indicated, according to the authors, that "private prayer might be less effective in eliciting a sense of purpose in life than spiritual activities that are shared with others" (p. 206).

McClain-Jacobson et al. (2004) assessed afterlife beliefs, spiritual well-being, and psychological functioning at the end of life among terminally ill cancer patients ($N=276$). Belief in afterlife appeared to be associated with lower levels of end-of-life despair (desire for death, hopelessness, and suicidal ideation) but not with levels of depression or anxiety. When controlled for spirituality, the effect of afterlife beliefs disappeared. The authors concluded that instead of beliefs held about afterlife, rather, it is spirituality that has a powerful effect on psychological functioning.

Lundh and Radon (1998) compared religious believers, atheists, and agnostics on a questionnaire measure of death anxiety (the Death Depression Scale) and a Stroop task with death-related words. Religious believers showed less death anxiety than atheists and agnostics; however, they did not differ on Stroop interference for death-related words. The Stroop task consisted of measurement of response latency of color naming of death-related, death-control, positive, and positive-control words. The authors warned against too much reliance on self-report measures of death anxiety and suggested that the Death Depression Scale and the Stroop task capture different aspects of death anxiety. Another interpretation would be that the Stroop task measures a less specific emotional response to the sudden appearance of death-related words on a screen.

Finally, Thorson (1998; Thorson et al. 1997) compared intrinsic religious motivation and death anxiety among samples from the United States, Kuwait, and Egypt. In general, Egyptian males and females both scored much higher on intrinsic religiosity, measured with the Hoge's scale for Intrinsic Religious Motivation. Death anxiety scores on the Revised Death Anxiety Scale were lower for Egyptians than for Americans, but not for Kuwaitis—a fact the author attributed to the experience of the Gulf War by the Kuwaitis. However, in contrast to this overall relationship Egyptian males scored higher than American males on items dealing with what happens to the body in the grave. Perhaps this is a result of the fear of what could happen to the body in the grave. According to Muslim faith, the body is visited by two angels immediately after burial, and after interrogation, they may inflict punishment to the body—the so-called *azab-e-qabr*. It might also be that American males feel more free to express their vulnerability with respect to death and dying. American females, however, score much higher than Egyptian females on items related to fear of decomposition and loss of bodily integrity. This may be a cultural artifact based on the societal pressure to look good, the author suggested.

Discussion

This overview of studies on the relationship between religious and spiritual issues and anxiety disorders and adjustment disorder leaves us with an imprecise and inconsistent picture. Research has found correlations between these issues and the presence of anxiety disorder. However, the findings were contradictory, and the measures (at least those assessing religion/spirituality) were often simplistic. Moreover, the majority of studies were correlational and did not allow any conclusion about causation. It is therefore not possible at the present moment to give an answer to the questions that were raised earlier in the chapter about the nature of the relationship between religious and spiritual issues and anxiety (disorders). Findings so far are compatible with all three interpretations—that is, that religious and spiritual issues do not affect the core of anxiety and/or adjustment disorder; that these issues are relevant for anxiety but not for the distinctness of different classes of anxiety disorder; and that religion/spirituality and anxiety disorder are related in a yet unknown way.

There was a tendency toward a negative relationship between intrinsic religiosity and level of anxiety or presence of anxiety disorder, but it is unclear whether this was a direct effect of religious belief or mediated by other factors. In fact, effects of religiosity sometimes disappeared after correction for age, marital status, and sociocultural and other extrinsic factors. In other studies religious and spiritual issues had more impact on general psychological well-being than on anxiety.

The majority of studies on anxiety disorders and religion/spirituality have been devoted to OCD. Much less work has been done on agoraphobia, panic disorder, social phobia, and specific phobias (posttraumatic stress disorder is reviewed elsewhere in this volume). Research on adjustment disorder is simply lacking. Instead of focusing on relationships between anxiety disorder and religiosity/spirituality in general, future research should focus on more specific and complex routes via which religious and spiritual issues may have an impact on anxiety and adjustment disorders. We may think of breaking up the constructs of religion and spirituality into several components or dimensions and of making distinctions between religious beliefs and practices as such and their embedding in the social and cultural practices of a certain group. Developmental parameters such as parenting, attachment style, religious socialization, and education may be related to domains of personal functioning and personality characteristics in later life (see Figure 4–1).

One promising approach aims at possible relations between the morality part of the thought-action fusion measure and religiosity. We saw that Protestant belief was related to the tendency to believe that thinking something wrong is morally equal to doing something wrong (Rassin and Koster 2003). Recently thought-action fusion has been related to work on the concept of metacognition. *Metacognition* is a concept that refers to knowledge about one's own cognitions (Garcia-Montes et al. 2006). In the field of psychopathology it has been developed in the context

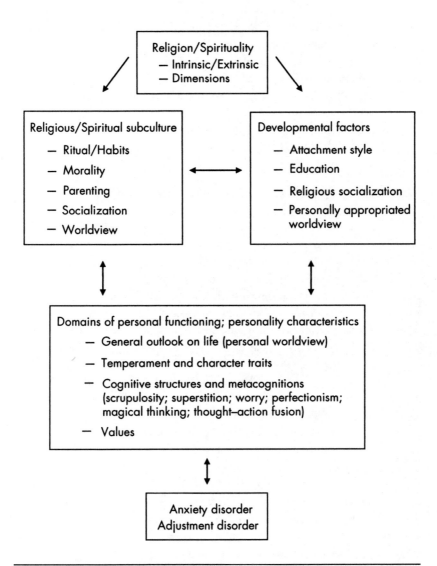

FIGURE 4–1. Conceptual map of possible relationships and causal routes between religion/spirituality and anxiety and adjustment disorder.

of the so-called Self-Regulatory Executive Function model. According to this model, certain types of metacognition would lead people to develop a response pattern to thoughts or other private events characterized by heightened self-awareness, activation of dysfunctional beliefs, and the use of self-regulation strategies that fail to restructure maladaptive beliefs. Studies of metacognitive beliefs in patients with hallucinations and with OCD have found that the superstition, punishment, and responsibility items of the Metacognitions Questionnaire are related to both hallucinations and OCD. Superstition entails, in this context, the false and magical belief that certain cognitive intrusions should be controlled as if they were occasioned by a factor or agent outside the person. Thought-action fusion and schizotypy have been shown to be related, and both are related to OCD. This type of research aims at establishing relationships between a particular subset of a person's cognitions and religious and/or spiritual variables.

Similar work could be done in the field of moral emotions and character as the study of Kroll et al. (2004) has shown.

Toward a Research Agenda for DSM-V

What can be concluded from this review for the research agenda for DSM-V? In general there is a need for standardized and more refined measurement instruments for religion (Brun 2005; Fetzer Institute 1999) and for research that relates different aspects of religion to phases (age), prognostic factors, and subtypes and/or aspects of anxiety disorders and adjustment disorders. We need, for instance, studies that relate subsets of religious cognitions to the course and prognosis of anxiety disorders (Kroll et al. 2004; Trenholm et al. 1998). Such more fine-grained studies should be combined with studies that aim at subthreshold and subsyndromal forms of anxiety. Study on subsyndromal anxiety could lead to the inclusion of this category in the section on "other conditions that may be focus of clinical attention." Subsyndromal anxiety could then be specified to different contexts (somatic disease for instance), phases of life (death anxiety), and religiously and spiritually significant experiences (conversion, induction of guilt, exorcistic ritual). Such research could also lead to the inclusion of death anxiety as a separate category in the section "other conditions that may be focus of clinical attention."

In view of the inconclusive results of studies on the relation between religious and spiritual issues and OCD, we have to conclude that more studies are needed that address the relationship between these issues and thought-action fusion, perfectionism, ritual, and doubt. With respect to adjustment disorders, we need studies that focus on the relationship between onset and subtypes of adjustment disorder on the one hand, and phase of life, existential and/or religious problems on the other hand.

Recommendations for DSM-V

Research

1. Fine-grained studies relating different aspects of religiosity/spirituality to phases (age), prognostic factors, and subtypes and/or aspects of anxiety and adjustment disorders
2. Studies relating different aspects of religiosity/spirituality to subthreshold and subsyndromal forms of anxiety

Include death anxiety in the section "Other conditions that may be focus of clinical attention"

Include subsyndromal and subthreshold anxiety in the section "Other conditions that may be focus of clinical attention"

References

Abramowitz JS, Huppert JD, Cohen AB, et al: Religious obsessions and compulsions in a non-clinical sample: the Penn Inventory of Scrupulosity (PIOS). Behav Res Ther 40:825–838, 2002

Abramowitz JS, Deacon BJ, Woods CM, et al: Association between Protestant religiosity and obsessive-compulsive symptoms and cognitions. Depress Anxiety 20:70–76, 2004

Allport G: The Individual and His Religion. New York, MacMillan, 1950

Allport G, Ross JM: Personal religious orientation and prejudice. J Pers Soc Psychol 5:432–443, 1967

Ardelt M, Koenig CS: The role of religion for hospice patients and relatively healthy older adults. Res Aging 28:184–215, 2006

Beard GM: A Practical Treatise on Nervous Exhaustion (Neurasthenia): Its Symptoms, Nature, Sequences, Treatment. Edited with notes and additions by Rockwell AD. London, England, HK Lewis, 1890

Berle D, Starcevic V: Thought-action fusion: review of the literature and future directions. Clin Psychol Rev 25:263–284, 2005

Berrios GE: The History of Mental Symptoms: Descriptive Psychopathology Since the Nineteenth Century. Cambridge, UK, Cambridge University Press, 1996

Boscaglia N, Clarke DM, Quinn MA: The contribution of spirituality and spiritual coping to anxiety and depression in women with a recent diagnosis of gynaecological cancer. Int J Gynecol Cancer 15:755–761, 2005

Brun WL: A proposed diagnostic schema for religious/spiritual concerns. J Pastoral Care Counsel 59:425–440, 2005

Fetzer Institute: Multidimensional Measurement of Religiousness/Spirituality for Use in Health Research. Kalamazoo, MI, Fetzer Institute, 1999

Freud S: Hemmung, Symptom und Angst. Gesammelte Werke, Band XIV, 1926, pp 111–205

Garcia-Montes JM, Pérez-Alvarez M, Soto Balbuena C, et al: Metacognitions in patients with hallucinations and obsessive-compulsive disorder: the superstition factor. Behav Res Ther 44:1091–1104, 2006

Glas G: A conceptual history of anxiety and depression, in Handbook on Anxiety and Depression, 2nd Edition. Edited by den Boer JA, Sitsen A. New York, Marcel Dekker, 2003, pp 1–48

Goldstein K: Zum Problem der Angst. Allgemeine ärztliche Zeitschrift für Psychotherapie und Psychische Hygiene, Band 2, 1929, pp 409–437

Greenberg D, Shefler G: Obsessive compulsive disorder in ultra-orthodox Jewish patients: a comparison of religious and non-religious symptoms. Psychology and Psychotherapy: Theory, Research and Practice 75:123–130, 2002

Hermesh H, Masser-Kavitzky R, Gross-Isseroff R: Obsessive-compulsive disorder and Jewish religiosity. J Nerv Ment Dis 191:201–203, 2003

Hybels CF, Blazer DG, Kaplan BH: Social and personal resources and the prevalence of phobic disorder in a community population. Psychol Med 30:705–716, 2000

Kaczorowski J: Spiritual well-being and anxiety in adults diagnosed with cancer. Hospital Journal 5:105–116, 1989

Kendler KS, Liu X-Q, Gardner CO, et al: Dimensions of religiosity and their relationship to lifetime psychiatric and substance abuse disorders. Am J Psychiatry 160:496–503, 2003

Kierkegaard S: The Concept of Anxiety: A Simple Psychologically Orienting Deliberation on the Dogmatic Issue of Hereditary Sin (1844). Edited and translated by Thomte R, Anderson AB. Princeton, NJ, Princeton University Press, 1980

Koenig HG: Religion and medicine, II: religion, mental health, and related behaviours. Int J Psychiatry Med 31:97–109, 2001

Koenig HG, Ford SM, George LK, et al: Religion and anxiety disorder: an examination and comparison of associations in young, middle-aged, and elderly adults. J Anxiety Disord 7:321–342, 1993

Konstam V, Moser DK, De Jong MJ: Depression and anxiety in heart failure. J Card Fail 11:455–463, 2005

Kraepelin E: Psychiatrie. Ein Lehrbuch für Studirende und Aertzte. Band I. Allgemeine Psychiatrie (sechste, vollständig umgearbeitete Auflage). Leipzig, Germany, Johann Ambrosius Barth, 1899

Kraepelin E, Lange J: Psychiatrie. Band I: Allgemeine Psychiatrie (neunte Auflage). Leipzig, Germany, Johann Ambrosius Barth, 1927

Kroll J, Egan E, Erickson P, et al: Moral conflict, religiosity, and neuroticism in an outpatient sample. J Nerv Ment Dis 192:682–688, 2004

Kronfeld A: Über angst. Nederlandsch Tijdschrift voor Psychologie 3:366–387, 1935

Loewenthal KM, Goldblatt V, Gorton T, et al: The social circumstances of anxiety and its symptoms among Anglo-Jews. J Affect Disord 46:87–94, 1997

Lundh L-G, Radon V: Death anxiety as a function of belief in afterlife: comparison between a questionnaire measure and a Stroop measure of death anxiety. Pers Individ Dif 25:487–494, 1998

May R: The Meaning of Anxiety. New York, The Ronald Press Company, 1950

May R: The Discovery of Being: Writings in Existential Psychotherapy. New York, WW Norton, 1983

McClain-Jacobson C, Rosenfeld B, Kosinski A, et al: Belief in afterlife, spiritual well-being and end-of-life despair in patients with advanced cancer. Gen Hosp Psychiatry 26:484–486, 2004

McCoubrie RC, Davies AN: Is there a correlation between spirituality and anxiety and depression in patients with advanced cancer? Support Care Cancer 14:379–385, 2006

Nelson LD, Cantrell CH: Religiosity and death anxiety: a multi-dimensional analysis. Rev Relig Res 21:148–157, 1980

Rassin E, Koster E: The correlation between thought–action fusion and religiosity in a normal sample. Behav Res Ther 41:361–368, 2003

Schapman AM, Inderbitzen-Nolan HM: The role of religious behaviour in adolescent depressive and anxious symptomatology. J Adolesc 25:631–643, 2002

Shreve-Neiger AK, Edelstein BA: Religion and anxiety: a critical review of the literature. Clin Psychol Rev 24:379–397, 2004

Tapanya S, Nicki R, Jarusawad O: Worry and intrinsic/extrinsic religious orientation among Buddhist (Thai) and Christian (Canadian) elderly persons. Int J Aging Human Dev 44:73–83, 1997

Tek C, Ulug B: Religiosity and religious obsessions in obsessive-compulsive disorder. Psychiatry Res 104:99–108, 2001

Thorson JA: Religion and anxiety: Which anxiety? Which religion?, in Handbook of Religion and Mental Health. Edited by Koenig HG. San Diego, CA, Academic Press, 1998, pp 147–160

Tillich P: The Courage to Be. New Haven, CT, Yale University Press, 1952

Thorson JA, Powell FC, Abdel-Khalek AM, et al: Constructions of religiosity and death anxiety in two cultures. J Psychol Theol 25:374–383, 1997

Trenholm P, Trent J, Compton WC: Negative religious conflict as a predictor of panic disorder. J Clin Psychol 54:59–65, 1998

Wink P, Scott J: Does religiousness buffer against the fear of death and dying in late adulthood? Findings from a longitudinal study. J Gerontol 60B:P207–P214, 2005

Yalom ID: Existential Psychotherapy. New York, Basic Books, 1980

Zohar AH, Goldman E, Calamary R, et al: Religiosity and obsessive-compulsive behavior in Israeli Jews. Behav Res Ther 43:857–868, 2005

Commentary 4A

COMMENTARY ON "RELIGIOUS AND SPIRITUAL ISSUES IN ANXIETY AND ADJUSTMENT DISORDERS"

A New Psychiatric Frontier?

H. M. Van Praag, M.D., Ph.D.

Professor Glas's informative exploration of the relationship between religious/spiritual variables and anxiety (disorders) induces me to make a few remarks.

1. In psychiatry the reality of religiosity and spirituality has been sorely neglected in the past century. By many professionals it was regarded, at best, as an anachronistic remnant of an infantile past not to be cherished but rather to be treated. This attitude has been seriously mistaken. Psychiatric diagnosing requires thorough scrutiny of the major domains that have shaped or might have shaped someone's life, such as upbringing, social conditions, educational experiences, relational development, and, last but not least, religiosity, or in more general terms, an individual's spiritual outlook on life. Concerning the latter domain, the question should be posited whether it has developed at all, and if so, what its salience is and to what extent it may have contributed to someone's personhood. Psychiatrists cannot with impunity ignore potentially important spheres of life, whatever their private convictions might be. This view implies that future psychiatrists should receive training in how to enter

97

and explore the spiritual realm, how to overcome personal biases, and how to assess its possible etiological relevance.

2. In studying the relationship between religious/spiritual variables and anxiety, I would not recommend using the subdivision of anxiety disorders as proposed by the DSM classificatory system as a starting point. Those categorical constructs are to a large extent manmade, not well validated, and broadly overlapping. The scientific study of the etiology of mental disturbances requires precise and detailed definition of the psychopathological variables one aspires to study. If that is not the case few relationships will be uncovered, or spurious ones. The dimensional approach therefore makes much more sense. It is the study of "pure" anxiety—anxiety as a discrete, definable and measurable state of mind—independent of the categorical entity in which it happens to occur (most often an anxiety disorder, a mood disorder, or a personality disorder). For a long time I have advocated and applied this strategy in pathophysiological studies of mental disturbances, and not without positive results (Van Praag 2001; Van Praag et al. 1987, 2004).

3. What should be studied in the spiritual sphere? First, we should ascertain whether a relationship is demonstrable between religiosity/spirituality and the anxiety dimension, and next, which components of religiosity/spirituality it concerns. Once a relationship has been made plausible, the question arises whether the religious/spiritual variables play a mere pathoplastic or an etiological role. Finally, one should try to answer the question whether the patient's belief system has had an ameliorating or provocative effect on the anxious mood state. In both cases the patient's religious/spiritual notions have to be studied in more depth. Do they represent an experiential world laden with fear and trepidation, or do they constitute a source of hope and relief? If the former seems to be the case, one has to explore whether the patient's troubled faith seems to be cause or consequence of the pathological mental condition.

4. The exploration of someone's religious/spiritual life requires, above all, the method of free interviewing. Rating scales and even the structured standard interview are insufficient, because they possess not enough "resolving power." The reliability of the data so derived can be checked by videotaping the interview and having it assessed by independent investigators.

5. Religious variables may be of etiological significance or may form part of the symptomatology. In clinical studies both aspects should be clearly discriminated. Moreover, because religiosity and spirituality are complex constructs, they should be dissected into component parts, and methods have to be developed to assess those reliably. I mention an analogy: stress. That construct, too, is used both in an etiological and a phenomenological sense. Both ways it shows considerable variability. Stress research often fails to take that into account, to the detriment of its significance.

6. In studying religiosity and psychopathology, in this case anxiety, data concerning different religions should, of course, be distinguished. Data concerning their orthodox and more liberal adherents should be analyzed separately as well. A key question to be raised is whether the various belief systems influence mental health differently or whether a common core is discernable. Such comparative studies might generate new insights into the impact human behavior and experience have on religious philosophies, and vice versa, into the way human behavior and experience influence the thinking of theologians.

7. Finally, the treatment issues. Should religious faith play a role in the treatment of anxiety (or any other psychopathological condition)? It might, provided evidence is emerging that faith issues have contributed to the state of anxiety, and/or if those issues seem to be applicable in the therapeutic process. The question of who should take the lead in this endeavor, pastor or psychiatrist, depends for the time being on qualifications, experience, and mindset of the potential therapists and on the patient's preference. Possibly a tandem approach would be preferable. Empirical studies should shed light on this question.

Fifty years ago, the study of brain and behavior relationships was a true frontier area in psychiatric research. Researchers succeeded to move that frontier far ahead. In the past century religion has been a taboo region for (many) research-oriented psychiatrists. Possibly the scene is changing by now. If true, rightly so. Religion and its relationship to both normal and abnormal human behavior seems (at least to me) a fascinating and novel field, well worth being studied in depth by psychiatrists with a pioneering spirit. I consider it to be a potential new frontier region in psychiatric research. May that become the conviction of many.

References

Van Praag HM: Anxiety/aggression-driven depression: a paradigm of functionalization and verticalization of psychiatric diagnosis. Prog Neuropsychopharmacol Biol Psychiatry 25:893–924, 2001

Van Praag HM, Kahn R, Asnis GM, et al: Denosologization of biological psychiatry or the specificity of 5-HT disturbances in psychiatric disorders. J Affect Disord 13:1–8, 1987

Van Praag HM, de Kloet T, van Os J: Stress, the Brain, and Depression. Cambridge, UK, Cambridge University Press, 2004

Commentary 4B

COMMENTARY ON "RELIGIOUS AND SPIRITUAL ISSUES IN ANXIETY AND ADJUSTMENT DISORDERS"

Dan J. Stein, M.D., Ph.D.

Professor Glas employs his considerable clinical and philosophical expertise to provide a thoughtful overview of the intersection between religious and spiritual issues and anxiety/adjustment disorders. He begins by noting that references to religious, spiritual, and existential aspects of anxiety are missing from current nosology and by providing three different interpretations. First, there is the possibility that these issues do not affect the core of anxiety and/or adjustment disorders. Second, there is the possibility that although religious and spiritual issues are relevant for anxiety they do not affect the distinctiveness of different classes of anxiety disorders. Third, there is the possibility that these issues and anxiety disorders are related in an unknown way.

After reviewing a range of studies, Glas concludes that the data are currently imprecise and inconsistent. Thus, it is not yet possible to decide among the three interpretations listed in his introduction. He goes on to provide a number of interesting suggestions for future research. In particular, he recommends fine-grained studies relating different aspects of religious and spiritual issues to phases (age), prognostic factors, and subtypes and/or aspects of anxiety disorders, as well as studies relating different aspects of theses issues to subthreshold and subsyndromal forms of anxiety. He also advocates for the inclusion of death anxiety and subsyndromal and subthreshold anxiety in the section "Other Conditions That May Be a Focus of Clinical Attention."

101

In the human sciences, including psychiatry, there is a long-standing tension between theories and methods focusing on *erklären* (explanation) versus those focusing on *verstehen* (understanding), between approaching humans as objects that must be detailed and accounted for, in terms of underlying mechanisms, and as subjects that must be described and accounted for, in terms of what is meaningful to them (Bhaskar 1979; Jaspers 1963; Stein 1991). Some of the same tension seems present in any consideration of the intersection between religion/spirituality and anxiety/adjustment disorders. On the one hand, a thorough understanding of any patient with an anxiety disorder requires an understanding of the person's religious, spiritual, and existential views and attitudes. On the other hand, a comprehensive explanation of such patients may include an account of both their religious, spiritual, and existential beliefs and of their anxiety symptoms, in terms of underlying psychobiological mechanisms.

A number of studies described by Glas are helpful in emphasizing the importance of understanding the religious, spiritual, and existential views and attitudes of those with anxiety disorders. The study by McCoubrie and Davies (2006), for example, emphasized that when one is faced with life-threatening illness, the ability to find meaning and purpose, rather than religious faith per se, affects one's psychological well-being. Similarly, Nelson and Cantrell (1980) concluded that consistency of beliefs and practices, rather than religiousness per se, buffers against death anxiety in old age. Certainly, in clinical practice, when a patient's explanatory model of illness differs from that of the standard psychiatric model, it is crucial to negotiate between the two (Kleinman 1988). In OCD with predominantly religious and spiritual concerns, a more medical model may well be appropriate (Fallon et al. 1990). However, on some occasions anxiety and stress are perhaps best conceptualized as an opportunity for growth (including spiritual growth; Tedeschi et al. 1998) and resilience (Stein et al. 2007).

Advances in cognitive-affective neuroscience in general, and of the anxiety disorders in particular, may also shed light on the psychobiology of religious and spiritual views. Moral reasoning, for example, like other kinds of reasoning, is increasingly viewed as open to empirical investigation (Johnson 1993). It is notable that in OCD, moral concerns in children and adolescents are fairly concrete (e.g., certain objects are viewed as contaminated), whereas in adulthood they become more abstract (e.g., certain ideas may be viewed as blasphemous) (Stein et al. 2001). This is consistent with the Piagetian notion in much cognitive-affective neuroscience today that the brain-mind is embodied and that complex abstract notions develop out of more basic sensorimotor and affective experience (Lakoff et al. 1999; Varela et al. 1991). It is notable that in posttraumatic stress disorder, forgiveness may be a key variable in determining prognosis (Kaminer et al. 2000). This is consistent with the Kendler et al. (2003) twin study reviewed by Glas and the notion that trauma therapy involves the articulation and working through of thoughts and feelings. Studies of the psychobiology of spiritual experience will surely continue to grow in the future, affecting our understanding of disorders such as obsessive-compulsive disorder and posttraumatic stress disorder (Stein and Kaminer 2006).

A key challenge for the human sciences, and indeed for the good practice of psychiatry, is the integration of explanation and understanding. Glas recommends that we undertake fine-grained studies relating different aspects of religious and spiritual issues to phases (age), prognostic factors, and subtypes and/or aspects of anxiety disorders as well as studies relating different aspects of these issues to subthreshold and subsyndromal forms of anxiety; such studies will surely contribute to such an integration. In addition, when working with patients with anxiety disorders, we need to pay close attention to the way in which their explanatory models of these disorders reflect their religious, spiritual, and existential views and to the possibility that some of these views are explicable in terms of their underlying psychobiology.

References

Bhaskar R: The Possibility of Naturalism. Hassocks, Sussex, UK, Harvester Press, 1979

Fallon BA, Liebowitz MR, Hollander E, et al: The pharmacotherapy of moral or religious scrupulosity. J Clin Psychiatry 51:517–521, 1990

Jaspers K: General Psychopathology. Chicago, IL, University of Chicago Press, 1963

Johnson M: Moral Imagination: Implications of Cognitive Science for Ethics. Chicago, IL, University of Chicago Press, 1993

Kaminer D, Stein DJ, Mbanga I, et al: Forgiveness: toward an integration of theoretical models. Psychiatry 63:344–357, 2000

Kendler KS, Liu X-Q, Gardner CO, et al: Dimensions of religiosity and their relationship to lifetime psychiatric and substance abuse disorders. Am J Psychiatry 160:496–503, 2003

Kleinman A: Rethinking Psychiatry: From Cultural Category to Personal Experience. New York, Free Press, 1988

Lakoff G, Johnson M: Philosophy in the Flesh: The Embodied Mind and Its Challenge to Western Thought. New York, Basic Books, 1999

McCoubrie RC, Davies AN: Is there a correlation between spirituality and anxiety and depression in patients with advanced cancer? Support Care Cancer 14:379–385, 2006

Nelson LD, Cantrell CH: Religiosity and death anxiety: a multi-dimensional analysis. Rev Relig Res 21:148–157, 1980

Stein DJ: Philosophy and the DSM-III. Compr Psychiatry 32:404–415, 1991

Stein DJ, Kaminer D: Forgiveness and psychopathology: psychobiological and evolutionary underpinnings. CNS Spectr 11:87–89, 2006

Stein DJ, Liu Y, Shapira NA, Goodman WK: The psychobiology of obsessive-compulsive disorder: how important is the role of disgust? Curr Psychiatry Rep 3:281–287, 2001

Stein DJ, Seedat S, Iversen A, et al: Post-traumatic stress disorder: medicine and politics. Lancet 369:139–144, 2007

Tedeschi RG, Park CL, Calhoun LG: Posttraumatic Growth: Positive Changes in the Aftermath of Crisis. Hillsdale, NJ, Lawrence Erlbaum, 1998

Varela FJ, Thompson E, Rosch E: The Embodied Mind: Cognitive Science and Human Experience. Cambridge, MA, MIT Press, 1991

5

RELIGION AND SPIRITUALITY IN THE DESCRIPTION OF POSTTRAUMATIC STRESS DISORDER

Samuel B. Thielman, M.D., Ph.D.

Although DSM-IV-TR (American Psychiatric Association 2000) alludes to one religious feature that may be associated with posttraumatic stress disorder (PTSD)—the emergence of "omen formation" in some patients with PTSD—in general it disregards religious and spiritual factors that may impinge on PTSD. The openness of the American Psychiatric Institute for Research and Education to inclusion of these factors in DSM-V should significantly enhance the usefulness of DSM-V and bring to the attention of the field the importance of considering religious and spiritual factors when assessing patients. Weaver et al. (2003) reviewed the research literature on the relationship of religion and trauma response in a major journal of trauma research between 1990 and 1999 and found that 4.1% of 467 articles dealt with religion/spirituality and that the number of articles addressing religion increased during the second half of the decade. A patient's religious or spiritual outlook shapes, and is shaped by, posttrauma symptoms in a number of

---

The opinions expressed in this paper are those of the author and do not represent the views of the U.S. Department of State or the U.S. government.

ways: through the influence of religion and spirituality on worldview; through making available otherwise inaccessible coping strategies; through its influence on the individual's perception of the moral meaning of the traumatic event; and through its influence on the social forces that contextualize the traumatic event.

PTSD and the Religious/Spiritual Worldview

PTSD, by its nature, involves consideration of *worldview*, and therefore of religion and spirituality, so considerations of religion and spirituality are important for accurate diagnosis of the condition. For an event to be traumatic, it must be interpreted by the patient as having been traumatic, and worldview plays a determining role in how a patient interprets a catastrophic event. Judith Herman, in *Trauma and Recovery*, portrayed the psychological response to trauma as one in which existential doubt and hopelessness lurk. She told of people who, in situations of terror, cry out for God or parents, but "when this cry is not answered, the sense of basic trust is shattered" (Herman 1997, p. 52). Herman wrote that traumatic events "undermine the belief systems that give meaning to human experience. They violate the victim's faith in a natural or divine order and cast the victim into a state of existential crisis" (p. 51). She cited examples of Vietnam veterans and Holocaust survivors who witnessed events they could not reconcile with their view of God. Yet many victims of trauma do not perceive their cries to God as going unanswered. As psychiatric knowledge has touched non-Western populations, it has become clear that the responses of victims described by Herman are not the responses of people throughout the world.

The range of assumptions throughout the world about the way the world is ordered means that there is also a range of interpretations of meaning of a traumatic event. If a patient believes events are random, due to luck, and occurring outside a larger "story," then anxiety may be increased. If they believe in destiny, they may have a more directed view of the world order, but one that is not always reassuring. When a traumatic experience is viewed within the context of a larger religious or spiritual narrative, its meaning may be less forbidding or anxiety provoking to the patient. Traditional Christians believe in providence, God's ultimately protective ordering of things. Hindus, Jains, Buddhists, and others believe in karma, the notion that the totality of a person's actions in this life and in past lives determine the course of events. The notion that there is a variety of interpretations of a particular trauma and that this may have an impact on response to trauma has not attracted much attention from psychiatric researchers. Nonetheless, evidence suggests that a religious or spiritual worldview is of great importance in the trauma response of large populations. And the list could continue. A study by Patel of Zimbabweans seeking care at a public health clinic found that half the subjects used spiritual models of illness and that patients who held the spiritual model had higher levels of mental disorder and were more likely to have a mental illness than those who did not. These subjects were more likely to consult a traditional medical provider (Patel 1995). Fox (2003) found that the Mandinka people have traditional names for trauma responses that do not correlate well with Western models and that incorporate notions of a spiritual etiology of trauma response. Niaz (2006) recently reported that after the October 8, 2005 earthquake in Pakistan that killed 100,000 people and left 35 million homeless, survivors looked to religion for consolation. They turned to God, "asking him for help and being thankful they were alive.... The underlying premise was that God gives and takes" (p. 205).

The importance of worldview, spirituality, and religion in shaping the response to trauma came home to me poignantly in what I was taught by patients I have treated who went through traumatic events in parts of the world very different from our own.

In a document distributed on the second anniversary of the August 7, 1998 bombing of the American Embassy in Nairobi, one Kenyan survivor, a Christian, wrote of the event:

> I was thrown down and covered with a lot of debris. I know of this because the Lord gave me a chance to live. So I found my self down and I could remember where I was lying. I thought I was having some nightmares.... When things in my mind were getting clearer that indeed something has happened and we were in danger. I started praying plural prayers. Lord please help us. Please Lord forgive us.... The Lord Jesus helped me wake up from the debris.... I was led to go out using the longest route from where I was. But God is so mighty, in that with the falling of the ceiling nothing hit my head when I was standing. ("Recollections of Foreign Service Nationals" 2000)

Another Kenyan, a 38-year-old office worker, took a more numerological approach:

> Seven has always been a lucky or sacred number and was given to all manner of grouping in the antiquity.... On the fateful day SEVENTH of August in 1998 we were a staff of SEVEN in my section: [six numbered names follow]; 7. Myself, and we all SURVIVED (Note "SURVIVE" is a SEVEN letter word.).... I do not want to be superstitious but I will keep asking them why it had to occur on the SEVENTH day of August. ("Recollections of Foreign Service Nationals" 2000)

This Kenyan, a member of the Kamba tribe, incorporating traditional Kamba notions of the meaning of the number seven, did not experience the event in the same way that a Westerner would have experienced it and probably would not respond to an unmodified psychological approach should he develop symptoms of PTSD (which, in fact, he had not developed) (Lindblom 1920).

In DSM-V, proposed wording for regarding the role of religious and spiritual factors would be included as a second paragraph in the PTSD section on "Specific Culture and Age Features" and would read as follows:

> Individuals in different parts of the world interpret traumatizing events in widely varying ways. Their interpretations may reflect deeply held religious views that can shape the experience of the traumatic event either positively or negatively. Clinicians should familiarize themselves with the worldview of the patient to maximize their ability to offer culturally sensitive care.

PTSD, Religious/Spiritual Coping, and DSM

A number of authors have looked at how religion and religious coping affect outcome in PTSD, and the results are mixed, a factor that should be incorporated into the prognostic considerations of the DSM. Religious faith sometimes positively affects the individual's ability to cope with trauma, and conversely, trauma may deepen the religious experience of some people. A study of survivors of the Dresden bombing found that there was a low rate of PTSD more than 50 years later, and that traumatic exposure was correlated with both PTSD *and* personal growth. The study further suggested that religious beliefs served as a moderator between exposure to trauma and the symptom of avoidance. A clinical understanding of the religious context of trauma for a given individual may help in formulating the prognosis of posttrauma symptoms (Maercker and Herrle 2003).

A systematic review by Shaw et al. (2005) found that religion and spirituality were often, although not always, a help to people who are dealing with traumatic events. They cited 6 case studies suggesting that religious and spiritual beliefs seemed to facilitate recovery from trauma, as well as five case studies documenting instances in which religious and spiritual beliefs had developed following traumatic events. Shaw et al. reviewed 11 empirical studies on religion and posttraumatic growth (4 quantitative and 7 qualitative). These studies suggested that multiply traumatized women found religion/spirituality to be a useful resource for dealing with the trauma's psychological effects. They also indicated that trauma survivors who were more committed to religious and spiritual goals more often said they had overcome the trauma and found meaning in it. In addition, their review found an association between posttraumatic growth and the traits of positive religious coping, religious openness, and readiness to face existential questions (Shaw et al. 2005). A recent study by Watlington and Murphy (2006) found that in African American women who had been victims of domestic violence, religious involvement was negatively correlated with posttraumatic stress symptoms.

Sometimes religious coping is a preferred method of coping but does not have the expected positive effect. Witvliet et al. (2004) studied 213 help-seeking veterans with PTSD and used two scales to determine the effect of forgiveness and religious coping style on anxiety, depression, and PTSD symptoms. They found that religious coping, both positive and negative, was associated with severity of PTSD symptoms. Positive religious coping meant seeking spiritual support, collaboration with God in solving the problem, and positive religious appraisal of the problem. Negative religious coping was interpersonal religious discontent, questioning God's power, and appraisal of the problem as God's punishment. Because several previous studies had found that positive religious coping had a beneficial impact on mental health in other types of patients, this group's finding that positive religious coping was associated with severity of PTSD symptoms was unexpected.

Fontana and Rosenheck (2004) found that among a large group of veterans (554 outpatient and 831 inpatient) attending specialized treatment programs for PTSD at the U.S. Department of Veterans Affairs (VA), veterans who had killed others or failed to prevent death often experienced weakened religious faith. Weakened religious faith and guilt contributed significantly to more extensive use of VA mental health services, whereas severity of PTSD symptoms and social functioning did not. They conceded that veterans' use of mental health services under these circumstances seemed to be connected with their search for meaning and purpose, suggesting a greater role for pastoral counseling or the inclusion of spiritual issues in traditional psychotherapy.

In other research, religiosity has seemed to have little or even negative impact. Connor et al. (2003) conducted a community survey of 1,200 people to measure resilience, spirituality, anger, forgiveness, and hatred. Of those who had been exposed to violent trauma, they found that those with greater acceptance of spiritual belief (e.g., reincarnation, existence of God, importance of spiritual forces, persistence after death, life purpose, life destiny) had poorer outcomes. A subsequent study of 1,969 people also found that in a U.S.-based group of subjects, those who endorsed a belief in karma experienced *more severe* intrusive thoughts and avoidant behaviors than those who did not, although the reason for this finding was unclear (Davidson et al. 2005).

As Herman (1997) indicated, trauma can cause a reassessment of worldview. In general, however, the literature indicates that this change is usually—but not always—in the direction of a more religiously oriented worldview. Falsetti et al. (2003), in a study of 120 participants in the DSM-IV Field Trial Study on PTSD, found that patients with PTSD were more likely to report changes in religious beliefs after a first trauma and that the change was in the direction of becoming less religious. This suggests that an extreme reaction to trauma can threaten religious beliefs as well as needed social support. By contrast, other literature indicates that clinicians should be aware of the possibility of existential reevaluation during trauma and that changes based on such a life reassessment may, in fact, result in an improved overall adjustment (Linley and Joseph 2004; Shaw et al. 2005).

In light of the body of literature indicating that for many who have experienced trauma, religious/spiritual coping is of benefit, wording in the "Course" section on PTSD could reflect this new knowledge by including the following language: *"There is evidence that, for religiously committed patients, religious and spiritual coping strategies may promote reduction of posttraumatic stress symptoms and promote personal growth."*

PTSD, Moral Context, and DSM

The *moral context* of traumatic events must be considered by the psychiatrist, and although he or she must avoid being judgmental, the psychiatrist cannot meaningfully hold a morally neutral stance in all circumstances (Shephard 2001). Clearly, patients who have witnessed gruesome events are more likely to develop PTSD symptoms than those who have not. Victims of torture suffer adverse psychological effects, and perpetrators of killing within a socially sanctioned context also experience adverse psychological consequences (Grossman 1996). DSM-IV-TR mentions guilt when it refers to "painful guilt feelings about surviving when others did not survive or about the things they had to do to survive" (p. 465), but it avoids the morally sensitive subject of those who have been killers or the perpetrators of atrocities.

Ben Shephard (2001), in his highly regarded history *A War of Nerves: Soldiers and Psychiatrists in the Twentieth Century,* wrote in detail about the difficulties therapists had in dealing with Vietnam veterans who had brutalized others. He recounted the professional experiences of Sarah Haley, author of the landmark paper "When the Patient Reports Atrocities." Although Haley advocated the classic stance of psychotherapeutic nonjudgmentalism, she found this approach extremely difficult to follow in practice. Shephard wrote that this stance, unmodified, devolves into absurdity when the therapist attempts to ignore the moral implications of the traumatic event that the patient both committed and experienced. He recounted in detail several well-documented and egregious examples of surreal clinical situations therapists created when they adopted this stance. He concluded that

> many therapists who have worked closely with chronic Vietnam cases emphasize the moral, spiritual side of [the veterans'] suffering, the way service in Vietnam involved, for many people, the 'undoing of character'....It is easy to mock [religious approaches]. What emerges from the strange mixture of psycho-babble and God-speak is that God has supplied many of the [veterans] with the authority figure they have been searching for and psychotherapists have failed to provide. (Shephard 2001, pp. 375–376)

Some research suggests that forgiveness, reconciliation, or witnessing justice for perpetrators has little psychological impact (Basoglu et al. 2005). Nonetheless, individual case studies indicate the value of religious belief in some veterans with PTSD. By way of example, Khouzam and Kissmeyer (1997) described a patient with PTSD and depression who was treated for concurrent depression and alcoholism. He responded to antidepressant treatment with markedly lessened depressive symptoms and attended a substance abuse treatment program that resulted in abstinence, but he continued to experience feelings of guilt. During the course of treatment, he attended Alcoholics Anonymous meetings and at some point committed his life to God and "accepted his survival as a heavenly gift." The survivor guilt resolved, and although he continued to experience posttrauma symptoms, he remained abstinent and free of the guilt (Khouzam and Kissmeyer 1997).

The moral context of the traumatic event, as well as the patient's moral stance during an event, should be taken into consideration when a diagnosis and prognosis are formulated. DSM's indication of the need for clinicians to consider the moral significance of a traumatic event may be vital in pointing the clinician in a therapeutic direction that may secure healing for the patient, although this is an issue that remains to be fully explored. At the very least, the DSM should acknowledge that PTSD is experienced by people who have committed morally reprehensible acts, with the implication that this guilt needs to be acknowledged and addressed in a therapeutically meaningful way. The PTSD section "Associated Features and Disorders: Associated Descriptive Features and Mental Disorders" could adopt the following change in wording: "Individuals with Posttraumatic Stress Disorder may describe painful guilt feelings about surviving when others did not survive or about things they had to do to survive. *Some may experience guilt related to the perpetration of a violent event and the moral implications of their actions.*"

PTSD and the Cultural Context of the Religious/Spiritual Narrative

Many cultures place little emphasis on individual psychological experiences, focusing instead on issues of family, religion, and meaning within a larger *social context* (Beiser 1985; Good 1987). Clinicians working in settings involving war, political uncertainty, or natural catastrophe should be circumspect when educating survivors about the emergence of PTSD and proposed remedies for traumatic stress. PTSD may not be as prevalent in non-Western settings as in the West, and the intact extended social networks that often exist in non-Western settings may be protective against the development of PTSD.

In a carefully thought out paper on psychological responses to civilian populations affected by war, Derek Summerfield (1999) observed that an excessive focus on individual psychological syndromes can detract from appreciation of the larger social contexts that lead to, cause, and perpetuate the alienation and anxiety associated with catastrophic events. He noted that in the West, the language of medicine and psychology have "displaced religion as the source of explanations for the vicissitudes of life, and of the vocabulary of distress" (p. 1449), and that this narrative language may be used by Western mental health professionals to substitute for local narratives that incorporate biblical, legal, ideological, humanist, or liberation themes. This insight helps us adopt a more humble approach toward our own knowledge base.

The DSM-V presentation of PTSD might profitably be framed in such a way that it does not facilitate the exportation to other cultures of a purely technological worldview that describes experiences of distress in technical terms and offers a technical solution. Such an approach will avoid draining local narratives of their meaning and will try to preserve alternative approaches to understanding that are steeped in local tradition and promote connectedness. In this way DSM will promote a way of understanding that helps those who have been traumatized to use readily available resources to grapple with and grow through the stressful circumstances. Although DSM focuses on the symptoms of the individual, these larger social considerations should also enter into the weight a clinician places on the likelihood of the PTSD diagnosis and the effectiveness of proposed treatments (i.e., securing basic needs such as food and shelter may be much more important than a decision on pharmacological treatment in some situations).

Future research directions in the relationship of PTSD to religious and spiritual concerns will need to include a focus on contextual factors that shape PTSD, use cross-cultural comparisons to highlight how divergent worldviews might affect the presentation and course of PTSD, and explore how religious and spiritual factors might ethically be included in treatment strategies.

References

American Psychiatric Association: Diagnostic and Statistical Manual of Mental Disorders, 4th Edition, Text Revision. Washington, DC, American Psychiatric Association, 2000

Basoglu M, Livanou M, Crnobaric C, et al: Psychiatric and cognitive effects of war in former Yugoslavia: association of lack of redress for trauma and posttraumatic stress reactions. JAMA 294:580–590, 2005

Beiser M: A study of depression among traditional Africans, urban North Americans, and Southeast Asian refugees, in Culture and Depression: Studies in the Anthropology and Cross-Cultural Psychiatry of Affect and Disorder. Edited by Kleinman A, Good B. Berkeley, CA, University of California Press, 1985, pp 272–298

Connor KM, Davidson JR, Lee LC: Spirituality, resilience, and anger in survivors of violent trauma: a community survey. J Trauma Stress 16:487–494, 2003

Davidson JR, Connor KM, Lee LC: Beliefs in karma and reincarnation among survivors of violent trauma: a community survey. Soc Psychiatry Psychiatr Epidemiol 40:120–125, 2005

Falsetti SA, Resick PA, Davis JL: Changes in religious beliefs following trauma. J Trauma Stress 16:391–398, 2003

Fontana A, Rosenheck R: Trauma, change in strength of religious faith, and mental health service use among veterans treated for PTSD. J Nerv Ment Dis 192:F579–F584, 2004

Fox SH: The Mandinka nosological system in the context of post-trauma syndromes. Transcult Psychiatry 40:488–506, 2003

Good CM: Ethnomedical Systems in Africa: Patterns of Traditional Medicine in Rural and Urban Kenya. New York, Guilford, 1987

Grossman D: On Killing: The Psychological Cost of Learning to Kill in War and Society, 1st Paperback Edition. Boston, MA, Little, Brown, 1996

Herman J: Trauma and Recovery: The Aftermath of Violence—From Domestic Abuse to Political Terror. New York, Basic Books, 1997

Khouzam HR, Kissmeyer P: Antidepressant treatment, posttraumatic stress disorder, survivor guilt, and spiritual awakening. J Trauma Stress 10:691–696, 1997

Lindblom G: The Akamba in British East Africa: An Ethnological Monograph, 2nd Edition. Uppsala, Sweden, Appelbergs Boktryckeri Aktiebolag, 1920

Linley PA, Joseph S: Positive change following trauma and adversity: a review. J Trauma Stress 17:11–21, 2004

Maercker A, Herrle J: Long-term effects of the Dresden bombing: relationships to control beliefs, religious belief, and personal growth. J Trauma Stress 16:579–587, 2003

Niaz U: Role of faith and resilience in recovery from psychotrauma. Pak J Med Sci 22:204–207, 2006

Patel V: Spiritual distress: an indigenous model of nonpsychotic mental illness in primary care in Harare, Zimbabwe. Acta Psychiatr Scand 92:103–107, 1995

Recollections of foreign service nationals of the August 7, 1998 bombing of the American Embassy in Nairobi. Distributed at the second anniversary memorial ceremony at the U.S. Ambassador's residence, U.S. Embassy, Nairobi, Kenya, 2000

Shaw A, Joseph S, Linley PA: Religion, spirituality, and posttraumatic growth: a systematic review. Mental Health, Religion, and Culture 8:1–11, 2005

Shephard B: A War of Nerves: Soldiers and Psychiatrists in the Twentieth Century. Cambridge, MA, Harvard University Press, 2001

Summerfield D: A critique of seven assumptions behind psychological trauma programmes in war-affected areas. Soc Sci Med 48:1449–1462, 1999

Watlington CG, Murphy CM: The roles of religion and spirituality among African American survivors of domestic violence. J Clin Psychol 62:837–857, 2006

Weaver AJ, Flannelly LT, Garbarina J, et al: A systematic review of research on religion and spirituality in the *Journal of Traumatic Stress*: 1990–1999. Mental Health, Religion, and Culture 6:215–228, 2003

Witvliet CV, Phipps KA, Feldman ME, et al: Posttraumatic mental and physical health correlates of forgiveness and religious coping in military veterans. J Trauma Stress 17:269–273, 2004

Commentary 5A

COMMENTARY ON "RELIGION AND SPIRITUALITY IN THE DESCRIPTION OF POSTTRAUMATIC STRESS DISORDER"

Carol S. North, M.D., M.P.E.

Dr. Thielman's chapter on religion and spirituality in the description of posttraumatic stress disorder (PTSD) is wonderfully conceived and executed. Importantly, his approach seeks available data to address what otherwise might seem to be unanswerable questions. Furthermore, Thielman applies his own experience with survivors of an extremely traumatic event, the 1998 bombing of the U.S. Embassy in Nairobi, Kenya, to this discussion.

Thielman astutely identifies the crux of the issue with PTSD, which is its unique potentially etiological basis (i.e., involving sufficient exposure to a qualifying traumatic event), a characteristic not included in other psychiatric diagnoses. The required trauma exposure characteristic of PTSD makes this disorder very difficult with which to study and work. It might seem that exposure should be a relatively cut and dried, clearly objective, matter. In reality, however, it is not. In affected populations, exposure seems to be in the eye of the beholder. One person nearly struck head-on by a semi-trailer truck might describe the experience as harrowing and terrifying, whereas another might merely dismiss the same experience as "It was nothing; it left not a scratch; I knew I would be all right." By DSM definition, the former individual might be a candidate for a diagnosis of PTSD if he or she developed the requisite number of symptoms in relation to it for more than a month, but the latter individual would not qualify for the diagnosis. This distinction is ultimately based on the individual's own perceptions. As Thielman points out, the individual's worldview is critical in determining whether the event is interpreted as traumatic by the individual, and cultural, spiritual, and religious factors have everything to do with one's worldview. Thus, religious and spiritual aspects of humanity are perturbing our notions of PTSD. The definition of PTSD was not designed to accommodate this particular wrinkle.

Issues of spiritual and religious coping with PTSD create yet another sticky wicket: determining causal associations and causal directionality. It is not obvious whether religious coping affects mental health, whether psychiatric problems affect ability or tendency to engage in religious coping, or whether some other factor associated with psychopathology and religious coping (such as family, educational, or socioeconomic background) is the apparent connection between these two variables. The variables may not necessarily be directly related to one another. Furthermore, the composite findings of the studies Thielman summarizes provide little agreement as to whether religious coping and psychopathology are positively or negatively associated or even unassociated. One cannot easily conduct prospective, randomized, controlled studies comparing groups instructed to cope religiously and nonreligiously, but such studies may be needed to clarify causalities.

An issue Thielman raises in the cross-cultural understanding of PTSD is the difficulty of comparing posttraumatic experience of populations in different parts of the world. If the expression of posttraumatic experience in different places varies with cultural influences, then it becomes impossible to compare prevalence rates of PTSD or other posttraumatic syndromes around the globe. Studies of PTSD would be comparing apples, oranges, and mangoes in different parts of the world. Other diseases have successfully been compared globally, including psychiatric diseases such as schizophrenia (Hendrie et al. 2006; Jablensky 2000; Rossler et al. 2005; Yusuf et al. 2001, 2004). Thus, PTSD would seem to diverge from other medical and psychiatric illness in this regard. Without a consistent global definition of PTSD, we cannot examine geographic variations in its presentation. Adding further complexity, prevalence rates for PTSD depend not only on expression of the related symptoms but also on the frequency and severity of traumatic events in different parts of the world.

Fortunately, systematic data can help to sort out many of these difficulties. We studied Kenyans who were exposed to the U.S. Embassy bombing in Nairobi and compared their experience with individuals similarly exposed to the 1995 Oklahoma City bombing, using consistent research methodology (North et al. 2005). We asked both groups of survivors the same set of questions (with some minor wording adjustments for cultural and language differences in symptom expression). We found remarkably similar rates of PTSD symptom reporting and similar symptom constellations among survivors of both bombings. What was remarkably different, however, was how the individuals in the two cultural settings coped with their traumatic experience. Oklahoma City survivors presented their needs to mental health professionals and physicians, but Nairobi survivors primarily sought help from their religious leaders and religious community. These findings suggest the likelihood of at least some transglobal consistency of symptomatic reporting among individuals with traumatic exposures, but how people of different cultures and religions conceptualize and manage their experience may vary to a much greater extent from place to place.

To better understand the effects of religious and spiritual aspects of PTSD, additional research is needed. Informed decisions will translate into better clinical care of those who experience emotional effects of trauma that is, unfortunately, so prevalent throughout the world.

References

Hendrie HC, Murrell J, Gao S, et al: International studies in dementia with particular emphasis on populations of African origin. Alzheimer Dis Assoc Disord 20(suppl):S42–S46, 2006

Jablensky A: Epidemiology of schizophrenia: the global burden of disease and disability. Eur Arch Psychiatry Clin Neurosci 250:274–285, 2000

North CS, Pfefferbaum B, Narayanan P, et al: Comparison of post-disaster psychiatric disorders after terrorist bombings in Nairobi and Oklahoma City. Br J Psychiatry 186:487–493, 2005

Rossler W, Salize HJ, van Os J, et al: Size of burden of schizophrenia and psychotic disorders. Eur Neuropsychopharmacol 15:399–409, 2005

Yusuf S, Reddy S, Ounpuu S, et al: Global burden of cardiovascular diseases, part II: variations in cardiovascular disease by specific ethnic groups and geographic regions and prevention strategies. Circulation 104:2855–2864, 2001

Yusuf S, Hawken S, Ounpuu S, et al: Effect of potentially modifiable risk factors associated with myocardial infarction in 52 countries (the INTERHEART study): case-control study. Lancet 364:937–952, 2004

Commentary 5B

COMMENTARY ON "RELIGION AND SPIRITUALITY IN THE DESCRIPTION OF POSTTRAUMATIC STRESS DISORDER"

Posttraumatic Stress Disorder, Life Threat, Religion, and Spirituality

Robert J. Ursano, M.D.
Jocelyn A. Kilgore, M.D.

Posttraumatic stress disorder (PTSD) and acute stress disorder are the potential outcome of exposure to death and the limitations of life. Although most who are exposed to traumatic events will do all right over time, for some the outcome may be psychiatric illness, distress, or altered health risk behaviors (Ursano et al. 2007). Much like life-threatening illness, the traumatic events of PTSD and acute stress disorder bring one to confront the limitations of life and of the future. To the extent that religion and spirituality are part of our grappling with the question of death and our wishes to experience life in the face of death, these disorders are the potential medical outcome of the often sudden experience of the risk of death to oneself or one's loved ones, which is is potentially life changing and always unexpected in its intensity and feelings.

Dr. Thielman thoughtfully addresses issues of clinical importance to practitioners working with patients with PTSD and important considerations for DSM-V and the diagnosis of PTSD. He proposes that the upcoming edition of DSM address and incorporate spirituality and religion in its comments on diagnosis, assessment, and treating PTSD. This in itself is an important issue.

Addressing religion and spirituality in DSM-V is a call for a more thorough consideration of culture and context in assessment, diagnosis, and treatment planning. What *constitutes* religion (and spirituality, an even more challenging concept) is a critical issue for an empirical approach such as DSM-V. To consider it, DSM-V requires a clear definition of what religion and spirituality are and are not. According to Wikipedia (2007), religion is "a set of common beliefs and practices generally held by a group of people, often codified as a prayer, ritual and religious law. Religion also encompasses ancestral and cultural traditions, writings, history and mythology as well as personal faith and mystic experience…and shared conviction."

Religion and spirituality are one part—not all—of culture and vary with cultures and subcultures. Of course, *religion* does not refer exclusively to Western religions, a consideration that is particularly important in PTSD, which spans the globe, and touches all nations and peoples. Religions of those who suffer traumatic events are as varied as the Hindu, Buddhist, Shinto, Christian, Judaism, Islamic, Sikh, Baha'i, and Jain faiths, to name only a few. To consider this in DSM-V will be challenging and valuable.

Dr. Thielman's chapter is divided into four main sections relating PTSD to religious/spiritual worldview, coping, moral context of traumatic events, and the cultural context of PTSD. The first two sections relate spirituality to the meaning of a traumatic event for the affected individual, his or her response, and how religious/spiritual coping may or may not be helpful. One's worldview, determined by multiple factors to include religion and spirituality, plays a determining role in how a person interprets and copes with a catastrophic event. In the discussion of PTSD and morality, Dr. Thielman notes that DSM-IV-TR (American Psychiatric Association 2000) does not address some extreme experiences of survivors, such as killing, highlighted by the Vietnam war and now the Iraq war. The importance of appreciating the patient's experience of the moral context of these situations—which may or may not be religious or spiritual—is important to treatment. Lastly, in addressing PTSD and cultural context, the cultural/social context in which the individual functions is important in the diagnosis and treatment of traumatic stress.

Although the existing literature on posttraumatic growth is limited, a number of authors document the importance of the individual's experience and religion for treatment and outcome. HIV patients with higher levels of support and spirituality and with greater levels of distress experienced the most growth (Cadell et al. 2003). Religious/spiritual coping styles have also been related to psychiatric symptoms (Fallot and Heckman 2005). For American Muslim women victims of interpartner violence, spirituality both served as an important means of coping at some times and inhibited their safety at others (Hassouneh-Phillips 2003). In war trauma, posttraumatic growth has been noted even in the most severe of traumatic events (Ursano and Benedek 2003). Veterans may pursue treatment to find meaning in their war experiences (Fontana and Rosenheck 2004).

In their community survey, Connor et al. (2003) noted that resilience was associated with health status and psychiatric symptom severity. Religious/spiritual themes such as reincarnation were not associated with outcome. In a relatively unique study of refugee Tibetan nuns, those who had been tortured experienced more long-term consequences than those who had been refugees (fleeing, living in exile) but not tortured. In both groups, spirituality was protective (Holtz 1998). After the Katrina hurricane as well, religion and spirituality were related to recovery. Nearly 69% of Katrina victims reported becoming more spiritual or religious after Katrina, and 75% reported finding a deeper meaning to life (Hurricane Katrina Community Advisory Group 2006).

Much of what is important in considering religion and spirituality in PTSD (and other psychiatric diagnoses) is part of the biopsychosocial model of disease, illness, and health. Religion and spirituality offer opportunities for care that are often thought of as part of psychological first aid: ensuring safety, connectedness, calming, practical and emotional skills for recovery, and hope for the future (Hobfoll et al. 2007). Using the patient's worldview in the assessment of PTSD as well as in consideration of treatment is tantamount to good care. Understanding an individual from the spiritual, moral, religious, and broader cultural context is integral to psychiatric assessment and care (American Psychiatric Association 2004). We can hope that what Dr. Thielman proposes is part of the training of all medical students and physicians, and in particular psychiatric physicians and other mental health caregivers. We need reminders, like Dr. Thielman's, to not lose our direction in the world of biomedical disease, illness, and treatment.

References

American Psychiatric Association: Diagnostic and Statistical Manual of Mental Disorders, 4th Edition, Text Revision. Washington, DC, American Psychiatric Association, 2000

American Psychiatric Association: Practice guideline for the treatment of patients with acute stress disorder and posttraumatic stress disorder. Washington, DC, American Psychiatric Association, 2004

Cadell S, Regehr C, Hemsworth D: Factors contributing to posttraumatic growth: a proposed structural equation model. Am J Orthopsychiatry 73:279–287, 2003

Connor KM, Davidson R, Lee LC: Spirituality, resilience and anger in survivors of violent trauma: a community survey. J Trauma Stress 16:487–494, 2003

Fallot RD, Heckman JP: Religious/spiritual coping among women trauma survivors with mental health and substance use disorders. Journal of Behavioral Health Sciences and Research 32:215–226, 2005

Fontana A, Rosenheck R: Trauma, change in strength of religious faith, and mental health service use among veterans treated for PTSD. J Nerv Ment Dis 192:579–584, 2004

Hassouneh-Phillips D: Strength and vulnerability: spirituality in abused American Muslim women's lives. Issues Ment Health Nurs 24:681–694, 2003

Hobfoll S, Watson P, Bell CC, et al: Five essential elements of immediate and mid term mass trauma intervention: empirical evidence. Psychiatry 70:283–315, 2007

Holtz TH: Refugee trauma versus torture trauma: a retrospective controlled cohort study of Tibetan refugees. J Nerv Ment Dis 186:24–34, 1998

Hurricane Katrina Community Advisory Group: Overview of Baseline Survey Results: Hurricane Katrina Community Advisory Group. Available online at http://hurricanekatrina. med.harvard.edu/pdf/baseline_report%208-25-06.pdf. Accessed January 20, 2008

Ursano RJ, Benedek DM: Prisoners of war: long-term health outcomes. Lancet 382:S22–S23, 2003

Ursano RJ, Fullerton CS, Weisaeth L, et al: Individual and community responses to disaster, In Textbook of Disaster Psychiatry. Edited by Ursano RJ, Fullerton CS, Weisaeth L, et al. London, England, Cambridge University Press, 2007

Wikipedia: Religion. Available at: http://en.wikipedia.org/wiki/Religion. Accessed October 8, 2007.

6

SPIRITUAL AND RELIGIOUS PERSPECTIVES ON CHILD AND ADOLESCENT PSYCHOPATHOLOGY

P. Alex Mabe, Ph.D.

Mary Lynn Dell, M.D., D.Min.

Allan M. Josephson, M.D.

The United States represents a religious country with about 40% of Americans worshipping at a church, synagogue, mosque, or temple weekly and about 20% attending monthly (Gallup 1996). It has been estimated that 95% of adults in the United States express a belief in God, and approximately 88% pray to God (Hoge 1996). Moreover, 90% of Americans indicate that they want some form of religious education for their children (Hoge 1996). In context of the family and the socialization of children, religion has played a key role in the United States since its Colonial days, and in many Christian denominations, the Bible is considered the most important parenting manual (Gershoff et al. 1999). In regard to our youth,

A portion of this material was adapted from Mabe PA and Josephson AM: "Child and Adolescent Psychopathology: Spiritual and Religious Perspectives." *Child Psychiatric Clinics of North America* 13:111–125, 2004. Copyright 2004 by copyright holder. Reprinted with permission.

95% of American teenagers believe in God, 42% pray frequently, 36% read scripture weekly, and 45% attend worship services weekly (Gallup and Bezilla 1992). Surprisingly, 27% of teens have reported that religious faith is more important to them than it is to their parents, and they indicated that they are more likely to attend worship services than adults (Gallup and Bezilla 1992).

Despite the commonality and importance of religion in most individuals' lives, however, examination of the consequences of such beliefs and practices on children's mental health and well-being has been quite limited. Systematic reviews of the empirical literature have indicated that religion and spirituality are understudied variables in health-related research, including child psychiatry. For example, Weaver et al. (2000) reported that in a review of 5 years of published research in five major adolescent research journals, only 11.8% of the studies included and assessed a religious variable. This lack of research attention appears to be changing, and current literature is increasing the understanding of the impact of religion and religious experience on children (in this article, the term *children* is used to include children and adolescents) and their families. Such information is likely to enhance our ability to understand and intervene in dealing with child psychopathology. Therefore, this article reviews some of the available research literature on religious and spiritual factors in psychopathology. It reviews the roles of religion and spirituality as risk and protective factors for psychopathology toward the goal of assisting the development of DSM-V.

Defining the Domain

Studying the relationships between children's religious beliefs and practices and psychopathology represents a formidable task for several reasons. First, religion and spirituality entail complex and diverse constructs. Religious terms encompass cognition (attributions, beliefs, knowledge), emotion (joy, hope, shame), behavior (church attendance, rituals, prayers, moral actions), and community affiliation (group interactions) (Holden 2001). Pargament (1990) distinguished between general measures of religiosity (e.g., church attendance and self-reported importance of religion) and measures of religious coping that could include specific religious practices of prayer, confessing one's sins, and seeking strength and comfort from God in response to a particular stressor. *Religious* has been differentiated from *spiritual,* in that the latter refers to believing in, valuing, or devoting oneself to some higher power without necessarily holding specific religious beliefs to be true (Worthington et al. 1996). It should be noted that being religious *could* involve an individual holding to certain doctrines within a religious organization without experiencing or expressing any devotion to a higher power other than intellectual assent to its existence. Thus, a person could be spiritual *and* religious, spiritual but not religious, religious but not spiritual, or none of these. Given the complexity and diversity of these constructs, it is likely that studies involving spirituality and religion will represent diverse psychosocial variables and therefore diverse outcomes in regard to child psychopathology would be anticipated.

Second, there is increasing heterogeneity in religious beliefs and practices in the United States, although the country remains overwhelmingly Judeo-Christian in tradition and numbers (Kosmin et al. 2001; U.S. Census Bureau 2000). Diverse religious groups, whether defined broadly or narrowly, have important differences in their beliefs and doctrines, practices, and community organization. Efforts to understand the impact of religious beliefs and practices on child and adolescent mental health outcomes will need to take into account the heterogeneity of religious affiliation.

Third, separating religious effects from psychological and cultural effects is often difficult. For example, adults who are more conventional are more likely to attend religious services. Thus, the association between religiosity and mental health outcomes in children may not be linked directly to religion per se but rather to other characteristics of families who regularly attend a church, synagogue, or mosque. Separating religious effects from cultural effects in the United States may be particularly difficult, given the religious heritage of this country and the considerable overlap between biblical and societal values (e.g., "The Golden Rule"—respecting others, treating others as you would want to be treated).

Links Between Child Psychopathology and Spiritual/Religious Perspectives: General Considerations

The literature is clear that religion/spirituality can be a risk factor or a protective factor for the onset of psychopathology (Mahoney et al. 2001). For adults, the link between religion and health has tended to emphasize either the psychosocial functions or the substantive elements of religion (Pargament 1997). The proposed *psychosocial functions* may serve independently of the content of religious beliefs and practices and involve religion and integration into the community, social support from people with similar attitudes, and participation in social activities. *Substantive elements,* on the other hand, refer to the specific contents of beliefs and practices promoted by different religions. Unfortunately, explanations for religious effects on mental health have been disjointed and fragmented, with few directed toward the functioning of children.

Discussion of the psychopathology of children and adolescents must be preceded by attention to family issues. In each aspect of the following review, family concerns are implicit, if not explicit. Parents influence their child's acquisition of social skills and developing cognitive percepts as well as the child's response to illness. The younger the child, the more this is so. This parental influence can ameliorate the symptoms of a disorder or give rise to a disorder. The remainder of this chapter focuses on individual psychopathology, but family functioning always must be considered (Diamond and Josephson 2005).

Empirical Data Pertaining to the Relationship Between Child Psychopathology and Spirituality/Religion: A Stimulus to DSM-V

Psychopathology in children is a product of multiple, interacting biopsychosocial factors. Study of these factors has consisted predominantly of correlational studies that can estimate the strength of association but not specify causality. This is especially true in the study of spiritual/religious variables and child psychopathology because controlled experiments of such phenomena are precluded by the freedom to choose one's religious beliefs and practices. Cause and effect regarding spiritual/ religious variables and child psychopathology is also difficult to study due to lack of construct consistency across studies, such that the construct of "religious" could pertain to such wide-ranging operations as self-reported statements of religious affiliation to accounts of church attendance to reports of using prayer when under stress. Consequently, the conclusions that can be drawn from the empirical data regarding the relationship between spiritual/religious variables and child psychopathology are limited and tentative.

Links Between Child Psychopathology and Spiritual/Religious Perspectives: Specific Conditions

It should be noted that the following four categories of empirical data do not utilize DSM nomenclature, because the research generally did not include such terms. The categories are nonetheless representative of DSM descriptive psychopathology.

DEPRESSION AND SUICIDE

On the whole, religious involvement appears to have an inverse relationship with depression and suicide among children (Weaver et al. 2000). Religious beliefs appear to be associated with lower levels of hopelessness and with less depression (Murphy et al. 2000). Furthermore, a lack of spiritual/religious support as denoted by low church attendance has been associated with higher rates of depression (Wright et al. 1993). The positive benefits of religion appear to be particularly robust for girls in regard to less depression (Miller et al. 2000) and within the African American community in regard to less suicide (Choi 2002). Although gender differences in the protective benefits of religiousness against depression have been consistently reported, the mechanism for these differences is not clearly understood. Researchers have shown, however, that adolescent boys compared with girls tend to report a more legalistic view of God and perhaps derive less comfort and support from this relationship (Miller et al. 2000). High levels of spiritual/religious belief in the African American community have been correlated with the particularly low suicide rate in this community (American Academy of Child and Adolescent Psychiatry 2001). Studies have suggested that African Americans are less accepting of suicide than white Americans, a difference that appears to be strongly linked to their high levels of orthodox belief and religious devotion, although not necessarily church attendance (Neeleman et al. 1998). The protective benefits of religion related to depression appear to be linked not only to measures of personal religious devotion but also to parental religiousness (Mahoney et al. 2001; Miller et al. 2000). It has been suggested that parental religiousness benefits children through improvement in parenting practices—a point to be further discussed (Mahoney et al. 2001).

An interesting example of this proposed link between religion and psychopathology is a longitudinal study by Miller et al. (2002) of adult religiousness and history of childhood depression. Their findings showed that adult "personal importance" of religion was associated with a decreased risk of depression in women without a history of childhood depression and an increased risk of depression in women with a history of childhood depression. The researchers hypothesized that perhaps severely depressed children gravitate to personal religiousness for comfort and support. Alternatively, they proposed that childhood depression could have a potentially mutagenic influence in the development of personal religiousness such that depressive symptoms in young girls could distort their understanding of religious beliefs and practices, resulting in excessive attention to self-effacing and guilt-induction aspects of religion. In turn, these distorted religious beliefs and practices could further shape children's thoughts and behaviors in depression-inducing ways. It is certainly evident that psychopathology in children can be expressed in the form of their religious beliefs and practices, but this notion—that dysfunctional thoughts and behaviors arising from psychopathology may have a reciprocal relationship with religious beliefs and practices—appears to be a cogent one.

SUBSTANCE ABUSE

In their review of 14 studies examining the relationship of substance abuse and religious variables, Weaver et al. (2000) depicted the findings as mixed. For example, they noted that in adolescents who had been arrested or admitted to a drug treatment program, religion appeared to have little influence on drug use (Bahr et al. 1993). Also, they observed that in a study of high school and college students, religious involvement and beliefs had only a moderate inverse relationship with illicit substance use (Free 1993). On the other hand, they also reported community studies in which religious involvement was associated with decreased alcohol and drug use among teenagers (Weaver et al. 2000). Studies of community samples of adolescents—measuring the personal importance of religions, church attendance, and religious affiliation—have consistently demonstrated beneficial effects of religion on reducing alcohol and drug consumption and abuse (Miller et al. 2000; Wills et al. 2003). For minority youths, religious involvement has been shown to be associated with increased participation rates in abstinence programs (McBride et al. 1996).

Interpretations of the links between religiosity and substance abuse have often emphasized religious coping that would seem to improve the management of stressful life events and, thus, reduce substance abuse (Miller et al. 2000). For example, using a latent growth analysis, Wills et al. (2003) reported that religiosity appeared to reduce the impact of life stress on initial level of substance abuse and on rate of growth of substance use over time. It has also been proposed that religious attitudes conveying a prohibition against drug use, as well as the social influence from a religious community (particularly with religious peers), may explain the lower rates of substance use/abuse among religious youth (D'Onofrio et al. 1999; Mullen and Francis 1995). Again, parental influences through parental religious beliefs and religious affiliations (particularly when the parent holds a position of authority within the religious organization) have been shown to influence substance use/abuse among adolescents (Merrill et al. 2001).

CONDUCT DISORDER AND ANTISOCIAL BEHAVIOR

Studies have consistently supported the position that religious beliefs and practices and strength of religion in the family and community are inversely related to antisocial and delinquent behavior among children (Blyth and Leffert 1995; Evans et al. 1996). For example, religious attendance among adolescents has been associated with fewer suspensions/expulsions from school, less theft, and less violent behavior (Ketterlinus et al. 1992). In a national study, Donahue and Benson (1995) reported that religious involvement among youth was associated with less likelihood of trouble with police, fighting, vandalism, gang violence, physically hurting someone, and use of a weapon to steal. Pearce (2004), in her analysis of the National Longitudinal Study of Adolescent Health, noted that although more-religious mothers and their adolescent children are less likely to have delinquent behaviors (in the children), the effect of one's religiosity depended on the other. That is, when both are religious, delinquency is less prevalent, but when either the mother or the child is very religious and the other is not, the child's delinquency increases. Thus religion can be cohesive and protective when shared among family members, but when not shared, higher adolescent delinquency results—a finding that may be particularly common with boys (Regnerus 2003).

SEXUALITY

Although sexuality is not a specific DSM entity, it is a domain that may shed considerable light into the child and adolescent diagnostic process. Sexual activity may be a sign of Axis I disorders, such as manic episodes or conduct disorder, or it may be a precipitant of other Axis I disorders, such as posttraumatic stress or other anxiety disorders. In some instances, it may be a signal of burgeoning Axis II psychopathology. Given these considerations, religion and spirituality as they pertain to child and adolescent sexuality are important to consider in any discussion of DSM.

Several negative consequences have been linked with adolescent sexual activity, including mood and behavioral disturbance, substance abuse, early pregnancy, and school dropout (Hallfors et al. 2005; Orr et al. 1991). Adolescents who are more religious, however, tend to have more negative attitudes toward premarital sexuality and, in turn, delay sexual intercourse (Weaver et al. 2000). Spilka et al. (1985) estimated that adolescents involved in religious life may be 50% less likely to engage in sexual intercourse than their nonreligious peers. Murray (1996) reported that frequent church attendance proved to be the second strongest predictor of coital timing among African American adolescent females, with only sexual knowledge being a stronger predictor. Again, the religious involvement of the family and of the individual appear to play an important role in delaying sexual intercourse (Murstein and Mercy 1994). On a negative note, one study found that sexually active church-going teenage girls were less likely to use contraceptives than non–church attendees, presenting a greater risk of unsafe sexual behavior and pregnancy (Studer and Thornton 1987).

Links Between Child Psychopathology and Spiritual/Religious Perspectives: Risk Factors

Although the preponderance of research findings has emphasized the benefits of spirituality and religion in promoting children's mental health, clinical practice reveals religion's and spirituality's negative effects. Most clinicians have had experiences with cases in which the child's religious beliefs have been associated with obsessions regarding some perceived sins. In addition, parents, under the mantle of religious faith, may engage in rigid and autocratic parenting practices that stifle healthy psychosocial development. The reality is that religion can be used to justify or maintain dysfunctional relationships or practices, although this may not be the normative experience in most religious families. In American culture, one notable exception is the negative association of Satanism/occult interests and adolescent mental health. Although only a few adolescent studies pertaining to Satanism/occult interests are available, the findings are indicative of associations with such adverse outcomes as low attachment to society (as represented by parents and school)

(Damphousse and Crouch 1992), low self-esteem (Tennant-Clark et al. 1989), low perceived control over one's life (Damphousse and Crouch 1992), alcohol and drug abuse (Burket et al. 1994; Damphousse and Crouch 1992), and self-mutilation (Burket et al. 1994). Again, Satanism may be a cause or an effect of these various aspects of psychopathology. Pfeifer (1994), in a critical evaluation of the notion of faith-induced pathology, made the point that empirical research and clinical experience suggest that psychopathology in religious patients must be seen against a background of their underlying pathology, their biography, and the way in which they integrate their faith into their lifestyles. The causal link between religious beliefs and spiritual practices and child psychopathology could point toward personal religious faith as a product of interacting personal variables.

Links Between Child Psychopathology and Spiritual/Religious Perspectives: Protective Factors

There is significant literature on the salutary effects of religion and spirituality. This has relevance to DSM-V in the discussion of protective factors in the natural course of disorders as well as informing Axis IV descriptors when these protective factors are absent, or their converse is present.

CORE BELIEFS ABOUT LIFE

Beliefs about the meaning of life, suffering, and moral order are central to spiritual perspectives and religious convictions. Answers to fundamental questions relating to the meaning of life and what one's life goals should be would certainly be expected to influence how children evaluate and respond to a variety of developmental tasks and life events. For example, religious beliefs could influence children's sense of responsibility for their own cognitive/academic and social development. Thus, a child who believes that his or her life purpose is to teach others about God's love by becoming a physician and caring for the health needs of others would likely work hard in school to succeed in this life goal. Perspectives on the meaning of suffering have long been considered important in determining how individuals interpret and respond to adverse events in their lives. Although children's abstract reasoning regarding suffering is initially primitive and evolves over the developmental years, their spiritual/religious mental representations of suffering may influence their coping with stress. For example, children who view suffering as an expected part of life that can (and will) be overcome by the divine presence and intervention of a higher being may well be more able to tolerate negative life events. Conversely, if children hold beliefs that suffering is punishment for negative behavior, then their tolerance for negative life events may be limited. Finally, all religious systems impose on their followers moral imperatives regarding many aspects of life (e.g., honesty, beneficence). Such injunctions would be expected to affect the development of children's attitudes and behaviors in a variety of intra-personal and interpersonal contexts that could lead to health-promoting or patho-genic behaviors. Positively, such moral imperatives could lead to the development of greater compassion, social responsibility, and even serve as protective factors in regard to psychiatric illnesses. On the other hand, extreme or overly rigid positions on moral imperatives could lead to a religious scrupulosity that could be highly guilt inducing for the individual or could lead to a moral/religious intolerance for others.

PRESCRIPTION FOR HEALTHY LIFESTYLES

Linked to religious moral imperatives are the religious prescriptions for a healthy lifestyle (Worthington et al. 1996). Most spiritual and religious traditions offer guidelines on how to live a healthy life. These religious injunctions relate to such matters as proper food and drink, personal hygiene practices, sexual behavior, re-ceptivity to instruction and authority, relationships with family and community, and social responsibility. Prescriptions for marital relationships and parenting are of particular importance in child mental health outcomes (Mahoney et al. 2001). Specifically, to the extent to which marriage is promoted and divorce is discour-aged, religion could increase marital stability and thus reduce exposure to the adverse effects of divorce on children (Wallerstein 1991). Carried to an extreme, religion could prohibit leaving an unhappy, even abusive marriage and, in so doing, main-tain an emotionally unhealthy family environment (Mahoney et al. 2001). In re-gard to parenting practices, religion could evoke such positive parental behaviors as valuing and nurturing of children, careful attention to the instruction/socializa-tion of children, shared social activities, and effective discipline. Conversely, reli-gion could evoke such negative parental behaviors as overly coercive discipline practices, excessive guilt induction in children, and parental control that discour-ages appropriate separation and individuation (Mahoney et al. 2001). Beyond the specific religious imperatives that guide family and parenting efforts, religion also may facilitate a certain confidence in family and parenting efforts that fosters a perception of efficacy. Theoretical and empirical work have pointed to self-efficacy beliefs as a promising area to consider in enhancing parenting behavior and child mental health outcomes (Coleman and Karraker 1997; Gondoli and Silverberg 1997). Also, it is proposed that religion may increase children's receptiveness to pa-rental authority by providing a context for parental instruction and discipline that helps the child interpret such parental behaviors as benevolent and appropriate. Therefore, with more confident parents and more child receptiveness to parental efforts, less parent–child conflict would be anticipated.

SOCIAL SUPPORT

Religious beliefs and practices generally do not occur in a context of social isolation; rather, they are taught and encouraged within a religious community. Families that regularly attend a church, synagogue, or mosque often have additional social contacts that maintain cohesiveness and support within their like-faith community (Dell 2004). This social environment may play an important role in the health and well-being of children. On a positive note, studies have suggested that religious communities provide a wide range of prevention- and treatment-oriented programs that could contribute significantly to the psychological and physical well-being of their congregants (Blank et al. 2002). This support has taken the forms of monetary aid, child care, educational classes in marital relationships and parenting, healthcare screening, substance abuse programs, and access to recreational facilities and activities. Religious communities have also provided social validation of marital and parenting beliefs and practices, emotional support around various child/ family stresses, and encouragement for health-conscious lifestyles. On a negative note, the religious community could have adverse effects on child mental health functioning because excessive demands to participate in religious activities detracts from the time and emotional energy of the family. Furthermore, religious communities could encourage malevolent responses toward child misbehavior or ostracize children and their families when they do not conform to group norms/expectations. Finally, religious communities could so emphasize cohesion and group norm adherence that children's opportunities for developmentally appropriate separation and individuation are hindered.

SKILL DEVELOPMENT OPPORTUNITIES

The religious training of children involves not only adult efforts to instruct children in their faith but also requirements for children to complete and provide evidence of progress in their religious education. Therefore, children often are expected to memorize and publicly recite passages from religious texts, recite and explain principles of the faith, and participate in formal ceremonies of commitment to their faith. In many religious communities, children also are encouraged to actively participate in leading a variety of the activities involving worship ceremonies and training of younger children. Thus, children may participate in drama or musical performances as part of worship, and they may be involved in assisting adults in teaching younger children. Moreover, in religious communities, children are often encouraged to participate in benevolent activities within the community. Consequently, religious communities often provide rich opportunities for skill development in academic-related skills (e.g., reading and studying skills), social skills (e.g., group cooperation, public speaking/performance), art/music skills, and skills relevant to social benevolence and activism. Of course, skill/performance activities tend to be a two-edged sword: skills can be developed, but deficits can also be revealed. Therefore, religious-oriented skill-developing opportunities could also be the opportunity for failure and embarrassment.

SPIRITUAL EXPERIENCE

Reflecting on American adolescents, Smith (2003) pointed out that spiritual experiences may have direct positive benefits on children. Similarly, Bergin and Payne (1993) suggested that a person's sense of the supernatural can certainly provide a psychological boost and may also entail a "spiritual boost" that cannot be measured phenomenologically. Although traditionally not considered in scientific contexts because of the transcendental nature of spiritual experience, people of religious faith consistently embrace a worldview that may include life-changing divine intervention and religious/spiritual influences on thought, behavior, and effort to deal with adversity. Children may also believe in divine activity in everyday life, and although science lends itself better to the study of the psychological effects of such beliefs, there is no logical basis to ignore the possibility that spiritual experiences may have direct effects on children's mental health.

CHILD SOCIAL COMPETENCIES/COPING SKILLS AND SPIRITUALITY/RELIGION

Research has indicated that religious involvement not only protects children from various forms of psychopathology but also seems to promote valuable social competencies. For example, religion appears to be positively related to school performance (Jeynes 2003; Regnerus 2000). Religious children appear to cope more effectively with a variety of stresses compared with their nonreligious peers (Mosher and Handal 1997). Wagener et al. (2003) reported that religiously active children had higher levels of personal restraint, positive values, school bonding and engagement, and social competence. Children with religious identification report having a clearer sense of personal meaning and more prosocial concerns (Furrow et al. 2004). Religious involvement has been associated with a higher propensity to help others and do volunteer work. Youth who practice their faith have higher levels of prosocial values and caring behaviors, and religious youth are more likely to serve as community volunteers and make charitable contributions (Weaver et al. 2000). Youniss et al. (1999) reported that children who were more religious were committed to their schooling, to bettering their communities, and to the development of personal identities that promote healthy lives. In addition, those children who rated religion as important to them were almost three times more likely to participate in community service than were those who did not believe religion was important. Taken together, research studies have suggested that involvement in religion can serve as a catalyst for positive social development. Using structural equation modeling, King and Furrow (2004) suggested that a significant mediating factor between child involvement in religion and the positive development of moral outcomes and social competence may be social capital in regard to increasing interactions with adults, friends, and parents whom they trust and with whom they share similar world views.

Religious coping skills entail cognitive or behavioral techniques that arise out of an individual's religion or spirituality and are used to address stressful life events (Tix and Frazier 1998). These techniques include but are not limited to beliefs about the controllability of negative life events, prayer and meditation, confession of one's wrongdoing or failures, religious counsel and instruction, and seeking strength and comfort from God in response to a stressful event (Pargament 1990). Although the extent to which children engage in such religious coping techniques has received little study, such practices could have important influences on child coping. Tix and Frazier (1998) pointed out that although religious coping has exhibited generally positive mental health outcomes, religious affiliation seems to moderate how stress is interpreted and, thus, how individuals respond to stress. For example, religious coping that emphasizes confession and forgiveness of sins (e.g., Catholicism) may be effective in dealing with negative life events perceived to be under the control of the individual. In contrast, religious coping that emphasizes faith in an all-powerful and benevolent God (e.g., Protestantism) may be more effective in dealing with life stresses that are perceived to be beyond one's control or influence. Consequently, the success of children's coping efforts may vary with their religious affiliation and the nature of the negative life event.

FAMILY FUNCTIONING AND SPIRITUALITY/RELIGION

Although Emery et al. (1990) appropriately cautioned that child psychopathology is multidetermined and that family risk factors should not be inferred to represent linear explanations of child problems, the weight of evidence would seem to take the parsimonious point of view that parents and family functioning can have direct positive and negative effects on children. Perhaps the most powerful impact of spirituality/religion on children is mediated through parent behaviors that are directly influenced and promoted by religion and spirituality. In this regard, the three most prominent family correlates of religious variables appear to be parenting behaviors, parental coping, and marital/family relationships.

Parenting Behaviors

Although critics of Christianity (in particular, conservative Protestantism) have expressed concern that parental religiousness is likely to produce excessively harsh parenting practices that in turn lead to mental health problems in children (Ellison 1996), greater parental religiousness generally has not been associated with such adverse outcomes, but instead has been associated with more effective parenting skills and positive child mental health outcomes (Mahoney et al. 2001). Conservative Protestant parents, however, consistently report having more positive attitudes toward and use of corporal punishment as a discipline approach to their children. Yet studies examining the link between parental religiousness and corporal punishment have suggested that religious parents tend to restrict corporal punishment to matters of serious moral transgression and with preadolescent children (Gershoff et al. 1999; Mahoney et al. 2001). Empirical research also has not substantiated concerns that conservative Christian affiliation or beliefs lead to heightened use of severe emotional or physical discipline (Gershoff et al. 1999; Mahoney et al. 2001). Greater Christian conservatism has been modestly correlated with placing a high priority on child conformity and obedience (Mahoney et al. 2001), and concerns have been raised regarding general authoritarian attitudes about childrearing among religious parents (Ellison et al. 1996). Yet again, the data reflect a picture that religious parents, even conservative Protestants, are no less enthusiastic about child intellectual autonomy (Ellison and Sherkat 1993) or the use of reasoning to assist in child socialization (Mahoney et al. 2001). Observations of dyadic problem-solving discussions between parents and their adolescents provide evidence that parents' religiousness may actually facilitate authoritative parenting (Gunnoe et al. 1999). Finally, Wilcox (1998) reported that parental endorsement of conservative Christianity and, in particular, frequency of church attendance were associated with more frequent hugging and praising of children.

Parental Coping

Religious parents may well rely on religion as a means of coping with a variety of family and child care stresses, including that of dealing with behaviorally or emotionally disturbed children. For example, religious parents may look to God for strength, support, and guidance in parenting; seek input from church members about parenting; perceive their role as parents and their children's stresses/problems as part of God's plan; and pray or attend religious services on behalf of their children. Studies related to parental religious coping have tended to focus more on general populations or on families experiencing various medical stresses (e.g., parents of children with medical or developmental disorders) than on families referred to mental health professionals. Nevertheless, studies that examine parental religious coping suggest that parents commonly use religion to help them cope with various problems in their children and generally find such religious coping to be helpful. Mahoney et al.'s (2001) review of the effects of religion in the home reported that greater religious coping was associated with better parental health, less parental stress and depression, more family cohesion, more support from outside the family, and fewer negative effects on parents or families in dealing with child health or developmental stresses. Carothers et al. (2005), following adolescent mothers over 10 years, found that religiosity among these mothers was associated with higher self-esteem, lower depression scores, less child abuse potential, and higher educational/ occupational attainment. Moreover, the children of the more religious mothers had less internalizing and externalizing problems. Interviews that have explored the role of religion in parenting children with special needs have suggested that religious families may accept their difficulties as gifts from God, as part of God's plan, and as opportunities for families to become closer and attain higher spiritual levels (Skinner et al. 1999). Such benefits of religious coping, however, have not been uniformly reported for parents dealing with children with developmental disabilities. Certain forms of religious coping appear to be problematic in parents' efforts to deal with their developmentally disabled children. Such negative religious coping involves beliefs that the child's disability is a punishment (or at least causes doubts about the benevolence of God), general feelings of discontent with God or the congregation for not being more helpful in their parenting efforts, and negative experiences with their disabled children during religious services or events (Tarakeshwar and Pargament 2001). These forms of negative religious coping have been associated with poorer mental status in parents and poorer resolution of negative events (Gershoff et al. 1999).

Marital/Family Relationships

Family stresses such as marital conflict and divorce have been consistently associated with adverse mental health outcomes in children. Conversely, a healthy family milieu with a high degree of marital commitment and instrumental and emotional support has been associated with many mental health benefits for children. Several research studies support a positive association between spiritually/religiosity and a supportive, cohesive family environment. It appears that individuals who report having an allegiance to a religious denomination or frequent church attendance have significantly lower divorce rates than those who have little to no religious affiliation (Mahoney et al. 2001). Furthermore, personal religiousness has been related to better couple communication, higher levels of marital satisfaction, and greater marital commitment (Mahoney et al. 2001). Ellison et al. (1999) reported that frequent church attendance was generally associated with much less aggression toward marital partners, although they also found that theologically conservative men married to more religiously liberal women were more likely to be physically aggressive than those married to women with similar views about the Bible. In two studies of African American parents' religiousness, Brody et al. (1994, 1996) found that self-reported religiousness (frequency of church attendance multiplied by importance of religion) was associated with less co-parenting conflict, better marital quality, greater observed family cohesion, and fewer child externalizing and internalizing behavior problems. Finally, Pearce and Axinn (1998), reporting data from an intergenerational panel study of mothers and children from 1962 to 1985, provided evidence that although religious affiliation per se had little impact on the mother–child relationship, religiosity (i.e., higher self-ratings of the importance of religion) had significant positive effects on mothers' and children's reports of the quality of their relationships. Furthermore, the congruence between mother–child religious attendance and religiosity predicted a more positive mother–child relationship. On the whole, it appears that commitment to one's religious beliefs has been consistently associated with a more cohesive and less conflictual family environment that predictably has been linked with fewer child mental health problems.

Clinical Implications

It is undeniable that religion and spirituality have a pervasive influence in our society and appears to play an important role in the socialization of our children. Thus, clinicians cannot afford to ignore this sphere of human experience as they diagnose and treat children with mental disorders. Unfortunately, the empirical data needed to guide the clinician in how to address issues of spirituality and religion in children and their families as they pertain to child psychopathology are limited.

There is evidence that significant links are present between spirituality and religious beliefs/practices and child psychopathology. On the whole, it appears that religion is primarily health promoting for children, although there are isolated exceptions. Therefore, the clinician should routinely assess for the presence of spirituality and religious beliefs/practices as potential resources toward the goal of treatment of child psychopathology. This assessment should be respectful of the diversity of beliefs and practices, and encouragement to use spiritual/religious resources should be cautiously weighed against the clinicians' understanding of the needs of the child and family.

There is evidence that spirituality and religious beliefs/practices play important roles in parenting and family functioning. Again, the valence appears to be primarily positive in regard to the relationship between religion and good parent/family functioning. The clinician needs to appreciate the influence that spirituality/religion has on family functioning and, in particular, on parenting practices. It is especially important to do this because prevailing views of parenting in professional psychiatry and psychology practice may not coincide with religious perspectives. In the service of establishing an effective collaborative relationship toward helping religious families address their children's problems, it would be best to view religion initially as a resource and to seek to establish commonalities and similarities between the religious and secular views of effective parenting and family functioning.

It is proposed that when spirituality and religious beliefs/practices have been associated with negative mental health outcomes in children or their families, evidence points to "poorness-of-fit," based on an interaction between the child's psychopathology and aspects of religious beliefs/practice. Clinically, there will be times when the family's religious beliefs/practices are not well suited to deal with the stresses at hand. If, for example, the parents are feeling punished by God because they have a mentally impaired child, then their coping efforts could be impeded by their religious beliefs. Also, it may be the case that a child's or family's psychopathology results in distorted religious beliefs/practices that could also impair child functioning. In either case, it is suggested that the clinician's dilemma lies in addressing issues of psychopathology and of distorted or dysfunctional religious faith. Such work may be possible for the clinician well versed in the religious beliefs/practices involved, but such work may be beyond the competencies of the average clinician. It would seem prudent for clinicians to begin building bridges to clergy and other religious leaders to establish additional therapeutic avenues for children and families with dysfunctional or distorted religious beliefs or practices.

Proposed Wording for DSM-V

Drawing on the range of issues covered in this chapter, we recommend the following specific wording for enhancement of the narrative of DSM-IV-TR. Recommendations are in italics, following a brief fragment of DSM-IV-TR text from the identified source page (American Psychiatric Association 2000).

1. Introduction—Ethnic and Cultural Considerations (p. xxxiv): "... communication, and coping mechanisms. *In childhood and adolescence, culturally shaped parental expectations of child behavior are influenced by the spiritual perspectives of faith traditions and communicated through family relationships.*"
2. Disorders Usually First Diagnosed in Infancy, Childhood, or Adolescence (p. 39): "...the text titled 'Specific Culture, Age, and Gender Features.' *This section also includes familial aspects of cultural significance (e.g., religious/spiritual) that place children at risk for, or protect from, disorder.*"
3. Conduct Disorder—Associated Features and Disorders (p. 96): "...certain kinds of familial psychopathology. *The family and relationship factors that predispose to the development of Conduct Disorder are influenced by cultural factors, such as the spirituality of parents.*"
4. Conduct Disorder—Specific Culture, Age, and Gender Features (p. 97): "...undesirable behaviors have occurred. *The early onset of risk behaviors (e.g., sexual behavior, drinking, illegal substance use) are strongly affected by family spiritual precepts.*"
5. Substance-Related Disorders—Specific Culture, Age, and Gender Features (p. 205): "...must take these factors into account. *Parental and family influences moderate early adolescent substance abuse, and these influences are broadranging (e.g., spiritual beliefs).*"

6. Mood Disorders—Specific Culture, Age, and Gender Features (p. 353): "...viewed as the 'norm' for a culture. *The predisposition to Depression may be influenced by a specific aspect of culture, namely religious and spiritual context.*"

7. Outline for Cultural Formulation and Glossary of Culture-Bound Syndromes (Appendix I, Page 898): "Cultural factors related to psychosocial environment and levels of functioning...instrumental, and informational support. *Parent behavior and decisions regarding childrearing may be directly influenced and promoted by religion and spirituality.*"

References

American Academy of Child and Adolescent Psychiatry: Practice parameters for the assessment and treatment of children and adolescents with suicidal behavior. J Am Acad Child Adolesc Psychiatry 40:24S–51S, 2001

American Psychiatric Association: Diagnostic and Statistical Manual of Mental Disorders, 4th Edition, Text Revision. Washington, DC, American Psychiatric Association, 2000

Bahr SJ, Hawk RD, Wang G: Family and religious influences on adolescent substance abuse. Youth Soc 24:443–465, 1993

Bergin AE, Payne IR: Proposed agenda for a spiritual strategy in personality and psychotherapy, in Psychotherapy and Religious Values. Edited by Worthington EL. Grand Rapids, MI, Baker, 1993, pp. 243–260

Blank MB, Mahmood M, Fox J, et al: Alternative mental health services: the role of the black church in the South. Am J Public Health 92:1668–1672, 2002

Blyth DA, Leffert N: Communities as contexts for adolescent development. J Adolesc Res 10:64–87, 1995

Brody GH, Stoneman Z, Flor D, et al: Religion's role in organizing family relationships: family process in rural, two-parent, African-American families. J Marriage Fam 56:878–888, 1994

Brody GH, Stoneman Z, Flor D: Parental religiosity, family processes, and youth competence in rural, two parent African American families. Dev Psychol 32:696–706, 1996

Burket RC, Myers WC, Lyles WB, et al: Emotional and behavioral disturbances in adolescents involved in witchcraft and Satanism. J Adolesc 17:41–52, 1994

Carothers SS, Borkowski JG, Lefever JB, et al: Religiosity and the socioemotional adjustment of adolescent mothers and their children. J Fam Psychol 19:263–275, 2005

Choi H: Understanding adolescent depression in ethnocultural context. Adv Nurs Sci 25:71–85, 2002

Coleman PK, Karraker KH: Self-efficacy and parenting quality: finding and future applications. Dev Rev 18:47–85, 1997

Damphousse KR, Crouch BM: Did the devil make them do it? Youth Soc 24:204–227, 1992

Dell ML: Religious professionals and institutions: untapped resources for clinical care. Child Adolesc Psychiatric Clin North Am 13:85–110, 2004

Donahue MJ, Benson PL: Religion and the well-being of adolescents. J Soc Issues 51:145–160, 1995

Diamond G, Josephson A: A ten year review of family intervention research. J Am Acad Child Adolesc Psychiatry 44:872–887, 2005

D'Onofrio BM, Murrelle L, Eaves LJ, et al: Adolescent religiousness and its influence on substance use: preliminary findings from the Mid-Atlantic School Age Twin Study. Twin Res 2:156–168, 1999

Ellison C: Conservative Protestantism and the corporal punishment of children: clarifying the issues. J Sci Study Relig 35:1–16, 1996

Ellison C, Sherkat DE: Obedience and autonomy: religion and parental values reconsidered. J Sci Stud Relig 32:313–329, 1993

Ellison C, Bartkowski JP, Segal ML: Conservative Protestantism and the parental use of corporal punishment. Soc Forces 74:1003–1028, 1996

Ellison C, Bartkowski JP, Anderson KL: Are there religious variations in domestic violence? J Fam Issues 20:87–113, 1999

Emery RE, Fincham FD, Cummings EM: Parenting in context: systemic thinking about parental conflict and its influence on children. J Consult Clin Psychol 60:909–912, 1990

Evans TD, Cullen FT, Burton VS, et al: Religion, social bonds, and delinquency. Deviant Behav 17:43–70, 1996

Free MD: Stages of drug use: a social control perspective. Youth Soc 25:251–271, 1993

Furrow JL, King PE, White K: Religion and positive youth development: identity, meaning, and prosocial concerns. Appl Dev Sci 8:17–26, 2004

Gallup GH: Religion in America: 1996. Princeton, NJ, Gallup Organization, 1996

Gallup GH, Bezilla R: The Religious Life of Young Americans. Princeton, NJ, George Gallup International Institute, 1992

Gershoff ET, Miller PC, Holden GW: Parenting influences from the pulpit: religious affiliation as a determinant of parental corporal punishment. J Fam Psychol 13:307–320, 1999

Gondoli DM, Silverberg SB: Maternal emotional distress and diminished responsiveness: the mediating role of parenting efficacy and parental perspective taking. Dev Psychol 33:861–868, 1997

Gunnoe ML, Hetherington EM, Reiss D: Parental religiosity, parenting style, and adolescent social responsibility. J Early Adolesc 19:199–225, 1999

Hallfors D, Waller M, Bauer D, et al: Which comes first in adolescence: sex and drugs or depression? Am J Prev Med 29:163–170, 2005

Holden GW: Psychology, religion, and the family: it's time for a revival. J Fam Psychol 15:657–662, 2001

Hoge DR: Religion in America, in Religion and the Clinical Practice of Psychology. Edited by Shafranske EP. Washington, DC, American Psychological Association, 1996, pp 21–41

Jeynes WH: The effects of religious commitment on the academic achievement of urban and other children. Educ Urban Soc 36:44–62, 2003

Ketterlinus RD, Lamb ME, Nitz K, et al: Adolescent nonsexual and sex-related problem behavior. J Adolesc Res 7:431–456, 1992

King PE, Furrow JL: Religion as a resource for positive youth development: religion, social capital, and moral outcomes. Dev Psychol 40:703–713, 2004

Kosmin BA, Mayer E, Keysar A: American Religious Identification Survey 2001. New York, Graduate Center of the City of New York, 2001

Mahoney A, Pargament KI, Tarakeshwar N, et al: Religion in the home in the 1980s and 1990s: a meta-analytic review and conceptual analysis of links between religion, marriage, and parenting. J Fam Psychol 15:559–596, 2001

McBride DC, Mutch PB, Chitwood DD: Religious belief and the initiation and prevention of drug use among youth, in Intervening With Drug-Involved Youth. Edited by McCoy CB, Metsch LR, Inciardi JA. Thousand Oaks, CA, Sage, 1996, pp 110–130

Merrill RM, Salazar DR, Gardner NW: Relationship between family religiosity and drug use behavior among youth. Soc Behav Personality 29:347–358, 2001

Miller L, Davies M, Greenwald S: Religiosity and substance use and abuse among adolescents in the National Comorbidity Survey. J Am Acad Child Adolesc Psychiatry 39:1190–1197, 2000

Miller L, Weissman M, Gur M, et al: Adult religiousness and history of childhood depression: eleven-year follow-up. J Nerv Ment Dis 190:86–93, 2002

Mosher JP, Handal PJ: The relationship between religion and psychological distress in adolescents. J Psychol Theol 25:449–457, 1997

Mullen K, Francis L: Religiosity and attitudes towards drug use among Dutch school children. J Alcohol Drug Educ 41:16–25, 1995

Murphy PE, Ciarrocchi JW, Piedmont RL, et al: The relation of religious belief and practices, depression, and hopelessness in persons with clinical depression. J Consult Clin Psychol 68:1102–1106, 2000

Murray VM: An ecological analysis of coital timing among middle-class African American adolescent females. J Adolesc Res 11:261–279, 1996

Murstein BI, Mercy T: Sex, drugs, relationships, contraception, and fear of disease on a college campus over 17 years. Adolescence 29:303–322, 1994

Neeleman J, Wessely S, Lewis G: Suicide acceptability in African- and white Americans: the role of religion. J Nerv Ment Dis 186:12–16, 1998

Orr DP, Beiter M, Ingersoll G: Premature sexual activity as an indicator of psychosocial risk. Pediatrics 87:141–147, 1991

Pargament KI: God help me: towards a theoretical framework of coping for the psychology of religion, in Research in the Social Scientific Study of Religion, Vol 2. Edited by Lynn ML, Moberg DO. Greenwich, CT, JAI Press, 1990, pp 195–224

Pargament KI: The Psychology of Religion and Coping: Theory, Research, Practice. New York, Guilford, 1997

Pearce L: Intergenerational religious dynamics and adolescent delinquency. Soc Forces 82:1553–1572, 2004

Pearce L, Axinn WG: The impact of family religious life on the quality of mother-child relations. Am Sociol Rev 63:810–828, 1998

Pfeifer S: Faith-induced neurosis: myth or reality? J Psychol Theol 22:87–96, 1994

Regnerus M: Shaping schooling success: religious socialization and educational outcomes in metropolitan public schools. J Sci Study Relig 39:363–370, 2000

Regnerus M: Linked lives, faith, and behavior: intergenerational religious influence on adolescent delinquency. J Sci Study Relig 42:189–203, 2003

Skinner D, Bailey DB, Correa V, et al: Narrating self and disability: Latino mothers' construction of identities vis-a-vis their child with special needs. Except Child 65:481–495, 1999

Smith C: Theorizing religious effects among American adolescents. J Sci Study Relig 42:17–30, 2003

Spilka B, Hood RW, Gorsuch RL: The Psychology of Religion. Englewood, NJ, Prentice-Hall, 1985

Studer M, Thornton A: Adolescent religiosity and contraceptive usage. J Marriage Fam 49:117–128, 1987

Tarakeshwar N, Pargament KI: Religious coping in families of children with autism. Focus Autism Dev Dis 16:247–260, 2001

Tennant-Clark CM, Fritz JJ, Beauvais F: Occult participation: its impact on adolescent development. Adolescence 24:757–772, 1989

Tix AP, Frazier PA: The use of religious coping during stressful life events: main effects, moderation, and mediation. J Consult Clin Psychol 66:411–422, 1998

U.S. Census Bureau: Statistical Abstract of the United States: The National Data Book. Washington, DC, U.S. Department of Commerce, 2000

Wagener LM, Furrow JL, King PE, et al: Religion and developmental resources. Rev Relig Res 44:271–284, 2003

Wallerstein JS: The long-term effects of divorce on children: a review. J Am Acad Child Adolesc Psychiatry 30:349–360, 1991

Weaver AJ, Samford JA, Morgan V, et al: Research on religious variables in five major adolescent research journals: 1992 to 1996. J Nerv Ment Dis 188:36–44, 2000

Wilcox WB: Conservative Protestant childrearing: authoritarian or authoritative? Am Sociol Rev 63:796–809, 1998

Wills TA, Yaeger AM, Sandy JM: Buffering effect of religiosity for adolescent substance use. Psychol Addict Behav 17:24–31, 2003

Worthington EL, Kurusu TA, McCullough ME, et al: Empirical research on religion and psychotherapeutic processes and outcomes: a 10-year review and research prospectus. Psychol Bull 119:448–487, 1996

Wright LS, Frost CJ, Wisecarver SJ: Church attendance, meaningfulness of religion, and depression symptomatology among adolescents. J Youth Adolesc 22:559–568, 1993

Youniss J, McLellan JA, Su Y, et al: The role of community service in identity development: normative, unconventional, and deviant orientations. J Adolesc Res 14:248–261, 1999

COMMENTARY ON "SPIRITUAL AND RELIGIOUS PERSPECTIVES ON CHILD AND ADOLESCENT PSYCHOPATHOLOGY"

Paramjit T. Joshi, M.D.

Drs. Mabe, Dell, and Josephson provide a very comprehensive review on the role of spirituality and religion on child and adolescent psychopathology and the impact on mental health outcomes. They carefully and thoughtfully examine the importance of religious practices and spirituality as they relate to the consequences of such beliefs and practice on children's emotional well-being and urge practitioners to consider the core concepts outlined in everyday clinical practice.

Religion plays a key role in the context of the family and the socialization of children, yet there is a paucity of literature on the impact of such beliefs and practices not only on children's mental health and well-being but also on other medical health-related conditions. In recent years there has been increased interest in including and exploring religious beliefs as a variable in research studies (Weaver et al. 2000). However, this remains challenging for a number of reasons: 1) religion and spirituality entail complex and diverse constructs and the two are not mutually exclusive; 2) health outcomes need to take into account the heterogeneity of various religions globally; 3) the interplay between religion and cultural values is difficult to tease apart in research studies; 4) because children do not choose their religion or related belief systems it is difficult to control for this in research studies; and

5) the lack of construct consistency across studies precludes studying religion as a variable.

This commentary explores both the protective and the risk factors that can be linked to one's religious practices and childhood psychopathology in several areas.

Depression

There is a body of literature exploring the strong link between religious practices and rates of depression and suicide. Several investigators have reported lower levels of depression and suicide in those who are more religious and further report on the more robust effect on girls and lower levels of suicide among African Americans (Choi 2002; Miller et al. 2000; Weaver et al. 2000). The only longitudinal study examining the link between religion and depression by Miller et al. (2002) showed that religious adults had higher rates of depression with a history of childhood depression.

The notion that depressed children are perhaps drawn to religion for comfort and support and hence become religious adults is not a proven construct but merely hypothesized by the authors. It is very possible that this is just an adaptive strategy by the individual rather than a direct clear link with a cause-and-effect relationship. Furthermore, it has been suggested that parental religiousness benefits children through improvement in parenting practices. However, it is extremely difficult to define the definitive research population to determine how a particular religious faith tradition, separate from its cultural context, influences the incidence and severity of depression in children that is not directly linked to their parents.

Substance Abuse

Mabe and colleagues report mixed findings in establishing a link between religion and substance abuse based on the review of the literature and propose that perhaps religion helps decrease life stresses or helps individuals cope with these stresses better, and that this in turn may reduce the degree of substance abuse and/or lead to better compliance with abstinence programs. On the other hand it has also been reported that parental religiosity has an impact on reduced substance abuse in adolescents (Merrill et al. 2001). What is not clear is whether there is a direct relationship between religious practices and use of substances or if this finding is compounded by religion being used as a coping mechanism with life stressors and hence a reduction in substance abuse. Although the use of alcohol is taboo among certain religions, the use of other substances, such as "hashish," although frowned upon, may not be taboo in the same way. Therefore in exploring this relationship further it would be important to make distinctions between the use of alcohol and other substances.

Sexuality

The authors address sexuality in more general terms and as part of other Axis I DSM diagnoses where hypersexuality can be considered—for example, as part of a manic episode. Several investigators have written about sexual conservatism among youth who are more religious and therefore at lower risk of the negative consequences of promiscuous behaviors such as substance abuse, teenage pregnancy, and school failure (Hallfors et al. 2005; Spilka et al. 1985; Weaver et al. 2000). At the same time the authors also address failure of use of premarital contraception leading to unsafe sexual practices or even teenage pregnancy (Studer and Thornton 1987). Although this may very well be the case in most parts of the world, it is important also to keep in mind certain groups of people in the world who are deeply religious and spiritual but do not necessarily have conservative sexual practices—leading to the practice of child brides or even prostitution. In such circumstances the prevailing culture may be more the link than religion or spirituality.

The protective aspects of religion and spirituality have to do with core beliefs of life, such as engendering a sense of purpose and responsibility, promoting altruism and coping with adverse life events, and enhancing resiliency that in turn may serve as a buffer in regard to psychiatric illness. Furthermore, these practices play an important role in family functioning and relationships, parenting styles, and coping. On the other hand, as the authors point out, extreme moral and religious rigidity can lead to intolerance and "poorness-of-fit" based on the interaction between the child's psychopathology and certain aspects of his or her particular beliefs and practices. Therefore it is important to discern the specific type of cognitive religious coping (positive or negative) employed by the individual and the difference in health outcomes between these two styles (Pargament et al. 2004). Both sides of this issue need to be factored into Axis IV not only to appreciate all of the variables that might exert an impact on a particular individual in formulating their treatment plan but also to gain a better appreciation of some of the therapeutic and supportive interventions that would be recommended.

As mental health professionals it is important for us in our clinical practice to be cognizant of these issues and also be mindful and respectful of the vast diversity of such beliefs and practices around the world, for only in so doing can we effectively treat our patients and advocate on their behalf. As the authors have pointed out, religious beliefs and practices can be generally viewed as health promoting and can certainly be a potential resource for our patients and their families as they struggle with any illness. Most acute healthcare facilities provide access to clergy of different faiths depending upon the needs and wishes of the patients, and this partnership needs to be fostered further.

Although it remains a challenge to include religious practices as a variable in any study, the authors eloquently argue the case for the inclusion of religion/spirituality as an important variable that should be further studied to achieve a better understanding of childhood psychopathology. Because religion and cultural beliefs are separate constructs, future studies should examine these as two separate variables in looking at health outcomes.

References

Choi H: Understanding adolescent depression in ethnocultural context. Adv Nurs Sci 25:71–85, 2002

Hallfors D, Waller M, Bauer D, et al: Which comes first in adolescence: sex and drugs or depression? Am J Prev Med 29:163–170, 2005

Merrill RM, Salazar DR, Gardner NW: Relationship between family religiosity and drug use behavior among youth. Soc Behav Pers 29:347–358, 2001

Miller L, Davies M, Greenwald S: Religiosity and substance use and abuse among adolescents in the National Comorbidity Survey. J Am Acad Child Adolesc Psychiatry 39:1190–1197, 2000

Miller L, Weissman M, Gur M, et al: Adult religiousness and history of childhood depression: eleven-year follow-up. J Nerv Ment Dis 190:86–93, 2002

Pargament KI, Koenig HG, Tarakeshwar N, et al: Religious coping methods as predictors of psychological, physical and spiritual outcomes among medically ill elderly patients: a two-year longitudinal study. J Health Psychol 9:713–730, 2004

Spilka B, Hood RW, Gorsuch RL: The Psychology of Religion. Englewood, NJ, Prentice-Hall, 1985

Studer M, Thornton A: Adolescent religiosity and contraceptive usage. J Marriage Fam 49:117–128, 1987

Weaver AJ, Samford JA, Morgan V, et al: Research on religious variables in five major adolescent research journals: 1992 to 1996. J Nerv Ment Dis 188:36–44, 2000

Commentary 6B

COMMENTARY ON "SPIRITUAL AND RELIGIOUS PERSPECTIVES ON CHILD AND ADOLESCENT PSYCHOPATHOLOGY"

Margaret L. Stuber, M.D.

Drs. Mabe, Dell, and Josephson have provided an overview of what is currently known about the relationship between child and adolescent psychopathology and religious and spiritual beliefs and practices. This is an area rife with contradictions and confusion, given the lack of uniformity of definitions of the major variables and the rather rudimentary nature of most of the measurement tools. However, as the authors point out, the growing influence of religious and spiritual groups on politics and public policy in the United States and around the world makes this an essential topic for researchers and clinicians alike.

The interest in this topic among clinicians has been evident in the Clinical Breakfasts on Religious and Spiritual Issues in Clinical Practice, chaired by Dr. Dell, which have been sold out each year for nearly a decade at the American Academy of Child and Adolescent Psychiatry's annual meetings. During these breakfasts, groups of psychiatrists have wrestled with topics such as how to work with faith-based organizations, how to utilize the social support offered by formal religious organizations, and how to help children and teens who are struggling with spiritual or religious issues in their lives. The growing national interest in complementary and alternative medicine or integrative medicine has also brought a focus on therapeutic uses of prayer, meditation, and yoga. The National Institutes of Health has a National Center for Complementary and Integrative Medicine (for more information see http://nccam.nih.gov/research), which includes a focus on religion and spirituality, and two journals devoted to complementary and alternative medicine are now listed on PubMed (*BMC Complementary and Alternative Medicine* and *Evidence Based Complementary and Alternative Medicine*).

At the same time, despite the growing heterogeneity in the United States, fears of terrorism have been used over the past few years to fan the flames of suspicions and xenophobia about people who are not from a Judeo-Christian background. In this setting, religious and cultural differences can become a focus for those with a variety of types of psychopathology, including the psychotic, anxiety, and personality disorders. People seeking security in a time of uncertainty may turn to charismatic leaders in the religious as well as political spheres. The resulting association between psychopathology and the religious fundamentalists of a variety of faiths can create an impression that leads psychologists and psychiatrists to be highly skeptical of the value of all religious beliefs.

To the extent that religion and spirituality are viewed as that which gives life meaning, two areas of research have suggested that religion and spirituality might be of psychological benefit. One is the area of *positive psychology*, described as "the scientific study of positive experiences and positive individual traits and the institutions that facilitate their development," one domain of which is meaning (Duckworth et al. 2005). Specific interventions, called "positive psychotherapy," have been recommended and found to be effective for treatment of depression (Seligman et al. 2006). In a study of "very happy people," the undergraduate students who were in the top 10% of happiness did not participate in religious activities significantly more (Diener and Seligman 2003). This suggests that if finding meaning generates happiness it has more to do with the *spiritual* than the *religious* as these concepts are defined in the Mabe, Dell, and Josephson chapter.

Another growing body of research on the psychological aspects of finding meaning in life events is the literature on posttraumatic growth. Although it has long been observed that religion and spiritual issues are more salient to those who face life-threatening illness or loss, the theoretical construct of posttraumatic growth goes beyond that. Posttraumatic growth is seen as a response to a traumatic event such that the individual reevaluates priorities and values and finds a new perspective of what is personally meaningful (Zoellner and Maercker 2006). Individuals can respond to a given traumatic event or events (such as war) in a number of ways—with resiliency, with symptoms of acute or posttraumatic stress, or with personal growth (Solomon and Dekel 2007). Although preexisting anxiety increases the likelihood of a posttraumatic stress response to trauma exposure, and certain interventions can help prevent chronic symptoms, it is not yet clear whether psychological health or illness contributes to the likelihood of posttraumatic growth. Nor is it yet known if and how growth might be promoted in response to a traumatic event, although this concept is a part of some faith backgrounds and is most notably present in some of the writings about responses to the Holocaust (Gerwood 1994).

Thus, a convergence of research findings, politics, and world events has made the relationship between psychopathology and religiosity or spirituality an important area for clinical consideration. This chapter provides a useful starting point for the ongoing discussion with psychology and psychiatry.

References

Diener E, Seligman ME: Very happy people. Psychol Sci 13:81–84, 2003

Duckworth LA, Steen TA, Seligman ME: Positive psychology in clinical practice. Annu Rev Clin Psychol 1:629–651, 2005

Gerwood JB: Meaning and love in Viktor Frankl's writing: reports from the Holocaust. Psychol Rep 75:1075–1081, 1994

Seligman ME, Rashid T, Parks AC: Positive psychotherapy. Am Psychol 61:774–788, 2006

Solomon Z, Dekel R: Posttraumatic stress disorder and posttraumatic growth among Israeli ex-POWs. J Trauma Stress 20:303–312, 2007

Zoellner T, Maercker A: Posttraumatic growth in clinical psychology: a critical review and introduction of a two component model. Clin Psychol Rev 26:626–653, 2006

7

RELIGIOUS AND SPIRITUAL ISSUES IN PERSONALITY DISORDERS

C. R. Cloninger, M.D.

Personality disorders are now defined in DSM-IV-TR (American Psychiatric Association 2000) as enduring patterns of inner experience and behavior that deviate markedly from the expectations of the individual's culture. They affect thoughts, feelings, relationships, and actions in ways that are maladaptive, inflexible, and pervasive, leading to distress or impairment for the individual and society. Before the 18th century, individuals with personality disorders were considered sinners and were censored or banished by religious, social, and family authorities. The very names of *psychology* and *psychiatry* are based on the word "psyche," which is Greek for the soul or spirit of a person. Psychology and psychiatry, therefore, refer to the study and treatment of the soul, but the importance of spiritual development is now often ignored or even actively avoided and rejected. The ignoring of spirituality in psychiatry is pervasive, even in the assessment and treatment of personality disorders in which deficits in spiritual perspective are at the crux of the disorder.

Before the 18th century and even now, spiritual and medical leaders have usually agreed that strengths of character can be described as "virtues" because they are associated with mental health and happiness. For example, the four "moral virtues" of Christianity are temperance, justice, prudence, and fortitude, whereas the three "theological virtues" are charity (love), hope, and faith. These seven virtues correspond well with healthy extremes of four dimensions of temperament and three dimensions of character that provide a comprehensive approach to variability in the personality of human beings regardless of their culture or religious preferences (Cloninger 2004). Similar systems of describing strengths of character from a contemporary psychological perspective based on psychometric work and a multicultural perspective produce similar descriptions regardless of culture or agnosticism (Cloninger 2005b; Peterson and Seligman 2004).

In contrast, faults in character leading to persistent patterns of maladaptive thoughts, feelings, and behavior are called *personality disorders* in the manual of mental disorders. Likewise, madadaptive patterns of thoughts, feelings, and behavior are also called "vices" or "sins." According to standard dictionaries, a *vice* is simply defined as a fault or failing in character and conduct leading to thoughts, feelings, and actions that are considered culturally and psychologically deviant, evil, sinful, or bad. For example, the seven "cardinal sins" of Christian religions are opposites of the seven virtues: they are lust (intemperance), gluttony (injustice), envy (imprudence), sloth (non-fortitude), hate (non-love), pride (non-faith), and greed (covetousness or non-hope).

Beginning in the 18th century, efforts were made to view these same individuals as sick rather than bad. The shift from viewing people with personality disorders as "sick" was intended to reduce judging and blaming as well as to improve treatment. However, the shift to viewing personality disorders as mental disorders with biological, psychological, and social roots has resulted in many mental health workers ignoring the important role of spiritual development in understanding and treating personality disorders. Ignoring spirituality in assessing the virtues and vices of individuals would be unthinkable except as a result of the anti-spiritual bias of modern psychiatry and psychology, which has its roots in the mindless reductionism of early behaviorists like Skinner, brainless cultural relativism of early anthropologists like Boas, and agnostic fears about wishful self-deception from Freud. The label of *personality disorder* has remained pejorative because individuals with personality disorders frequently elicit strong emotional responses from others (Cloninger and Svrakic 2000).

Regardless of the label, individuals with personality disorders involve persistent patterns of thought, feeling, and action produced by immature coping styles. In other words, these individuals have deficits in working, loving, and being happy. In order to understand these individuals and their psychological deficits, it is essential to consider these individuals in an integrative fashion that includes biological, psychological, sociocultural, and spiritual perspectives. Ignoring the substantial contributions of each of these perspectives to understanding the assessment, development, and treatment of personality disorder limits the adequacy of the classification of personality disorders and the full range of psychopathology that is related to underlying personality deviations.

Moral Insanity and Enlightenment

James Pritchard's description of "moral insanity" in 1835 may be the first description of what is now called antisocial personality disorder. He described moral insanity in this way:

> The intellectual faculties appear to have sustained little or no injury, while the disorder is manifested principally or alone in the state of the feelings, temper, or habits. In cases of this description the moral and active principles of the mind are strongly perverted and depraved, the power of self government is lost or impaired and the individual is found to be incapable...of conducting himself with decency and propriety. (Pritchard 1835, p. 6)

Similarly, in 1812 Benjamin Rush described individuals with good intellect and a lifelong history of irresponsibility without capacity for guilt or empathy for the suffering of others as having "derangement of the moral faculties" (Rush 1962). In other words, they had persistent patterns of vice, such as the cardinal sins of pride, hate, and greed. In modern terms, individuals with antisocial personality disorder or "psychopathy" have pathological narcissism (i.e., pride), impulsive-aggression (i.e., anger and hate), and poor impulse control (i.e., covetousness, craving for immediate gratification) (Cloninger 2005a).

More generally, different subtypes of personality disorders can be understood as having different profiles of personality traits and spiritual deficits. The correspondence between personality traits and various virtues and vices is summarized in Table 7–1. The correspondence between virtues, vices, and personality traits is apparent using the seven-factor model developed by Cloninger, but these relationships are obscure in other dimensional systems that do not distinguish temperament and character. Here my goal is to describe the spiritual aspects of personality disorders so I primarily use the terminology of DSM and the seven-factor model of personality.

Virtues are not merely the opposites of vices. *Virtues* are sublimations of emotional drives that otherwise predispose to vices when character development is immature: high novelty-seeking predisposes to gluttony, which in modern terminology is usually called *addiction* or *substance dependence,* whereas low novelty-seeking predisposes not to justness and fairness but to maladaptive rigidity; harm avoidance predisposes to anxiety when high and to lust when low; and reward dependence predisposes to envy when high and to aloofness when low. For example, people with histrionic personality disorders are high in novelty-seeking, low in harm avoidance, and high in reward dependence, so they are predisposed to addictions (irritability and gluttony from high novelty-seeking), lust (from low harm avoidance), and envy (from high reward dependence). According to current diagnostic criteria, such individuals are often unjustly demanding, seductive, and attention seeking.

What is most important to note is that it is not the particular emotional style that defines a personality disorder. The features that are diagnostic of the presence of a personality disorder are the style of self-government defined by the character traits of self-directedness (i.e., responsible and purposeful vs. irresponsible and aimless), cooperativeness (i.e., tolerant and helpful vs. prejudiced and hostile), and self-transcendence (i.e., insightful and intuitive vs. conventional and materialistic). These character traits quantify individual differences in executive, legislative, and judicial functions of self-government, as described in depth elsewhere (Cloninger 2004). Individuals who are low in all three of these character traits have a depressive character profile or worldview like that of Thomas Hobbes: life is hard, people are mean, and then you die. This depressive worldview predisposes people to be greedy, hateful, and proud and leads its adherents to attribute such dark motives to the vast majority of people, if not all. On the other hand, individuals who are high in all three of these character traits have an enlightened worldview like that of Plato and other positive philosophers (Cloninger 2004). Individuals with this positive worldview are predisposed to be hopeful, loving, and faithful. They are happy to work in the service of others so that everyone may develop their innate potential for similar characteristics by growing in self-awareness.

Essentially personality disorders are deficits in insight and judgment derived from the perspective an individual takes on his or her life and personhood. *Personality* is the interaction between the inner perspective of an individual and the external situation in which they exist and function. People's responses to a situation depend not only on the external context but also on the perspective they have of themselves in that situation. As a result of the unique human potential for self-awareness, a human being has the potential to be aware of the shifts in perspective that are elicited by different circumstances and to adapt his or her perspective so as to participate in life as a humble, loving, and peacemaking component of the whole. To ignore the immaterial connections that bind all components of life is to be deficient in one's spiritual perspective. A spiritual perspective is one that allows the individual to transcend the narrow viewpoints of both egocentricity and dogmatic authorities. Accordingly, the most effective treatments of personality disorders ultimately involve methods of expanding a person's self-awareness so they can function with deeper insight and flexible judgment.

Implications of Correspondence Between Personality Disorders and Spiritual Deficits

The effect sizes of nonspiritual approaches to the treatment of personality disorders are moderate. For example, in antisocial and borderline personality disorders, the effect size of treatment is moderate (Cohen's $d=0.4$) when there is a helpful working alliance (Cloninger 2005a). Such moderate effect sizes are comparable with the effect of antidepressants in the treatment of major depressive disorders (Cloninger

TABLE 7–1. Correspondence between specific dimensions of personality, virtues, and vices

Personality dimensions	Virtues	Vices (vs. conflict)
Temperament	Moral faculty	
Harm avoidance	Temperance	Lust (vs. anxiety)
Novelty seeking	Justice	Gluttony (vs. rigidity)
Reward dependence	Prudence	Envy (vs. aloofness)
Persistence	Fortitude	Sloth (vs. perseveration)
Character	Theological faculty	
Self-directedness	Hope	Greed
Cooperativeness	Love	Hate
Self-transcendence	Faith	Pride

Source. Adapted from Cloninger 2004.

2006). These moderate effects have been obtained with cognitive-behavioral and psychodynamic therapy methods.

More recent work suggests that spiritually augmented therapy methods may improve outcomes in the treatment of personality disorders. Randomized, controlled trials show that character development can be facilitated by use of meditation to enhance self-awareness, mindfulness, compassion, and happiness (Cloninger 2006). For example, Linehan's dialectical behavior therapy for patients with severe personality disorders uses behavioral and mindfulness techniques that reduce rates of suicide attempts and hospitalization (Linehan 1993).

Low self-directedness on the Temperament and Character Inventory is a strong indicator of vulnerability to both personality disorders (Svrakic et al. 1993) and major depressive disorders (Farmer et al. 2003). Self-directedness is a predictor of rapid and stable response to both antidepressants (Cloninger 2000; Tome et al. 1997) and cognitive-behavioral therapy (CBT; Bulik et al. 1998). Encouragement of problem solving leads to increases in autonomy and the sense of personal mastery, which facilitate greater hope and well-being in ways that are common in effective psychotherapies, including CBT (Beck 1996; Beck and Freeman 1990; Burns 1980) or CBT augmented with modules for awareness of positive emotions (Fava et al. 1998a, 1998b, 2005), mindfulness (Teasdale et al. 2000, 2002), or spiritual meaning (Burns 1980; D'Souza and Rodrigo 2004; Fava et al. 1998). The addition of modules for cultivating positive emotions, mindfulness, and/or spiritual meaning reduces dropouts, relapse, and recurrence rates substantially. For example, in the treatment of patients with recurrent depression, additional work on positive emotions lowered relapse and recurrence rates in 40 patients with recurrent depression over 2 years (25% vs. 80%) (Fava et al. 1998a, 1998b). Likewise, mindfulness training reduced the relapse rate from 78% to 36% at 60 weeks in depressed patients with three or more episodes (Ma and Teasdale 2004; Teasdale et al. 2000, 2002). The patients with recurrent depressive episodes who responded to mindfulness training also had histories of adverse childhood experiences typical of patients with comorbid personality disorders. Finding of spiritual meaning through self-transcendent values also reduces relapse and improves well-being in randomized, controlled trials of patients with depression, schizophrenia, and terminal diseases (D'Souza and Rodrigo 2004).

It has long been known that patients who remit from a personality disorder often attribute their improvement to a religious conversion or illumination experience (Cloninger 2005a; Robins 1966). Systematic treatment studies of meditation show that radical transformations of a person's character depend on increasing self-awareness to experience a more sublimated or spiritual worldview (Alexander and Langer 1990; Alexander et al. 1990; Cloninger 2004). These systematic studies indicate that people with personality disorders can be taught how to develop in character and spirituality and that spiritual development can be evaluated in a scientific manner (Cloninger 2004).

Overall the major implication of the correspondence between personality traits, virtues, and vices is that character development is another way of describing the development of self-awareness and spirituality. In fact, the three stages of self-aware consciousness correspond to the three stages of spiritual development.

Stages in the Path to Well-Being

There are three major stages of self-awareness along the path to well-being, as summarized in Table 7–2, based on extensive work by many people described elsewhere (Cloninger 2004). The absence of self-awareness occurs in severe personality disorders and psychoses in which there is little or no insightful awareness of the preverbal outlook or beliefs and interpretations that automatically lead to emotional drives and actions. Lacking self-awareness, people act on their immediate likes and dislikes, which is usually described as an immature or "child-like" ego state.

The first stage of self-awareness is typical of most adults today. Ordinary adult cognition involves a capacity to delay gratification in order to attain personal goals but to remain egocentric with frequent distress when attachments and desires are frustrated. Hence the average person can function well under good conditions but may frequently experience problems under stress. At this stage a person is able to make a choice to relax and let go of their negative emotions, thereby setting the stage for acceptance of reality and movement to higher stages of coherent understanding. This stage of self-awareness is usually described as the "purgative" phase of spiritual development because individuals still have many emotional problems that they are actively trying to eliminate.

The second stage of self-aware consciousness is typical of adults when they operate like a "good parent." A good parent is allocentric in perspective—that is, he or she is "other-centered" and capable of calmly considering the perspective and needs of his or her children and other people in a balanced way that leads to satisfaction and harmony. This state is experienced when a person is able to observe his or her own subconscious thoughts and consider the thought processes of others in a similar way to their observing their own thoughts. Hence the second stage is described as "meta-cognitive" awareness, mindfulness, or "mentalizing." The ability of the mind to observe itself allows for more flexibility in action by reducing dichotomous thinking (Teasdale et al. 2002). At this stage, a person is able to observe him- or herself and others for understanding, without judging or blaming. This stage of self-awareness is usually called the "illuminative" stage of spiritual development because in this stage a person is increasing in passive self-acceptance to allow infusion of enlightening insights. Nevertheless, this stage of awareness still involves a lack of humility because the person views him- or herself as an authority who intellectually controls what is right, which is effortful.

The third stage of self-awareness is called "contemplation" because it is direct perception of one's initial perspective—that is, the preverbal outlook or schemas that direct one's attention and provide the frame that organizes our expectations, attitudes, and interpretation of events. Direct awareness of our outlook allows the enlarging of consciousness by accessing previously unconscious material, thereby letting go of wishful thinking and the impartial questioning of basic assumptions and core beliefs about life, such as "I am helpless," "I am unlovable," or "faith is an illusion." Direct perception of one's own perspective has been described as listening to one's own soul (Cloninger 2004). This stage of self-awareness is characteristic of individuals in the "unitive" stage of spiritual development. This stage is described as "unitive" because it is nondualistic and eliminates any sense of separateness, which is the ultimate basis for all fears and psychopathology. In other words, the "soulful perspective" of the unitive stage provides a fully "spiritual perspective," which is a sublimated view of life regardless of external conditions.

Extensive empirical work has shown that movement through these stages of development can be described and quantified in terms of steps in character development or psychosocial development, as in the work of Vaillant on Erikson's stages of ego development (Vaillant and Milofsky 1980). Such development can be visualized as a spiral of expanding height, width, and depth as a person matures or increases in coherence of personality. Likewise, the movement of thought from week to week or month to month has the same spiral form regardless of the time scale. Such "self-similarity" in form regardless of time scale is a property characteristic of complex adaptive systems, which are typical of psychosocial processes in general (Cloninger 2004). The clinical utility of this property is that therapists can teach people to exercise their capacity for self-awareness, moving through each of the stages of awareness just described. Their ability to do so, and the difficulties they have, reveal the way they are able to face challenges in life. I have developed an exercise, called the "Silence of the Mind" meditation, with explicit instructions to take people through each of the stages of awareness as well as they can (Cloninger 2004; see pages 84–95). Using this and a way of observing thought during mental status examination, mental health professionals can assess a person's thought and its level of coherence in a way that is constructive, easy, and precise without being judgmental or dogmatic.

In summary, spiritual development is a psychological process, not an intellectual set of religious dogmas to be imposed or judged by authority figures. Recognition of the psychological nature of spirituality as a cognitive process is important to respect the freedom of all people to understand and follow their own minds and souls. The respect for individual freedom in the pursuit of happiness is not the same as ignoring the importance of each person finding a way to express their spirituality in religious freedom. People spend more time in prayer or meditation on average than they do in sexual activity (Cloninger et al. 1993).

TABLE 7–2. Three stages of self-awareness on the path to well-being

Stage	Description	Psychological characteristics
0	Unaware	Immature, seeking immediate gratification ("child-like" ego-state)
1	Average adult cognition	Purposeful but egocentric; able to delay gratification, but has frequent negative emotions (anxiety, anger, disgust) ("adult" ego-state)
2	Meta-cognition ("mindful perspective")	Mature and allocentric; aware of own subconscious thinking; calm and patient, so able to supervise conflicts and relationships ("parental" ego-state)
3	Contemplation ("soulful perspective")	Effortless calm, impartial awareness; wise, creative, and loving by listening to one's soul; able to access what was previously unconscious as needed without effort or distress ("spiritual state," "state of well-being")

Source. Adapted from Cloninger 2004.

Personality Disorders and Religious Activity

Religious activity, such as attendance at churches and temples, is frequently associated with lower rates of personality disorder (Cloninger et al. 1997). Individuals with any type of personality disorder attended church less often than those without personality disorder in a survey in the general population around St. Louis, Missouri. Two-thirds of those with antisocial and borderline personalities reported that they rarely or never attended church, whereas two-thirds of those without personality disorder reported attending church at least monthly. One-third of people without any personality disorder attended church at least weekly. People with antisocial personality disorder were also less likely than any other personality group to say they were affiliated with any religion (30% vs. 10% unaffiliated).

These findings indicate that individuals with personality disorders are less religiously active on average, as well as having lower levels of spiritual development and self-awareness. All three clusters of DSM personality disorders are associated with lower levels of positive emotions and higher levels of negative emotions (Cloninger et al. 1997; Tsuang et al. 2002). The association of personality disorder with depression and other negative emotions is expected because major depression is associated with low self-directedness, which is the core character deficit in personality disorder (Cloninger et al. 1993). Likewise, vulnerability to substance dependence is strongly related to personality traits and disorders, particularly Cluster B personality disorders (Cloninger 1987, 1999; Cloninger et al. 1988). These findings about religious activity and vulnerability to personality disorder and related psychopathology provide additional evidence supporting treatment studies in which religious activity and spiritual development play a helpful role in the treatment of personality disorder.

Recommendations for DSM-V

It is important for psychiatrists and other mental health workers to realize that the psychiatric terminology describing personality disorders corresponds to a much older and still meaningful language describing the moral and spiritual characteristics of people. Efforts to remove pejorative implications from the diagnostic criteria are good in their intentions but obscure the qualities that evoke strong emotions in others without actually eliminating the emotional responses themselves. The problem of stigma against personality disorders is actually rooted in the unjustified assumption that these individuals have untreatable defects. In contrast, much available data from randomized, controlled trials indicate that personality disorders are treatable when clinicians are properly trained and focus on problems of interest to the individual with personality disorder. In addition, recovery from personality disorders involves developments in character, self-awareness, spirituality, virtue, and well-being. The treatment of personality disorders involves the facilitation of a change in a person's worldview and lifestyle, just as the diagnosis rests on an assessment and understanding of the person's worldview and lifestyle. Consequently, religious activity and spiritual development are crucial components of the diagnosis and treatment of personality disorders. Accordingly, biological, psychological, sociocultural, and spiritual perspectives are complementary in assessment and treatment. There need be no competition or incompatibility between contributions that can be made to the evaluation and treatment of personality disorders by psychiatrists, other mental health workers, and experts in spiritual development.

Regarding the general diagnostic criteria for a personality disorder (American Psychiatric Association 2000), it is noteworthy that the criteria systematically avoid reference to spirituality despite the crucial feature of a personality disorder being a deficit in the person's character. The manifestations listed are each *nonessential* indicators of an underlying lack of integration in the perspective taken on life. The criteria suggest an anti-spiritual bias in describing disorders that are essentially spiritual deficits. The general criteria are most important because the most commonly diagnosed personality disorder in clinical practice is "not otherwise specified." The avoidance of the spiritual features of personality disorders limits the utility of the criteria for both diagnosis and treatment, which are key motivations for DSM.

A conservative solution to this deficiency in DSM-IV-TR would be to note that a personality disorder is

A. An enduring pattern of *perspective,* inner experience, and behavior that deviates markedly from the expectations of the individual's culture....
B. The enduring pattern is inflexible and pervasive across a broad range of personal and social situations *as a consequence of the person's perspective on life not integrating sexual, material, emotional, and intellectual situations into a coherent spiritual whole in his or her self-aware consciousness.*
C. The enduring pattern leads to clinically significant distress or impairment in social, occupational, *religious, spiritual,* or other important areas of functioning.
D, E, F. (no change)

Psychiatrists with a personal agnostic bias may be uncomfortable being reminded that their anti-spiritual attitudes are actually deviations from the expectations of their culture. Most psychiatric patients want their therapist to be aware of their spiritual beliefs and needs, but many psychiatrists and other scientists have a bias against spirituality that is inconsistent with this cultural expectation (D'Souza and Rodrigo 2004). Furthermore, "spiritual perspective" is the awareness that our best scientific understanding of nature must be informed by quantum physics. In other words, a person's spiritual perspective is deficient unless he or she recognizes that all things are inseparably interdependent parts of a whole, even though he or she can also recognize and respect the individual identity of the component parts. This holistic spiritual perspective is different from the egocentric view that is consistently found in patients with personality disorders: individuals with personality disorders think of themselves as fundamentally separate, like Newtonian billiard balls, and consequently are vulnerable to fears that lead to psychopathology.

Regarding individual subtypes, more specific comments about particular vices and resistance to religious and spiritual activities could be offered. However, these are cosmetic details until the essential issues about the general criteria are faced.

Introducing these proposed simple changes in the diagnostic criteria will acknowledge the compatibility of biopsychosocial approaches with spiritual approaches to diagnosis and treatment of mental health. It could refocus treatment on the development of well-being, including happiness, love, and virtues. Such a change would move DSM along with the developments in the third generation of psychotherapies that now emphasize the importance of the cultivation of strengths of character and self-awareness by use of meditation, mindfulness, and other activities that facilitate positive mental health (Cloninger 2004; Hayes et al. 2004; Linehan 1993). The facilitation of well-being can be accomplished in ways that are compatible with fundamental psychobiological principles of spirituality without entering into subjective judgments about religious dogma. The investigation of the psychobiology of self-aware consciousness is an important challenge in modern neuroscience. Personality disorders can play a key role in psychiatry's learning to understand and to appreciate the mystery of self-aware consciousness (Cloninger 2004; Davidson 2003; Kandel et al. 2000) if the criteria are allowed to reflect the central issues about self-awareness and spirituality (Cloninger 2004). It is essential that the field dedicated to the "healing of the soul" recognize the importance of self-awareness and a spiritual perspective in the disorders that are essentially spiritual deficits regardless of what terminology may be used.

References

Alexander CN, Langer EJ (eds): Higher Stages of Human Development. New York, Oxford University Press, 1990

Alexander CN, Davies JL, Dixon CA, et al: Growth of higher stages of consciousness: Maharishi's Vedic psychology of human development, in Higher Stages of Human Development. Edited by Alexander CN, Langer EJ. New York, Oxford University Press, 1990, pp 286–341

American Psychiatric Association: Diagnostic and Statistical Manual of Mental Disorders, 4th Edition, Text Revision. Washington, DC, American Psychiatric Association, 2000

Beck AT: Beyond belief: A theory of modes, personality, and psychopathology, in Frontiers of Cognitive Therapy. Edited by Salkovskis PM. New York, Guilford, 1996, pp 1–25

Beck AT, Freeman A: Cognitive Therapy of Personality Disorders. New York, Guilford, 1990

Bulik CM, Sullivan PF, Joyce PR, et al: Predictors of 1-year treatment outcome in bulimia nervosa. Compr Psychiatry 39:206–214, 1998

Burns DD: Feeling Good: The New Mood Therapy. New York, William Morrow, 1980

Cloninger CR: Neurogenetic adaptive mechanisms in alcoholism. Science 236:410–416, 1987

Cloninger CR: Genetics of substance abuse, in Textbook of Substance Abuse Treatment, Edited by Galanter M, Kleber HD. Washington, DC, American Psychiatric Press, 1999, pp 59–67

Cloninger CR: A practical way to diagnose personality disorder: a proposal. J Pers Disord 14:99–108, 2000

Cloninger CR: Feeling Good: The Science of Well Being. New York, Oxford University Press, 2004

Cloninger CR: Antisocial personality disorder: a review, in Personality Disorders: Evidence and Experience in Psychiatry, Vol 8. Edited by Maj M, Akiskal HS, Mezzich JE, et al. London, Wiley, 2005a, pp 125–129

Cloninger CR: Book review of Peterson and Seligman's Character and Human Virtues. Am J Psychiatry 162:820–821, 2005b

Cloninger CR: Fostering spirituality and well-being in clinical practice. Psychiatr Ann 36:156–167, 2006

Cloninger CR, Svrakic DM: Personality disorders, in Comprehensive Textbook of Psychiatry. Edited by Sadock BJ, Sadock VA. Philadelphia, PA, Lippincott Williams & Wilkins, 2000, pp 1723–1764

Cloninger CR, Sigvardsson S, Bohman M: Childhood personality predicts alcohol abuse in young adults. Alcohol Clin Exp Res 12:494–505, 1988

Cloninger CR, Svrakic DM, Przybeck TR: A psychobiological model of temperament and character. Arch Gen Psychiatry 50:975–990, 1993

Cloninger CR, Bayon C, Przybeck TR: Epidemiology and Axis 2 comorbidity of antisocial personality, in Handbook of Antisocial Behavior. Edited by Stoff DM, Breiling J, Maser JD. New York, Wiley, 1997, pp 12–21

Davidson RJ: Investigating the Mind: Studies of Emotion. Mind and Life Conference, Massachusetts Institute of Technology, Cambridge MA, September 2003

D'Souza RF, Rodrigo A: Spiritually augmented cognitive behavioral therapy. Australas Psychiatry 12:148–152, 2004

Farmer AA, Mahmood A, Redman K, et al: A sib-pair study of the Temperament and Character Inventory in major depression. Arch Gen Psychiatry 60:490–496, 2003

Fava GA, Rafanelli C, Grandi S, et al: Prevention of recurrent depression with cognitive behavioral therapy: preliminary findings. Arch Gen Psychiatry 55:816–820, 1998a

Fava GA, Rafanelli C, Cazzaro M, et al: Well-being therapy: a novel psychotherapeutic approach for residual symptoms of affective disorders. Psychol Med 28:475–480, 1998b

Fava GA, Ruini C, Rafanelli C, et al: Well-being therapy of generalized anxiety disorder. Psychother Psychosom 74:26–30, 2005

Hayes SC, Follette VM, Linehan MM (eds): Mindfulness and Acceptance: Expanding the Cognitive-Behavioral Tradition. New York, Guilford, 2004

Kandel ER, Schwartz JH, Jessell TM: Principles of Neural Science. New York, McGraw-Hill, 2000

Linehan MM: Cognitive-Behavioral Treatment of Borderline Personality Disorder. New York, Guilford, 1993

Ma SH, Teasdale JD: Mindfulness-based cognitive therapy for depression: replication and exploration of differential relapse prevention effects. J Consult Clin Psychol 72:31–40, 2004

Peterson C, Seligman MEP: Character Strengths and Virtues: Handbook and Classification. New York, American Psychological Association and Oxford University Press, 2004

Pritchard JC: A Treatise on Insanity and Other Disorders Affecting the Mind. London, Merchant, 1835

Robins LN: Deviant Children Grown Up: A Sociological and Psychiatric Study of Sociopathic Personality. Baltimore, MD, Williams and Wilkins, 1966

Rush B: Medical Inquiries and Observations upon the Diseases of the Mind. New York, Hafner, 1962

Svrakic DM, Whitehead C, Przybeck TR, et al: Differential diagnosis of personality disorders by the seven factor model of temperament and character. Arch Gen Psychiatry 50:991–999, 1993

Teasdale JD, Segal ZV, Williams JM, et al: Prevention of relapse/recurrence in major depression by mindfulness-based cognitive therapy. J Consult Clin Psychol 68:615–623, 2000

Teasdale JD, Moore RG, Hayhurst H, et al: Metacognitive awareness and prevention of re-
    lapse in depression: empirical evidence. J Consult Clin Psychol 70:275–287, 2002

Tome MB, Cloninger CR, Watson JP, et al: Serotonergic autoreceptor blockade in the re-
    duction of antidepressant latency: personality and response to paroxetine and pin-
    dolol. J Affect Disord 44:101–109, 1997

Tsuang MT, Williams WM, Simpson JC, et al: Pilot study of spirituality and mental health
    in twins. Am J Psychiatry 159:486–488, 2002

Vaillant GE, Milofsky E: Natural history of male psychological health, IX: empirical evi-
    dence for Erikson's model of the life cycle. Am J Psychiatry 137:1348–1359, 1980

Commentary 7A

COMMENTARY ON "RELIGIOUS AND SPIRITUAL ISSUES IN PERSONALITY DISORDERS"

Stephen Strack, Ph.D.

Professor Cloninger's (2004) recent monograph *Feeling Good: The Science of Well Being* established him as psychiatry's foremost integrative thinker on the biopsychosocial basis of self-transcendence, or spirituality, including how deficits in psychological maturity and self-aware consciousness lead to a wide variety of pathological conditions (e.g., depression, substance abuse, personality disorders). Drawing on that work, Cloninger here offers a simple way to correct a major problem in the current definition of personality disorders: namely, to recognize that these ingrained and dysfunctional patterns of thinking, feeling, and behaving are spiritual maladies rooted in an individual's dualistic world view of separateness, egocentricity, and fear.

Researchers and clinicians have long voiced dissatisfaction with the definition of personality disorders in the last four diagnostic manuals (Livesley 2001; Strack 2006). Beginning with DSM-III (American Psychiatric Association 1980), personality disorders were separated from other mental disorders to distinguish them as pervasive, maladaptive patterns of conduct that evolve from, and are inextricably linked with, an individual's culture. Theoretical assumptions were dropped in an effort to move past the psychoanalytic thinking that had been dominant in the early 20th century, and so the personality disorders that can be diagnosed do not represent a coherent taxonomy, nor are specific etiologies presumed. Diagnostic criteria focus on prototypical behavior patterns, attitudes, and feeling states, but inevitable overlap and low specificity have led practitioners to use the "not otherwise specified" category more often than any other (Livesley 2001).

Perhaps even more problematic than the diagnostic criteria themselves is that individuals labeled as having personality disorders are frequently viewed as troublemakers who overutilize mental health services and are essentially untreatable (Cloninger and Svrakic 2000). Personality disorders do not lend themselves to single-mode, short-term therapies. People with personality disorders are puzzling and exasperating to most clinicians, in part because the rigid defenses they utilize are interpersonal in nature, designed to elicit specific responses that will perpetuate and reinforce the person's negative world view, or schema.

Cloninger offers a means by which to clarify personality disorder diagnosis and help with treatment. He argues that mental health professionals should reclaim their roots as healers of the psyche and define these disorders as spiritual disorders that result in moral weakness and a preference for vice over virtue. He notes that early psychiatrists such as Rush and Pritchard recognized the central moral flaws in persons with antisocial personality disorder but that by the end of the 19th century the mental health field had abandoned such concepts in favor of a disease model: "The shift from viewing people with personality disorders as 'sick' was intended to reduce judging and blaming, as well as to improve treatment. However,…[this] has resulted in many…ignoring the important role of spiritual development in understanding and treating personality disorders." Cloninger believes that an "anti-spiritual bias" in modern science is largely to blame for this shift in thinking.

Cloninger's thesis is that personality disorders result from a worldview, or perspective, that life is inherently fraught with pain and suffering, that there is no light (happiness) at the end of the tunnel, and the best one can do is grab for whatever sustenance and pleasure is available and not be concerned with others or long-term consequences. He believes that all forms of personality disorder demonstrate the same flaw: "[I]t is not the particular emotional style that defines a personality disorder. The features that are diagnostic…are the style of self-government defined by the character traits of self-directedness (i.e., responsible and purposeful vs. irresponsible and aimless), cooperativeness (i.e., tolerant and helpful vs. prejudiced and hostile), and self-transcendence (i.e., insightful and intuitive vs. conventional and materialistic)." A negative worldview causes a devaluation of the elements that make a person happy, for example, trust and the virtues of love and hope. It makes attractive a lifestyle that destroys self-esteem and dignity, that is, the world of vice.

Although many biopsychosocial elements contribute to the adoption of a negative worldview, it is the failure of self-aware consciousness that is central to the development of personality disorder. People with these disorders are essentially unaware of themselves and others. They are immature, childlike, and seek immediate gratification. They are pawns to incoherent thoughts, feelings, and desires that prompt them to act, and they feel cheated and hurt when their needs are unmet.

To obtain desired ends, they adopt rigid, maladaptive coping strategies such as cloying dependence, histrionic displays, aggressiveness, avoidance, and withdrawal.

In Cloninger's view the key to treating personality disorders is in helping afflicted persons expand their self-aware consciousness. He believes that all people have an indelible connection to the universal unity of being, or God. As people with personality disorder become more self-aware, they begin to discover for themselves that they possess dignity and a right to be happy. Once oriented to a positive worldview, these individuals can learn to sublimate conflicting needs and desires. They will, with proper guidance, seek to expand their connection to God, which results in more virtuous behavior and increased happiness and well-being.

As a clinician with 25 years of experience working with personality disorders I welcome Professor Cloninger's recommendations. Like alcoholic persons who have lost all self-respect in their addiction, people with personality disorders have lost their spiritual selves. They live in a chaotic world with no hope of things getting better. Change requires a radical shift in thinking. Cloninger's recognition of the loss of spiritual self in a lack of self-aware consciousness sets the stage for clear treatment avenues. His own *coherence therapy* (Cloninger 2004), based on mindfulness meditation that builds self-awareness, works very well with a variety of personality disorder clients.

A survey of my colleagues and students informs me that many in the psychiatric community are not ready to embrace spirituality as an explanatory variable in the etiology and treatment of personality disorders. Cloninger is aware of this. He knows that scientists fear going back to a prescientific past where religious doctrine substituted for the truth. However, those who are courageous enough to entertain a role for spirituality in understanding these disorders will find that Cloninger's (2004) own work offers an intriguing conceptual and empirical base for his claims. Cloninger's spiritual model is areligious, holding sacred the belief that all persons need freedom to explore their minds and souls as they see fit: "[S]piritual development is a psychological process, not an intellectual set of religious dogmas to be imposed or judged by authority figures." As such, it offers the mental health community a science-based definition of a universal individual differences variable that needs to have a place in 21st century psychiatry, including the diagnostic criteria for personality disorders.

References

American Psychiatric Association: Diagnostic and Statistical Manual of Mental Disorders, 3rd Edition. Washington, DC, American Psychiatric Association, 1980

Cloninger CR: Feeling Good: The Science of Well Being. New York, Oxford University Press, 2004

Cloninger CR, Svrakic DM: Personality disorders, in Comprehensive Textbook of Psychiatry. Edited by Sadock BJ, Sadock VA. New York, Lippincott Williams and Wilkins, 2000, pp 1723–1764

Livesley WJ: Conceptual and taxonomic issues, in Handbook of Personality Disorders. New York, Guilford, 2001, pp 3–38

Strack S: Introduction, in Differentiating Normal and Abnormal Personality, 2nd Edition. Edited by Strack S. New York, Springer, 2006, pp xvii–xxvii

Commentary 7B

COMMENTARY ON "RELIGIOUS AND SPIRITUAL ISSUES IN PERSONALITY DISORDERS"

George E. Vaillant, M.D.

Dr. Cloninger's chapter on the role of spirituality in the classification of personality disorders reflects a bold proposal by a psychiatrist distinguished for his innovative work in both genetics and personality disorders. Cloninger points out that the 20th-century shift from viewing people with personality disorders as "bad" to "sick" was intended to reduce judging and blaming as well as to improve treatment. However, the shift to viewing personality disorders as mental disorders with biological, psychological, and social roots has resulted in many mental health workers ignoring the important role of spiritual development. Cloninger suggests that "ignoring spirituality in assessing the virtues and vices of individuals would be unthinkable except as a result of the anti-spiritual bias of modern psychiatry and psychology…" This is unfortunate because a spiritual perspective is one that allows the individual to transcend the narrow viewpoints of both his or her own egocentricity and dogmatic authorities. Accordingly, the most effective treatments of personality disorders ultimately involve "spiritual" methods of expanding a person's self-awareness so that he or she can function with deeper insight and flexible judgment.

Cloninger cites work by several investigators (D'Souza and Rodrigo 2004; Hayes et al. 2004; Linehan 1993) that suggests that spiritually augmented therapy methods may improve outcomes of personality disorders. Alcoholics Anonymous, of course, reflects another successful example. For example, in the treatment of patients with recurrent depression, additional work focusing upon positive emotions (another way of discussing spirituality) lowered relapse and recurrence rates in 40 patients with recurrent depression over 2 years (25% vs. 80%; Fava et al. 1998).

In Cloninger's view healthy character can be defined not only by the dimensions of harm avoidance, reward dependence, novelty-seeking, and persistence but also by three additional character traits of self-directedness (hope—i.e., responsible and purposeful vs. irresponsible and aimless), cooperativeness (love—i.e., tolerant and helpful vs. prejudiced and hostile), and self-transcendence (faith—i.e., insightful and intuitive vs. conventional and materialistic). Because people's responses to a situation depend not only on the external context but also on the perspective they have of themselves in that situation, Cloninger suggests that deficits in the three "theological" or spiritual virtues of faith, hope, and love need to be taken into account. In view of the importance of such positive emotions in the recovery from personality disorders, it may be important to emphasize that spiritual development is more limbic than neocortical (Vaillant 2008); and as Alcoholics Anonymous members well understand, individuals with personality disorders develop spiritually through "the language of the heart," not just from cognitive therapy.

I have nothing but praise for Cloninger's rewriting the definition of personality disorders, except in Section B I would cut the word "spiritual," which may grate on the ears of some readers. In addition, Cloninger (2005) refers to "spiritual deficits" as "deficits in the coherence of their fundamental assumptions and schemas about life." This is a rather unusual definition of *spiritual*. (In revising his recommendations, Cloninger might do well to review the important works by Newberg and D'Aquilli [2001] and the Fetzer Institute [2003] that are missing from his bibliographies.)

References

Cloninger CR: Book review of Peterson and Seligman's Character and Human Virtues. Am J Psychiatry 162:820–821, 2005

D'Souza RF, Rodrigo A: Spiritually augmented cognitive behavioral therapy. Australas Psychiatry 12:148–152, 2004

Fava GA, Rafanelli C, Grandi S, et al: Prevention of recurrent depression with cognitive behavioral therapy: preliminary findings. Arch Gen Psychiatry 55:816–820, 1998

Fetzer Institute: Multidimensional Measurement of Religiousness/Spirituality for Use in Health Research. Kalamazoo, MI, John E. Fetzer Institute, 2003

Hayes SC, Follette VM, Linehan MM (eds): Mindfulness and Acceptance: Expanding the Cognitive Behavioral Tradition. New York, Guilford, 2004

Linehan MM: Cognitive-Behavioral Treatment of Borderline Personality Disorder. New York, Guilford, 1993

Newberg A, D'Aquilli E: Why God Won't Go Away: Brain Science and the Biology of Belief. New York, Ballantine Books, 2001, p 37

Vaillant GE: Spiritual Evolution: A Scientific Defense of Faith. New York, Doubleday Broadway, 2008

8

DSM-IV RELIGIOUS AND SPIRITUAL PROBLEMS

David Lukoff, Ph.D.

Francis G. Lu, M.D.

C. Paul Yang, M.D., Ph.D.

Background

In 1994, DSM-IV (American Psychiatric Association 1994) included a new V code entitled "Religious or Spiritual Problem":

> V62.89: This category can be used when the focus of clinical attention is a religious or spiritual problem. Examples include distressing experiences that involve loss or questioning of faith, problems associated with conversion to a new faith, or questioning of other spiritual values which may not necessarily be related to an organized church or religious institution. (p. 685; see also American Psychiatric Association 2000, p. 1393)

The acceptance of this new category by the American Psychiatric Association Task Force on DSM-IV was based on a proposal documenting the extensive literature on the frequent occurrence of religious and spiritual issues in clinical practice, the lack of training provided to mental health professionals, and the need for a diagnostic category to support training and research in this area of clinical practice (Lukoff et al. 1992a).

Religion and spirituality have been distinguished in a multitude of ways, including definitions in which religion subsumes spirituality and vice versa (Koenig et al. 2001; Shafranske and Sperry 2005). The scientific and healthcare databases such as Medline and PsycInfo distinguish between religion and spirituality along

171

the lines delineated in the DSM-IV definition of religious or spiritual problem. The *Thesaurus of Psychological Index Terms* (Walker 1991) defines *religion* as "associated with religious organizations and religious personnel" (p. 184), whereas *spirituality* refers to the "degree of involvement or state of awareness or devotion to a higher being or life philosophy. Not always related to conventional religious beliefs" (p. 208). Thus religious problems involve a person's conflicts over the beliefs, practices, rituals, and experiences related to a religious belief system or community. In contrast, spiritual problems involve distress associated with a person's personal relationship to a higher power or transcendent force that may or may not be related to a religious worldview.

In this chapter we present a typology for religious problems and a separate one for spiritual problems. These typologies are based on systematic and ongoing literature reviews of PubMed (Medline) and PsycInfo as well as theology and anthropology reference databases to identify case studies and other research as well as clinical articles that address religious and spiritual problems (Lukoff et al. 1992b, 1993, 1999). In the latter part of this chapter, we also discuss the co-occurrence of religious and spiritual problems with mental disorders, provide general guidelines for treatment of religious and spiritual problems, and conclude with suggestions for DSM-V.

Typology of Religious Problems

The original definition proposed to the Task Force on DSM-IV and published in the *Journal of Nervous and Mental Disease* (Lukoff et al. 1992a) included four types of religious problems based on literature reviews conducted through 1991:

1. Loss or questioning of faith
2. Change in denominational membership
3. Conversion to a new faith
4. Intensification of adherence to religious practices and orthodoxy

In the final definition of "Religious or Spiritual Problem" published in DSM-IV, only two of the four types were included: 1) loss or questioning of faith, and 2) conversion to a new faith. The typology of religious problems that follows has been updated in this chapter to reflect new studies reported in the databases of health-care and scientific literature since 1991:

- Loss or questioning of faith
- Changes in membership, practices, and beliefs (including conversion)
- New Religious Movements and cults
- Life-threatening and terminal illness

LOSS OR QUESTIONING OF FAITH

Loss of faith is specifically mentioned in the DSM-IV definition as a religious problem. There are several forms that loss of faith can take. Shafranske (1991) described a psychotherapy case involving a man of professional accomplishment whose life was founded upon the conservative bedrock of Roman Catholic Christianity. He came to doubt the tenets of his religion and, in so doing, felt he had lost the vitality to live. Some crises of faith are recognized as part of spiritual development. James Fowler (1995), building on the work of Piaget, Kohlberg, and other developmental theorists, has proposed that there is an invariant order of faith development involving six distinct stages. Problems may arise in the transition from one stage to another, and these are often experienced as a crisis of faith.

A similar problem can occur when a person is ostracized by his or her religious community. One such crisis was precipitated when a Jehovah's Witness cardiac patient elected to have a medically necessary heart transplant despite his family's and religious community's objections on religious grounds: "His family and church community subsequently refused to have any contact with him. Ultimately, the patient became suicidal and required psychiatric hospitalization" (Waldfogel and Wolpe 1993, p. 474). Loss of faith can involve a person questioning his or her whole way of life, purpose for living, and source of meaning.

In addition, a person's social world can be affected because religion is for many an important part of their social network. Barra et al. (1993) conducted a survey study and also reviewed the anthropological, historical, and contemporary perspectives on loss and grief. They found that loss of religious connectedness,

> whether in relation to traditional religious affiliation or to a more personal search for spiritual identity, frequently resulted in individuals experiencing many of the feelings associated with more "normal" loss situations. Thus, feelings of anger and resentment, emptiness and despair, sadness and isolation, and even relief could be seen in individuals struggling with the loss of previously comforting religious tenets and community identification. (p. 292)

Because this type of loss is typically not acknowledged by others, it is a "disenfranchised grief." The authors cited one case of a graduate student who stopped believing in her religion of origin. She reported feeling alienation, fear, anxiety, anger, hopelessness, and even suicidal ideation, the common sequelae of a grief reaction. The American Psychiatric Association's "Guidelines Regarding Possible Conflict Between Psychiatrists' Religious Commitments and Psychiatric Practice" (American Psychiatric Association 1990) mentioned a case in which a psychiatrist provided interpretations to a devoutly religious man. "In doing this, however, she denigrated his long-standing religious commitments as foolishly neurotic. Because of the intensity of the therapeutic relationship, the interpretations caused great distress and appeared related to a subsequent suicide attempt" (p. 542). This is an iatrogenic religious problem triggered by culturally insensitive treatment.

Therapy can focus on the change as a turning point in faith that offers the potential for personal exploration and discovery:

> If, later in life, we suffer a profound disillusionment in our experience of the world, we may find ourselves turning back towards psychic resources that previously we had repressed. This is the beginning of what I have called "regression in the service of transcendence," which I think most people would know better using the term of St. John of the Cross, "the dark night of the soul." It can be a very long, difficult, and trying period. (Washburn 1998, p. 2)

Loss of faith can serve as an opportunity for the patient to grow into a new relationship to the mystery of life. Referral to a religious professional can help some to reconnect with their faith. Others may not want to become involved with an organized religion again but would explore alternative spiritual practices and use of spirituality as a source of personal meaning and of social connection.

CHANGES IN MEMBERSHIP, PRACTICES, AND BELIEFS (INCLUDING CONVERSION)

Changes in Membership

Due to intermarriage, mobility, and the breakdown of geographic limitations to church membership, more than one-third of people convert to new religions or change their denominational membership during their lifetime. When people move to a community that does not have a branch of their original religious group, the change may be experienced as forced rather than voluntary. They may experience a loss associated with separation from a previously valued religious community (Hoge 1996).

Intensification of Belief

Another type of religious problem can occur when a person intensifies adherence to religious practices and orthodoxy, especially when the person does not feel free to talk about the change in their religious beliefs to family or friends who may not be supportive. Intensification of religious practice and conversion can be misdiagnosed as mental disorders. Greenberg and Witztum (1991), Israeli psychiatrists who work with orthodox Jewish patients, have developed criteria for distinguishing normative strict orthodox religious beliefs and practices from psychotic symptoms that include religious content. They propose that symptoms of mental disorder

- are more intense than normative religious experiences in their religious community,
- are often terrifying,

- are often preoccupying,
- are associated with deterioration of social skills and personal hygiene, and
- often involve special messages from religious figures.

At times devout religious practices can be viewed as extreme and result in conflict with the law, as with genital mutilation, a practice associated with several religions (Abu-Sahlieh 1994).

If the patient is newly religious, the therapist needs to help identify and work on conflicts between the patient's former and current lifestyle, beliefs, and attitudes. Spero (1987) described the case of a 16-year-old adolescent from a reform Jewish family who underwent a sudden religious transformation to orthodoxy. The dramatic changes in her life, including long hours studying Jewish texts, avoidance of friends, and sullenness at meals, led her parents to schedule an appointment with a psychiatrist. A mental status examination determined that neither schizophrenia nor any other disorders were present. The therapy then dealt with the impact of religious transformation on her identity and object relations. "The process of religious change challenges important areas of stability, and can represent a crisis for all nouveau-religionists" (Spero 1987, p. 69).

Intensification may also be one of the coping mechanisms used to deal with trauma and is associated with the need to find meaning in the distressing event in order to avoid a breakdown of identity. Yet such intensification may also occur as an attempt to deal with feelings of guilt.

Conversion Experiences

Conversion refers to the adoption of a new religious identity or a change from one religious identity to another, based on an experience that involves a huge displacement and rearrangement of the convert's personality (James 1902/1958). Conversion occurs not only from one religion to another but also between different sects, such as the various Protestant denominations. Cultural and social factors play an important role in the conversion process, and religious groups view conversion differently, from welcoming to questioning converts.

> These changes in beliefs and practices quite often do in fact disrupt peoples' lives. It does disrupt families. Even though we may give a theology of conversion that can soft pedal all those issues, the truth is, the issue is controversial because it is disruptive...a disorientation, and something that has caused a lot of complications in many peoples' lives. (Malony 1992, p. 95)

NEW RELIGIOUS MOVEMENTS AND CULTS

Clinical understanding of the impact of intense religious groups has been complicated by the legal implications of labeling a group a *cult*. *New Religious Movement* is the term that sociologists often use to refer to the multitude of small religious groups that are not destructive. In the mental health field, "cult" carries the implication that the group uses intimidation, coercion, and indoctrination to systematically recruit, initiate, and influence inductees. Some genuinely dangerous and destructive cults do arise under the banner of religion. A recent example is the Branch Davidians.

However, *cult* also carries the nonpejorative meaning of a group of people who gather for some religious purpose. All religions originally began as cults and were originally perceived as a threat to the status quo in society. Mental health professionals may need to distinguish socially controversial New Religious Movements from cults. In assessing whether the group shows the signs of pathology that distinguish a misguided cult from wholesome spiritual communities, Wellwood (1987) lists these characteristics of pathological communities:

- The leader has total power to validate or negate the self-worth of the devotees and uses this power extensively.
- The group is held together by allegiance to a cause, a mission, and ideology.
- The leader keeps his followers in line by manipulating emotions of hope and fear.
- "Groupthink" is used to knit followers together.
- Cult leaders are usually self-styled prophets who have not studied with great teachers or undergone lengthy training or discipline.

Nine factors have been associated with recruitment into cults (Curtis and Curtis 1993):

1. Generalized ego-weakness and emotional vulnerability
2. Propensities toward dissociative states
3. Tenuous, deteriorated, or nonexistent family relations and support systems
4. Inadequate means of dealing with exigencies of survival
5. History of severe child abuse or neglect
6. Exposure to idiosyncratic or eccentric family patterns
7. Proclivities toward or abuse of controlled substances
8. Unmanageable and debilitating situational stress and crises
9. Intolerable socioeconomic conditions

The assumption that cult involvement induces psychopathology has been disputed. Galanter (1983) studied members of the Unification Church and found that they had had a significantly higher degree of distress before conversion when compared with a control group, thus showing that symptoms of psychopathology had not been caused by cult involvement—30% had sought professional help for emotional problems before conversion. This finding may account for reports of abnormal behavior among ex-members. Galanter (1999) has proposed viewing con-

temporary cults and zealous self-help movements as charismatic groups characterized by 1) a high level of social cohesiveness, 2) an intensely held belief system, and
3) a profound influence on its members' behavior.

> It is "charismatic" because of the commitment of members to a fervently espoused,
> transcendent goal; indeed, this goal is frequently articulated by a charismatic leader
> or ascribed to the progenitor of the group...charismatic groups can relieve certain
> symptoms associated with psychopathology, although they can precipitate psychi-
> atric symptoms as well. (Galanter 1999, pp. 81–84)

Membership in cults is not uniformly oppressive or detrimental to mental
health. For the vast majority, such "radical religious departures" are part of adolescent or young adult identity exploration. People join cults as part of a search for
community and a spiritual quest (Galanter 1990; Hoge 1996). One study found
that the majority of all defectors or ex-members (67%) looked back on their experience as something that made them wiser for the experience, rather than feeling
angry or duped or showing other ill effects (Wright 1987). Vaughan (1986) also
reported that many individuals who joined and then left destructive groups
believed that the experience contributed to their wisdom and maturity through
a sense of having met the challenge by restoring their integrity. Because more
than 90% of persons who join New Religious Movements leave within 2 years,
Post (1993) pointed out that "if brainwashing goes on, it is extremely ineffective"
(p. 373).

In 1989, the American Psychiatric Association's Committee on Psychiatry and
Religion called upon psychiatrists to help temper the anti-cult fanaticism that often develops in families who are concerned about a family member's involvement
with a New Religious Movement. After the Jonestown massacre, there were attempts to sanction the forcible deprogramming and involuntary hospitalization of
religious seekers who were "turning East." There are reports of posttraumatic stress
disorder being induced by such aggressive deprogramming (Ikemoto and Nakamura 2004). However, "exit counseling," which is less coercive, has largely re-
placed "deprogramming."

People transitioning from the "culture of embeddedness" with New Religious
Movements and cults into more independent functioning sometimes seek psychotherapeutic help. Vaughan (1986) described a psychotherapeutic approach that
focuses on the psychological consequences of joining a movement that purport-
edly offers spiritual self-realization. Her client-centered approach does not evaluate the relative merit of alternative spiritual practices or try to determine whether
the "teacher" is a true spiritual authority. Individuals may have any of a number of
motivations for joining a group, ranging from difficulty supporting themselves, to
loneliness, to actualizing their potential by progressing along a path of spiritual development. With someone who has left, or who is considering joining or leaving

a movement or cult, the therapy could be focused on helping the client explore the following issues:

- What attracts me to this person?
- Am I attracted to his or her power, showmanship, cleverness, achievements, glamour, ideas?
- Am I motivated by fear or love?
- Is my response primarily physical excitement, emotional activation, intellectual stimulation, or intuitive resonance?
- What would persuade me to trust him or her more than myself?
- Am I looking for a parent figure to relieve me of the responsibility for my life?
- Am I looking for a group where I feel I can belong and be taken care of in return for doing what I am told?
- What am I giving up?
- Am I moving toward something I am drawn to, or am I running away from my life as it is?

TERMINAL AND LIFE-THREATENING ILLNESS

Although listed here as a religious problem, both religious and spiritual beliefs and practices can influence the ways patients cope with serious illnesses. This is particularly true in the case of terminal illnesses that raise fears of physical pain, the unknown aspects of the dying process, the threat to integrity, and the uncertainty of life after death (Doka and Morgan 1993). In addition, religious and spiritual changes often occur during terminal illness related to feelings of loss, alienation, abandonment, anger, suffering, and dependency. Issues such as forgiving others, finding peace, discussing death, grieving, and planning the funeral often involve religion (Sulmasy 2006). Loss of hope and a sense of meaning become problems for some patients.

Religious beliefs, participation in religious rituals, and affiliation with a religious community can all be affected by serious illness. Loss or questioning of faith, anger at God, guilt over "sins," and discontinuation of religious practices have been reported with terminal and life-threatening illness (Miovic 2007). The nursing diagnostic nomenclature specifically notes that spiritual distress in a patient can be related to the patient's inability to practice religious rituals and conflict between religious or spiritual beliefs and prescribed medical care (Carpenito 1983).

Religious coping is one of the main strategies used to address fears about facing death (Pargament et al. 2004). In her research on narrative life story therapy with the elderly, Viney (1993) found that prayer was particularly helpful for dying persons: "Talking with God can provide opportunity to make the pain meaningful, confront the risks, confirm the integrity and give more certainty about life after death" (p. 165).

The Joint Commission (2007) has set accreditation standards that mandate spiritual care be a component of hospice care. Spirituality can be useful in addressing "Why me?" questions that patients frequently raise, so therapists and caregivers should actively support and facilitate religious and spiritual thinking in terminally ill patients. Millison (1988) maintained that "The caregiver needs to understand the power of spiritual beliefs in helping the patient cope with dying, and needs to be aware of the ways that spiritual striving can be helped, hindered, or undermined" (p. 37).

The transitions from living to dying are essentially spiritual, and clearly not solely physiological, psychological, or social (Millison 1988). Many terminal patients return to their childhood religious beliefs and practices, whereas others search for new forms of spirituality. Treatment often includes working with or consulting with a religious professional (Doka and Morgan 1993). For many with a serious or life-threatening illness, the same questions and concerns arise. Being diagnosed with HIV or AIDS often initiates a reexamination of spiritual and religious issues and a person's connection to the sacred (Ironson et al. 2006). Religious and spiritual competency in being able to address the diversity of beliefs in increasingly multicultural clinical settings is an essential skill (Richards and Bergin 2000). Conducting a religious and spiritual history is an important component of clinical work in this area (Puchalski and Romer 2000).

CASE EXAMPLE

A woman hospitalized with a spinal injury after an automobile accident showed symptoms consistent with a depressive disorder. The psychiatrist called in to consult found that she missed the religious and spiritual practices that were part of her life before the hospitalization. The consultant recommended psychotherapy to explore her religious beliefs in light of her accident and helped her obtain a tape player so she could listen to religious music. A clergy member of her faith was contacted and made several hospital visits to provide support. The authors concluded, "Although religious interventions are not substitutes for therapeutic interventions, 'religious prescriptions' are ethically sound and may complement more traditional therapies." (Waldfogel and Wolpe 1993, p. 475)

Another case example is of a Hodgkin's disease survivor with metastatic prostate cancer and severe coronary artery disease (Penson et al. 2001). He complained that he was "losing God." His caregivers were able to provide the sense of community in which he could reestablish his faith. The authors concluded that healthcare providers do not have to be religious in order to help patients deal with a spiritual crisis: "The clinical skills of compassion need to be deployed to diagnose and respond to spiritual suffering. Acknowledging and addressing anger or guilt, common sources of suffering, are essential to adjustment. Simply being there for the patient and being open to their hurt can help resolve their spiritual crisis" (Penson et al. 2001, p. 286).

Pargament et al. (2004) found that people struggling with religious beliefs or whose faith is shaken when they fall ill are at greater risk of dying. They studied 596 patients aged 55 years or older on medical inpatient units. Patients who reported that they felt alienated from or unloved by God and attributed their illness to the devil or said they felt abandoned by their church community had a 19%–28% increase in the risk of dying within the next 2 years compared with those who had no such religious doubts, even after controlling for the patients' health, mental health, and demographic status. Specifically, those who indicated that they "Wondered whether God had abandoned me" and "Questioned God's love for me" had a higher mortality rate. The authors indicated that these results highlight the need for spiritual assessment and pastoral interventions for patients whose faith is shaken by illness.

Typology of Spiritual Problems

The original definition proposed to the Task Force on DSM-IV included two types of spiritual problems that had been identified through literature searches: 1) near death experiences and 2) mystical experiences. DSM-IV adopted a more general definition for spiritual problems: "questioning of other spiritual values which may not necessarily be related to an organized church or religious institution." The typology that follows reflects recent studies reported in the databases of healthcare and scientific literature:

- Mystical experiences
- Near-death experiences
- Psychic experiences
- Alien abduction experiences
- Meditation and spiritual practice-related experiences
- Possession experiences

Polls have shown a dramatic increase in the percentages of people who report mystical and near-death experiences, contact with the dead, extrasensory perception, visions, out-of-body experiences, UFO abductions, and other unusual experiences. About 75% of Americans hold some form of belief in the paranormal, such as extrasensory perception, ghosts, telepathy, clairvoyance, astrology, communicating with the dead, witches, reincarnation, or channeling (Gallup 2002). During the past 25 years there has also been a significant increase in participation in spiritual practices such as meditation, tai chi, yoga, sweat lodges, drumming circles, and other spiritually oriented new age groups, all of which can induce intense spiritual experiences (Gallup and Jones 2000). The majority of these experiences are not problematic, do not disrupt psychological/social/occupational functioning, and do not lead to mental health treatment. However, with increased participation in practices and in groups that induce intense spiritual experiences, it can be expected that the incidence of spiritual problems seen in treatment is likely to increase (Lukoff 2007b).

Anomalous experiences include a variety of unusual experiences that appear to challenge our understanding of the world, such as mystical experiences, near-death experiences, alien encounters, psychic experiences, lucid dreaming, and psychedelic drug experiences. These non-ordinary experiences have often been ignored or ridiculed by mainstream psychology, even though interest in exceptional mental states dates back to William James on *Exceptional Mental States: The 1896 Lowell Lectures* (Taylor 1983). The more recent *Varieties of Anomalous Experiences: Examining the Scientific Evidence,* published by the American Psychological Association (Cardena et al. 2000), examined 10 types of anomalous experiences and found little relationship between anomalous experiences and psychopathology. Indeed, many of these experiences have been associated with claims of positive life changes following the experience.

Anomalous experiences such as mystical, psychic, and near-death experiences often include religious and spiritual content. Yet they can be distressing and lead to contact with mental health professionals. Four anomalous experiences are included as spiritual problems in the typology in this chapter: mystical experiences, near-death experiences, alien abduction experiences, and psychic experiences.

MYSTICAL EXPERIENCE

Studies of this phenomenon date back to William James, who considered such experiences to be at the core of religion and maintained that such experiences led to the founding of the world's religions (James 1902/1958). Definitions used in research and clinical publications vary considerably, ranging from "upheaval of the total personality" (Neumann 1964) to those that include "everyday mysticism" (Scharfstein 1973). For clinical purposes, a *mystical experience* can be defined as a transient, extraordinary experience marked by

- Feelings of unity
- Sense of harmonious relationship to the divine
- Euphoria
- Sense of noesis (access to the hidden spiritual dimension)
- Loss of ego functioning
- Alterations in time and space perception
- Sense of lacking control over the event

Surveys assessing the incidence of mystical experience in the general population show that it has been rising over the past few decades. For more than 30 years, the Gallup Poll has posed the question: "Have you ever been aware of, or influenced by, a presence or a power—whether you call it God or not—which is different from your everyday self?" Affirmative answers have continuously increased: 27% in 1973, 42% in 1986, 54% in 1990, and 70% in 2001 (Gallup 2002). Considering that most American adults report having mystical experiences, they are clearly normal rather than pathological phenomena.

Yet historically, psychological theory and diagnostic classification systems have tended to either ignore or pathologize such intense spiritual experiences. Some clinical literature has described the mystical experience as symptomatic of ego regression, borderline psychosis, a psychotic episode, or temporal lobe dysfunction (Lukoff 1985). Freud reduced the "oceanic experience" of mystics to "infantile helplessness" and a "regression to primary narcissism" (Freud 1989).

However most clinicians do not currently view mystical experiences as pathological (Allman et al. 1992). To some degree, this may reflect a change that is partly attributable to Abraham Maslow. His studies of peak experiences, which he considered religious experiences for many individuals, validated their importance and nonpathological nature. In addition, studies have found that people reporting mystical experiences scored lower on psychopathology scales and higher on measures of psychological well-being than control subjects (Wulff 2002).

The mystical experience is one type of spiritual problem that therapists regularly encounter in therapy. In a survey, psychologists reported that 4.5% of their clients over the past 12 months brought such an experience into therapy (Lannert 1991). Mystical experiences can be overwhelming for individuals who do not have a strong sense of ego. In addition, another risk observed following an ecstatic mystical experience is ego inflation, in which the individual develops highly grandiose beliefs or even delusions about their own spiritual stature and attainment (Rosenthal 1990). Individuals in the midst of intense mystical experiences have been hospitalized and medicated when less restrictive interventions could have been utilized (Chapman and Lukoff 1996; Lukoff and Everest 1985).

DSM-IV and DSM-IV-TR (American Psychiatric Association 2000) highlight the need for cultural sensitivity when clinicians assess for schizophrenia in socioeconomic or cultural situations different from their own: "Ideas that may appear to be delusional in one culture (e.g., sorcery and witchcraft) may be commonly held in another. In some cultures, visual or auditory hallucinations with a religious content may be a normal part of religious experience (e.g., seeing the Virgin Mary or hearing God's voice)" (American Psychiatric Association 2000, p. 306).

NEAR-DEATH EXPERIENCE

The near-death experience is a subjective event experienced by persons who come close to death or who confront a potentially fatal situation and escape uninjured. Since 1975, when Raymond Moody (1975) first focused public attention on near-death experiences in his book *Life After Life,* they have been the focus of considerable scientific research (Greyson 1993, 1997; Ring 1990). Near-death experiences typically follow a characteristic temporal sequence of stages, including

- Peace and contentment
- Detachment from physical body
- Entering a transitional region of darkness
- Seeing a brilliant light
- Passing through the light into another realm of existence
- Strong positive affect
- Dissociation from the physical body
- Transcendental or mystical elements

The person often feels unconditionally accepted and forgiven by a loving source. Life review is also common, and the person returns with a mission or "vision," believing that there is still more to be done in this life.

Modern medical technology has resulted in many persons having near-death experiences. They are reported by 35% of individuals who come close to death. Gallup Polls estimated that about 5% of the adult American population, approximately 13 million American adults, have had a near-death experience with at least some of the features described earlier, making it a clinically significant and pervasive phenomenon (Gallup 2002).

The non-pathological nature of the near-death experience is documented by the growing literature on its after effects—in particular, positive attitude and value changes, personality transformation, and spiritual development. Ring (1990) has conducted studies on these experiences and found these changes to occur within 5 years of the experience and to remain stable over time.

Despite generally positive outcomes, significant intrapsychic and interpersonal difficulties frequently arise in the wake of a near-death experience. Intrapsychic problems include

- Anger or depression related to losing the near-death state
- Difficulty reconciling the event with previous religious beliefs, values, or lifestyle
- The fear that the experience might indicate a mental disorder

Interpersonal problems associated with near-death experiences (Greyson 1997) include

- Difficulty reconciling attitudinal changes with the expectations of family, friends, and colleagues at work
- A sense of isolation from those who have not had a similar experience

- A fear of ridicule or rejection from others
- Difficulty communicating the meaning and impact of the experience

The many published scientific articles and first person accounts of near-death experiences have resulted in greater sensitivity to these experiences. They are recognized as fairly common occurrences in modern intensive care units (ICUs), as is the need to differentiate between near-death experiences and ICU psychoses (which do occur often as a side effect of medical treatments). With this increased awareness of near-death experiences, ICU staff are less likely to misdiagnose and inappropriately "treat" patients with these experiences with antipsychotic medication. According to Greyson (1997), "The inclusion of this new diagnostic category in the DSM-IV permits differentiation of [near-death experiences] and similar experiences from mental disorders and may lead to research into more effective treatment strategies" (p. 327).

Some near-death experiences become very distressing and meet the criteria for DSM-IV-TR adjustment disorder (Greyson and Bush 1992). However, the level of distress often warrants the diagnosis of a V Code rather than of a mental disorder.

PSYCHIC EXPERIENCES

Psychic experiences are extrasensory occurrences such as clairvoyance (visions of past, future, or remote events); telepathy (communication without apparent physical means); poltergeist phenomena (physical disturbances in a house with no apparent physical cause); precognition (visions or dreams that provide formerly unknown information); synchronistic events (meaningful coincidences of two apparently unrelated events); and after-death communications. Extrasensory perception has been the subject of scientific research for more than 100 years, continuing to the present (Krippner 1991; Ullman et al. 2003). Although the scientific status of psychic experiences has been the subject of much debate, there is no question that most people have such experiences. Gallup polls show that a majority of American adults have extrasensory experiences, and the percentage is increasing (from 58% in 1973 to 67% in 1986; Gallup 2002). Unfortunately, both sensationalism in tabloid media and commercialism (e.g., fee-based psychic hotlines) are associated with this topic.

A study of 212 adults and 91 high school students found that reports of psychic experiences were correlated with reports of transcendental spiritual experiences, and more than 90% of the respondents with transcendent experiences considered them valuable (Kennedy and Kanthamani 1995). Psychic experiences are considered to be genuine abilities by many, including the influential theorist of psychotherapy, Jerome Frank, who considered it a skill possessed by the best therapists (Frank and Frank 1991). Psychic experiences are associated with many spiritual practices and altered states of consciousness, but practitioners in most spiritual traditions are taught that these are distractions from the true path of spiritual development (Caplan 1999). Although claims of psychic abilities and experiences are not, in themselves, evidence of mental disorder (Targ and Hastings 1987), psychic experiences are also reported by people in psychotic and dissociative states. Thus, differential diagnosis is a key issue.

Confusion and the fear that "I'm going crazy" are common reactions to spontaneous psychic experiences (Tart 1995). Some people report feeling isolated from others because they are afraid to talk about these experiences with their friends and family. Most people who have psychic experiences are able to integrate them without any professional help, but some do seek assistance from a therapist in understanding such events and coping with their reactions to them (Targ et al. 2002). Hastings (1983) suggested that "[t]he focus of this counseling, given therapeutic purposes, rather than research purposes only, should be to assist the person to a experience of balance, integration, and judgment relating to apparent or genuine parapsychological experience" (p. 143). He described seven steps for working with someone who has had a disturbing psychic experience:

1. Ask the person to describe the experience or events.
2. Listen fully and carefully, without judging.
3. Reassure the person that the experience is not "crazy" or "insane" (if this is appropriate).
4. Identify or label the type of event.
5. Give information about what is known about this type of event.
6. Where possible, develop reality tests to discover if the event is genuine or if there are nonpsychic alternative explanations.
7. Address the psychological reactions that result from the experience.

ALIEN ABDUCTION EXPERIENCES

The chapter on alien abduction experiences in *Varieties of Anomalous Experience* included this definition: *alien abduction experiences* are characterized by "subjectively real memories of being taken secretly and/or against one's will by apparently non-human entities, usually to a location interpreted as an alien spacecraft (i.e., a UFO)" (Appelle et al. 2000, p. 254). In addition to reports from the United States, accounts from England, Mexico, Brazil, Chile, and Australia show the same content themes: capture, examination, communication with aliens, otherworldly journey, theophany (receipt of spiritual messages), and return to earth (Mack 1999).

Gallup polls reveal how widespread beliefs are in UFO-related phenomena. Fifty percent of a representative sample of the U.S. population taken in 1999 reported that they believe there is life on other planets, which is up from 34% in 1966 (Gallup and Jones 2000). UFO sightings are also reported by millions of people in the United States. When the Gallup Poll asked a representative national sample: "Have you, yourself, ever seen anything you thought was a UFO?" 12% answered "Yes." In 1997, a Time/CNN poll found that 22% of Americans believe that the earth has been visited by space aliens (Time/CNN 1997). There are now thousands of cases of alien encounters published, and researchers have studied more than 1,700 cases. Extrapolating from findings with a group of students, another researcher suggested that 15 million Americans may have had such experiences. However, after citing these statistics, Apelle et al. (2000) concluded, "Even if the numbers are much lower than some of these estimates, it is clear that many thousands of Americans believe they have been abducted by aliens" (p. 256).

Both positive and problematic effects have been reported by individuals with alien abduction experiences, including a range of physical and psychological after-effects such as injuries, eye problems, skin burns, gastrointestinal distress, and equilibrium and balance problems. Anxiety and recurring nightmares have also frequently been reported. Other symptoms and potential problems include irritability, intrusive thoughts about aliens and abduction, labile mood, disorientation, derealization, and depersonalization (Bullard 1989b).

Although psychopathology is present in some people who report alien abduction experiences (Lukoff 1988), assessment by both clinical examination and standardized tests has found that, as a group, abduction experiencers are not different from the general population in terms of prevalence of psychopathology. Many report that their lives have been radically altered on a deep spiritual level by their encounters with aliens. They have developed a heightened reverence for nature and human life and transformed their lives in ways similar to what happens after a near-death experience (Ring 1990; Spanos et al. 1993).

Some individuals who have had alien abduction experiences seek therapy to help them integrate their anomalous experiences. Hypnotizing patients to obtain a fuller account of the experience is controversial, and aggressive use of suggestive memory recovery procedures can increase distress and feelings of helplessness (Bullard 1989a).

> The risk of providing therapy can be minimized, and positive outcomes best assured, when the focus of treatment deals with educating clients about possible explanations for the [experience], encouraging them to understand [it] in terms of its meaning in their life, and otherwise working on coping strategies that transcend the inevitable inconclusiveness about the [experience's] objective reality. (Appelle et al. 2000, p. 271)

MEDITATION AND SPIRITUAL PRACTICE–RELATED EXPERIENCES

Beginning in the 1960s, interest in Asian spiritual practices such as yoga, meditation, qigong, and tai chi increased. Intensive meditation practices can involve meditating for 12 or more hours a day over a period of weeks or months. Asian traditions recognize a number of pitfalls associated with intensive meditation practice, such as altered perceptions that can be frightening, and "false enlightenment" associated with delightful or terrifying visions (Kornfield 1993). Teachers of these practices are aware of risks for problems associated with these practices (Caplan 1999): "Whereas spiritual masters have been warning their disciples for thousands of years about the dangers of playing with mystical states, the contemporary spiritual scene is like a candy store where any casual spiritual 'tourist' can sample the 'goodies' that promise a variety of mystical highs" (p. 17).

People can and do make use of books and audiovisual material to practice on their own without the supervision of a knowledgeable teacher. Anxiety, dissociation, depersonalization, agitation, and muscular tension have been reported in Western meditation practitioners (Walsh and Roche 1979). Transient psychotic-like episodes associated with qigong practice are well documented as a culture-bound syndrome that is similar to conditions associated with intensive practice of yoga and meditation (Shan 2000).

DSM-IV and DSM-IV-TR emphasize the need to distinguish between psychopathology and meditation-related experiences: "Voluntarily induced experiences of depersonalization or derealization form part of meditative and trance practices that are prevalent in many religions and cultures and should not be confused with Depersonalization Disorder" (p. 488). Stanislav and Christina Grof coined the term "spiritual emergency" and founded the Spiritual Emergency Network in 1980 to identify individuals experiencing psychological distress associated with spiritual practices and spontaneous spiritual experiences (Grof and Grof 1989). Treatment typically involves discontinuation of the spiritual practice, at least temporarily, and engaging in alternative "grounding" activities such as taking walks in nature, hot baths, and working in a garden (Kornfield 1993).

POSSESSION

In possession states, a person enters an altered state of conscious and feels taken over by a spirit, power, deity, or other person who assumes control over his or her mind and body. Generally, the person has no recall of these experiences in the waking state. The deliberate induction of possession states has been part of valued religious rituals in many cultures (Behrend and Luig 2000) and is probably the most popular form of union with the divine throughout human history. The deliberate induction of possession states is part of valued religious rituals in many ancient cultures, including ancient Egypt and Greece (where the Delphi oracle spoke through women possessed by spirits) and the earliest forms of Kabbalistic practice. Possession is a central feature of Haitian voodoo ceremonies in which specific deities are invited to "ride" the bodies of the worshipers during ceremonies. Possession also appears in early Christianity in a positive light, particularly in the form of "speaking in tongues." Many contemporary forms of evangelical Christianity consider it desirable to be possessed by the Holy Spirit, with physical manifestations that include shaking and speaking in tongues. Bizarre behavior such as choking, projectile vomiting, frantic motor behavior, wild spasms, and contortions along with grotesque vocalizations can be a frightening experience both for the person possessed and for others witnessing it.

The oldest theories about the etiology of mental disorders identify spirit possession as the causal agent, and many religions offer rituals and healings to protect participants from unwanted possession. One of the signs of Christ's divinity was his ability to cast out demons from people who were possessed.

Possession experiences can be pathological when there is impairment in social or occupational functioning or marked distress. Some people reporting possession feel their behavior is beyond their control. Possession and possession trance are listed under the diagnosis dissociative disorder not otherwise specified: "Possession trance involves replacement of the customary sense of personal identity by a new identity, attributed to the influence of a spirit, power, deity, or other person" (American Psychiatric Association 2000, p. 532).

Although possession is a common experience in many cultures (Prince 1992), in Western industrialized societies such experiences are not normative. A patient's report of possession experiences can lead to an inappropriate diagnosis of a dissociative or psychotic disorder, particularly among members of immigrant groups (Cardena et al. 1994). Treatment should include social integration of the experience within their community. If the individual is connected with a group whose practices include possession, then collaboration with leaders of that religious community should be part of the treatment plan.

Spiritual and Religious Problems Concurrent With Mental Disorders

Some people with psychotic and other mental disorders have religious and spiritual experiences and beliefs that can also become a focus of treatment. Addressing the religious and spiritual beliefs and experiences of a patient with a psychotic disorder can have therapeutic benefit. Particularly during the postpsychotic phase, therapists may help patients explore the spiritual contents of their hallucinations and delusions to find personal insights and archetypal patterns that have growth potential (Bradford 1985; Lukoff and Lu 2005; Silverstein 2007). Jerome Stack (1997), a Catholic chaplain for 25 years at Metropolitan State Hospital in Norwalk, California, observed that many people with mental disorders do have genuine religious experiences:

> Many patients over the years have spoken to me of their religious experiences and I have found their stories to be quite genuine, quite believable. Their experience of

the divine, the spiritual, is healthy and life-giving. Of course, discernment is important, but it is important not to presume that certain kinds of religious experience or behavior are simply "part of the illness." (p. 23)

The movement of consumers of mental health services has embraced spirituality as an essential component of recovery (Lukoff 2007a).

The *Handbook of Religion and Health* (Koenig et al. 2001) reviewed more than 1,600 studies and found that across mental and physical disorders, religion is overwhelmingly associated with positive outcomes such as ameliorating the distress and problems of severe illness, including serious mental disorders. Studies have shown that many people coping with persistent mental disorders utilize spiritual practices such as meditation and reading sacred literature (Fallot 1998, 2001; Sullivan 1993). In DSM-IV-TR, the diagnosis of religious or spiritual problem is listed in the section for "Conditions That May be a Focus of Clinical Attention," an Axis I diagnosis that can be assigned along with a coexisting Axis I disorder such as bipolar and psychotic disorder diagnoses.

There is evidence for a type of brief psychotic disorder that is related to a religious or spiritual problem. During a first psychotic episode, some individuals may be undergoing a visionary spiritual experience (Lukoff 2007b) in which components of their personality are undergoing rapid change: "There is every indication that this process emerges as the psyche's own way of dissolving old states of being and of creatively...forming visions of a renewed self and of a new design of life with revivified meanings in one's world" (Perry 1974, p. 38). Many of these patients have explicit religious themes in their psychotic process (Clarke 2001; Lukoff and Everest 1985).

Some residential settings, including Soteria (Mosher et al. 2004) and Diabysis (Perry 1998), based their treatment approaches on this perspective. They treated first-onset patients with minimal use of medication and a supportive psychosocial milieu to foster a natural recovery. A study of Soteria found that most of the patients recovered in 6–8 weeks without medication (Mosher et al. 2004). A recent meta-analysis of data from two carefully controlled studies of Soteria found better 2-year outcomes for the randomly assigned Soteria patients in the domains of psychopathology, work, and social functioning than for the patients with newly diagnosed schizophrenia spectrum psychoses who were treated in a psychiatric hospital. Only 58% of Soteria subjects received antipsychotic medications during the follow-up period, and only 19% were continuously maintained on antipsychotic medications (Bola and Mosher 2003).

Criteria for identifying such visionary spiritual experiences have been proposed (Agosin 1992; Grof and Grof 1989; Lukoff 1985, 2007b), and there is considerable overlap among the proposed criteria. The criteria that follow are based on outcome studies of recovery from psychotic episodes that have identified good prognostic signs and could be useful in identifying individuals who are in the midst of a tumultuous spiritual problem that has a possibility of a positive outcome without medication (Buckley 1981; Lukoff 2007b).

1. Cognitions and speech thematically related to religious or spiritual traditions or anomalous experiences
2. Good prognostic signs
   A. Good pre-episode functioning
   B. Acute onset of symptoms during a period of 3 months or less
   C. Stressful precipitants to the psychotic episode
   D. A positive exploratory attitude toward the experience
   E. No conceptual disorganization

Treatment of Religious and Spiritual Problems

Although each type and each individual case of religious or spiritual problem presents unique therapeutic challenges, there are some basic principles that apply to all cases. Rather than trying to determine whether the experiences actually occurred or are "real," the most important task is to provide patients with a positive context for their experiences. If they express fears of "going crazy" or are having anxiety about the experience, this would include sharing the diagnostic assessment and normalizing the experience for the patient by providing background information. Therapy should allow, even facilitate, full exploration of the experience and release of emotions. Interventions can include referral to a spirituality group (Kehoe 2007), support for a time-limited crisis, intensive psychotherapy, and the involvement of relatives and friends (Lukoff and Lu 2005). Collaboration with religious professionals and spiritual teachers should be considered, as well as referrals. In cases related to intensive religious and spiritual practices and experiences, therapy can make use of the following nine interventions:

- Normalize the experience
- Create a therapeutic container
- Help patient reduce environmental and interpersonal stimulation
- Have patient temporarily discontinue spiritual practices
- Use the therapy session to help ground the patient
- Suggest the patient eat a diet of "heavy" foods and avoid fasting
- Encourage the patient to become involved in simple, grounding, calming activities
- Encourage the patient to express his or her inner world through drawing, journal writing, movement, and so forth
- Evaluate for medication

Use of Religious or Spiritual Problem V Code

One study of 258 psychologists found that 44.7% were familiar with the criteria for the category of religious or spiritual problem, whereas 55.3% were not; 11.2% reported using the diagnosis within the past year; and 19.2% had used it at some time in the past (Scott et al. 2003). Another survey of 333 psychologists found that 6.2% had used religious or spiritual problem as part of a diagnosis: 4.5% of those in independent practice; 0% at university specialty clinics; and 75% in military settings (Hathaway et al. 2004). Hartter (1995) surveyed 100 psychologists (60 women and 40 men, 84% of whom were in private practice) as to their experiences with religious and spiritual problems in psychotherapy. She found that the psychologists studied tended to consider the DSM-IV category a necessary and valuable contribution to their diagnostic practices. Sixty-five percent indicated that they would use the V-code religious or spiritual problem more frequently but that third party reimbursement was a barrier.

Although these statistics are low, the researchers also found an increase in training from 1990, when almost no psychologists reported training in religious and spiritual issues (Shafranske and Maloney 1990), to 2003, when 34% reported such training. Medical schools and psychiatric residencies have also increased their level of training in religious and spiritual issues (Boston et al. 2006; Larson et al. 1996).

Conclusion

With interest in spiritual practices and reports of intense spiritual experiences increasing (Fuller 2001; Gallup and Jones 2000) and individual spirituality gaining prominence on the cultural landscape (Shafranske and Sperry 2005), it seems likely that the incidence of spiritual problems could be increasing. It is imperative that psychotherapists improve their clinical competence in diagnosing and treating clients with religious and spiritual problems (Pargament 2007). Training in diagnosis and treatment of religious and spiritual problems has not been found to be part of the curriculum in most clinical programs (Russell and Yarhouse 2006).

The introduction of the V code for religious or spiritual problem allows researchers to further understand the psychosocial correlates that may lead to development of more comprehensive and effective treatment. For instance, one recent survey of religious and spiritual concerns among 5,472 college students from 39 universities found that nearly one-third of the college students seeking help from university counseling centers report experiencing some distress from religious or spiritual problems (Johnson and Hayes 2003). Researchers found that students with spiritual or religious concerns were nearly twice as likely as those who did not have spiritual problems to be confused about their beliefs and values, 25% were more likely to have sexual concerns, and 29% were more likely to have problems related to relationships with peers. They also found that students who struggled with religion and spirituality were more likely to be homesick, suicidal, victims of sexual assault, or distressed over a break-up. Furthermore, some students experienced personal and social conflicts with roommates, friends, or classmates over religious and spiritual differences.

Religious and spiritual problems need to be subjected to more research to better understand their prevalence, clinical presentation, differential diagnosis, outcome, treatment, relationship to the life cycle, ethnic factors, and predisposing intrapsychic factors. Although defining discrete religious and spiritual problems clearly presents challenges, such as the frequent overlap in the categories (e.g., mystical experience with psychic experiences), the extensive and rigorous research on the phenomenology, prevalence, outcome, clinical sequelae, and treatment of near-death experiences serves as a model demonstrating that the obstacles are not insurmountable (Greyson and Harris 1987; Ring 1990).

RECOMMENDATION FOR DSM-V

The acceptance of religious or spiritual problem as a new diagnostic category in DSM-IV and DSM-IV-TR is a reflection of increasing sensitivity to cultural diversity and worldview (Josephson and Peteet 2004) in the healthcare professions that can be enhanced in DSM-V. The definition for the V code category of religious or spiritual problem should be updated to reflect current peer-reviewed research on religious and spiritual problems by including mention of the additional types of problems identified in the literature:

> V62.89: This category can be used when the focus of clinical attention is a religious or spiritual problem. Examples include distressing experiences that involve loss or questioning of faith; *changes in membership, practices, and beliefs (including conversion); New Religious Movements and cults; and life-threatening and terminal illness. Examples of spiritual problems include mystical experiences, near-death experiences, psychic experiences, alien abduction experiences, meditation and spiritual practice-related experiences, possession experiences, and* questioning of other spiritual values that may not necessarily be related to an organized church or religious institution.

References

Abu-Sahlieh S: To mutilate in the name of Jehovah or Allah: legitimization of male and female circumcision. Med Law 13:575–622, 1994

Agosin T: Psychosis, dreams and mysticism in the clinical domain, in The Fires of Desire. Edited by Halligan F, Shea J. New York, Crossroad, 1992

Allman LS, De La Roche O, Elkins DN, et al: Psychotherapists' attitudes towards clients reporting mystical experiences. Psychotherapy 29:564–569, 1992

American Psychiatric Association: Guidelines regarding possible conflict between psychiatrists' religious commitments and psychiatric practice. Am J Psychiatry 147:542, 1990

American Psychiatric Association: Diagnostic and Statistical Manual of Mental Disorders, 4th Edition. Washington, DC, American Psychiatric Association, 1994

American Psychiatric Association: Diagnostic and Statistical Manual of Mental Disorders, 4th Edition, Text Revision. Washington, DC, American Psychiatric Association, 2000

American Psychiatric Association Committee on Psychiatry and Religion: Cults and New Religious Movements. Washington, DC, American Psychiatric Association, 1989

Appelle S, Lynn S, Newman L: Alien abduction experiences, in Varieties of Anomalous Experience: Examining the Scientific Evidence. Edited by Cardena E, Lynn S, Krippner S. Washington, DC, American Psychological Association, 2000, pp 253–282

Barra D, Carlson E, Maize M: The dark night of the spirit: grief following a loss in religious identity, in Death and Spirituality. Edited by Doka K, Morgan J. Amityville, NY, Baywood, 1993

Behrend Ha, Luig U (eds): Spirit Possession, Modernity, and Power in Africa. Madison, WI, University of Wisconsin Press, 2000

Bola JR, Mosher LR: Treatment of acute psychosis without neuroleptics: two-year outcomes from the Soteria Project. J Nerv Ment Dis 191:219–229, 2003

Boston P, Puchalski CM, O'Donnell JF: Spirituality and medicine: curricula in medical education. J Cancer Educ 21:8–12, 2006

Bradford D: A therapy of religious imagery for paranoid schizophrenic psychosis, in Psychotherapy of the Religious Patient. Edited by Spero M. Springfield, IL, Thomas, 1985

Buckley P: Mystical experience and schizophrenia. Schizophr Bull 7:516–521, 1981

Bullard T: Hypnosis and UFO abductions: a troubled relationship. Journal of UFO Studies 1:3–42, 1989a

Bullard T: The influence of investigators on UFO abduction reports: results of a survey, in Alien Discussions: Proceedings of the Abduction Study Conference held at MIT. Edited by Pritchard A, Pritchard D, Mack J, et al. Cambridge, MA, North Cambridge Press, 1989b, pp 571–619

Caplan M: Halfway Up the Mountain: The Error of Premature Claims to Enlightenment. Prescott, AZ, Hohm Press, 1999

Cardena E, Lewis-Fernandez R, Bear D, et al: Dissociative disorders, in Sourcebook for DSM-IV. Edited by Frances A. Washington, DC, American Psychiatric Press, 1994

Cardena E, Lynn S, Krippner S (eds): Varieties of Anomalous Experience: Examining the Scientific Evidence. Washington, DC, American Psychological Association, 2000

Carpenito L: Nursing Diagnosis: Application to Clinical Practice. Philadelphia, PA, JB Lippincott, 1983

Chapman J, Lukoff D: The social safety net in recovery from psychosis: a therapist's story. Hosp Community Psychiatry 47:69–70, 1996

Clarke I: Cognitive behavior therapy for psychosis, in Psychosis and Spirituality: Exploring the New Frontier. Edited by Clarke I. London, Whurr, 2001, pp 15–26

Curtis J, Curtis M: Factors related to susceptibility and recruitment by cults. Psychol Rep 73:451–460, 1993

Doka K, Morgan J: Death and Spirituality (Death, Value and Meaning). Amityville, NY, Baywood Publishing Company, 1993

Fallot R: Spiritual and religious dimensions of mental illness recovery narratives, in Spirituality and Religion in Recovery From Mental Illness. Edited by Fallot R. Washington, DC, New Directions for Mental Health Services, 1998, pp 35–44

Fallot R: Spirituality and religion in psychiatric rehabilitation and recovery from mental illness. Int Rev Psychiatry 13:110–116, 2001

Fowler J: Stages of Faith: The Psychology of Human Development. New York, HarperCollins, 1995

Frank JD, Frank JB: Persuasion and Healing: A Comparative Study of Psychotherapy, 3rd Edition. Baltimore, MD, Johns Hopkins Press, 1991

Freud S: The Future of an Illusion. New York, WW Norton and Co, 1989

Fuller R: Spiritual, but not Religious: Understanding Unchurched America. New York, Oxford University Press, 2001

Galanter M: Unification Church ("Moonie") dropouts: psychological readjustment after leaving a charismatic religious group. Am J Psychiatry 140:984–989, 1983

Galanter M: Cults and zealous self-help movements: a psychiatric perspective. Am J Psychiatry 147:543–551, 1990

Galanter M: Cults: Faith, Healing, and Coercion. New York, Oxford University Press, 1999

Gallup G: The 2001 Gallup Poll: Public Opinion. Wilmington, DE, SR Books, 2002

Gallup G, Jones T: The Next American Spirituality: Finding God in the Twenty-First Century. Colorado Springs, CO, Chariot Victor Publishing, 2000

Greenberg D, Witztum E: Problems in the treatment of religious patients. Am J Psychother 65:554–565, 1991

Greyson B: Varieties of near-death experience. Psychiatry 56:390–399, 1993

Greyson B: The near-death experience as a focus of clinical attention. J Nerv Ment Dis 185:327–334, 1997

Greyson B, Bush N: Distressing near-death experiences. Psychiatry 55:95–110, 1992

Greyson B, Harris B: Clinical approaches to the near-death experience. Journal of Near-Death Studies 6:41–52, 1987

Grof S, Grof C (eds): Spiritual Emergency: When Personal Transformation Becomes a Crisis. Los Angeles, CA, Tarcher, 1989

Hartter DK: The identification of spiritual emergencies in the practice of clinical psychology by frequency and ability of therapist to recognize. Doctoral dissertation, The Union Institute, Cincinnati, OH, 1995

Hastings A: A counseling approach to parapsycholgical experience. Journal of Transpersonal Psychology 15:143–167, 1983

Hathaway W, Scott S, Garver S: Assessing religious/spiritual functioning: a neglected domain in clinical practice? Prof Psychol Res Pract 35:97–104, 2004

Hoge D: Religion in America: the demographics of belief and affiliation, in Religion and the Clinical Practice of Psychology. Edited by Shafranske E. Washington, DC, American Psychological Association, 1996, pp 21–42

Ikemoto K, Nakamura M: Forced deprogramming from a religion and mental health: a case report of PTSD. Int J Law Psychiatry 27:147–155, 2004

Ironson G, Kremer H, Ironson D: Spirituality, spiritual experiences, and spiritual transformations in the face of HIV, in Spiritual Transformation and Healing: Anthropological, Theological, Neuroscientific, and Clinical Perspectives. Edited by Koss-Chioino J, Hefner P. Lanham, MD, AltaMira Press, 2006

James W: The Varieties of Religious Experience (1902). New York, New American Library of World Literature, 1958

Johnson C, Hayes J: Troubled Spirits: Prevalence and predictors of religious and spiritual concerns among university students and counseling center clients. J Couns Psychol 50:409–419, 2003

The Joint Commission: 2007 Requirements Related to the Provision of Culturally and Linguistically Appropriate Health Care. Oakbrook Terrace, IL, The Joint Commission, 2007

Josephson A, Peteet J: Handbook of Spirituality and Worldview in Clinical Practice. Washington, DC, American Psychiatric Publishing, 2004

Kehoe N: Spirituality groups in serious mental illness. South Med J 100:647–648, 2007

Kennedy JE, Kanthamani H: Association between anomalous experiences and artistic creativity and spirituality. J Am Soc Psych Res 89:333–343, 1995

Koenig H, McCullough M, Larson D (eds): Handbook of Religion and Health. New York, Oxford University Press, 2001

Kornfield J: A Path with Heart: A Guide through the Perils and Promises of Spiritual Life. New York, Bantam Books, 1993

Krippner S: Advances in Parapsychological Research. Jefferson, NC, McFarland and Co, 1991

Lannert J: Resistance and countertransference issues with spiritual and religious clients. Journal of Humanistic Psychology 31:68–76, 1991

Larson D, Lu F, Swyers J: Model Curriculum for Psychiatry Residency Training Programs: Religion and Spirituality in Clinical Practice. Rockville, MD, National Institute for Healthcare Research, 1996

Lukoff D: The diagnosis of mystical experiences with psychotic features. Journal of Transpersonal Psychology 17:155–181, 1985

Lukoff D: Transpersonal therapy with a manic-depressive artist. Journal of Transpersonal Psychology 20:10–20, 1988

Lukoff D: Spirituality in the recovery from persistent mental disorders. South Med J 100:642–646, 2007a

Lukoff D: Visionary spiritual experiences. South Med J 100:635–641, 2007b

Lukoff D, Everest HC: The myths in mental illness. Journal of Transpersonal Psychology 17:123–153, 1985

Lukoff D, Lu F: Spiritual and Transpersonal Approaches to Psychotic Disorders in Spiritually Oriented Psychotherapy. Edited by Sperry L, Shafranske E. Washington, DC, American Psychological Association, 2005

Lukoff D, Lu F, Turner R: Toward a more culturally sensitive DSM-IV: psychoreligious and psychospiritual problems. J Nerv Ment Dis 180:673–682, 1992a

Lukoff D, Turner R, Lu F: Transpersonal psychology research review: psychoreligious dimensions of healing. Journal of Transpersonal Psychology 24:41–60, 1992b

Lukoff D, Turner R, Lu FG: Transpersonal psychology research review: psychospiritual dimensions of healing. Journal of Transpersonal Psychology 25:11–28, 1993

Lukoff D, Provenzano R, Lu F, et al: Religious and spiritual case reports on MEDLINE: a systematic analysis of records from 1980–1996. Altern Ther Health Med 5:64–70, 1999

Mack J: Passport to the Cosmos: Human Transformation and Alien Encounters. New York, Crown Publishers, 1999

Malony HN (ed): Handbook of Religious Conversion. Birmingham, AL, Religious Education Press, 1992

Millison M: Spirituality and the caregiver: developing an underutilized facet of care. Am J Hosp Care 5:37–44, 1988

Miovic M: Spirituality, OCD, and life-threatening illness. South Med J 100:649–650, 2007

Moody R: Life after Life. New York, Bantam, 1975

Mosher L, Hendrix V, Fort D: Soteria: Through Madness To Deliverance. Philadelphia, PA, Xlibris Corp, 2004

Neumann E: Mystical man, in The Mystic Vision. Edited by Campbell J. Princeton, NJ, Princeton University Press, 1964

Pargament K: Spiritually Integrated Psychotherapy: Understanding and Addressing the Sacred. New York, Guilford, 2007

Pargament K, Koenig HG, Tarakeshwar N, et al: Religious coping methods as predictors of psychological, physical and spiritual outcomes among medically ill elderly patients: a two-year longitudinal study. J Health Psychol 9:713–730, 2004

Penson RT, Yusuf RZ, Chabner BA, et al: Losing God. Oncologist 6:286–297, 2001

Perry J: The Far Side of Madness. Englewood Cliffs, NJ, Prentice Hall, 1974

Perry J: Trials of the Visionary Mind: Spiritual Emergency and the Renewal Process. Albany, NY, State University of New York Press, 1998

Post SG: Psychiatry and ethics: the problematics of respect for religious meanings. Cult Med Psychiatry 17:363–383, 1993

Prince RH: Religious experience and psychopathology: cross-cultural perspectives, in Religion and Mental Health. Edited by Schumacher JF. New York, Oxford University Press, 1992, pp 281–290

Puchalski C, Romer A: Taking a spiritual history allows clinicians to understand patients more fully. J Palliat Med 3:129–137, 2000

Richards PS, Bergin A: Towards religious and spiritual competency for mental health professionals, in Handbook of Psychotherapy and Religious Diversity. Edited by Richards PS, Bergin A. Washington, DC, American Psychological Association, 2000

Ring K: Life at Death: A Scientific Investigation of the Near-Death Experience. New York, Coward, McGann and Geoghegan, 1990

Rosenthal J: The meditative therapist. The Family Therapy Networker 14:38–43, 1990

Russell S, Yarhouse M: Training in religion/spirituality within APA-accredited psychology predoctoral internships. Prof Psychol Res Pract 37:430–436, 2006

Scharfstein B: Mystical Experience. New York, Bobbs-Merrill, 1973

Scott S, Garver S, Richards J, et al: Religious issues in diagnosis: the V-Code and beyond. Mental Health, Religion and Culture 6:161–173, 2003

Shafranske E: Beyond countertransference: on being struck by faith, doubt and emptiness. Presented at the annual meeting of the American Psychiatric Association, New Orleans, LA, May 1991

Shafranske E, Maloney H: Clinical psychologists' religious and spiritual orientations and their practice of psychotherapy. Psychotherapy 27:72–78, 1990

Shafranske E, Sperry L: Addressing the spiritual dimension in psychotherapy: introduction and overview, in Spiritually Oriented Psychotherapy. Edited by Sperry L, Shafranske E. Washington, DC, American Psychological Association, 2005, pp 11–29

Shan H: Culture-bound psychiatric disorders associated with Qigong practice in China. Hong Kong Journal of Psychiatry 10:12–14, 2000

Silverstein S: Integrating Jungian and self-psychological perspectives within cognitive-behavior therapy for a young man with a fixed religious delusion. Clinical Case Studies 6:263–276, 2007

Spanos N, Cross P, Dickson K, et al: Close encounters: an examination of UFO experiences. J Abnorm Psychol 102:624–632, 1993

Spero MH: Identity and individuality in the nouveau-religious patient: theoretical and clinical aspects. Psychiatry 50:55–71, 1987

Stack J: Organized religion is but one of the many paths toward spiritual growth. The Journal 8:23–26, 1997

Sullivan W: "It helps me to be a whole person": the role of spirituality among the mentally challenged. Psychosoc Rehabil J 16:125–134, 1993

Sulmasy D: Spiritual issues in the care of dying patients. JAMA 296:1385–1392, 2006

Targ E, Schlitz M, Irwin H: Psi-related experiences, in Varieties of Anomalous Experience: Examining the Scientific Evidence. Edited by Cardena E, Lynn S, Krippner S. Washington, DC, American Psychological Association, 2002, pp 219–252

Targ R, Hastings A: Psychological impact of psychic abilities. Psychological Perspectives 18:38–51, 1987

Tart C: Parapsychology and spirituality. ReVision 18:2–10, 1995

Taylor E: William James on Exceptional Mental States: The 1896 Lowell Lectures. New York, Scribner, 1983

Time/CNN: Poll: U.S. hiding knowledge of aliens. Available at: http://www.cnn.com/US/9706/15/ufo.poll/index.html. Accessed April 7, 2010.

Ullman M, Krippner S, Vaughan V: Dream Telepathy: Experiments in Nocturnal Extrasensory Perception. Charlottesville, VA, Hampton Roads Publishing, 2003

Vaughan F: The Inward Arc: Healing and Wholeness in Psychotherapy and Spirituality. Boston, MA, Shambala, 1986

Viney L: Life Stories: Personal Construct Therapy with the Elderly. Chichester, UK, Wiley, 1993

Waldfogel S, Wolpe P: Using awareness of religious factors to enhance interventions in consultation-liaison psychiatry. Hosp Community Psychiatry 44:473–477, 1993

Walker A (ed): Thesaurus of Psychological Terms, 2nd Edition. Washington, DC, American Psychological Association, 1991

Walsh R, Roche L: Precipitation of acute psychotic episodes by intensive meditation in individuals with a history of schizophrenia. Am J Psychiatry 136:1085–1086, 1979

Washburn M: Life's Three Stages: Infancy, Ego, and Transcendence. Michael Washburn interviewed by Paul Bernstein, 1998. Available at: http://pbernste.tripod.com/lifethre.pdf. Accessed February 28, 2008.

Wellwood J: On spiritual authority: genuine and counterfeit, in Spiritual Choices: The Problem of Recognizing Authentic Paths to Inner Transformation. Edited by Anthony D, Ecker B, Wilber K. New York, Paragon House, 1987, pp 283–304

Wright S: Leaving Cults: The Dynamics of Defection. Storrs, CT, Society for the Scientific Study of Religion, 1987

Wulff D: Mystical experience, in Varieties of Anomalous Experience: Examining the Scientific Evidence. Edited by Cardena E, Lynn S, Krippner S. Washington, DC, American Psychological Association, 2002, pp 397–440

Commentary 8A

COMMENTARY ON "DSM-IV RELIGIOUS AND SPIRITUAL PROBLEMS"

Bruce W. Scotton, M.D.

Drs. Lukoff and Lu and their group have done our profession a tremendous service in perceiving and making great strides to correct what was previously a gaping inconsistency in our diagnostic thinking and nomenclature. Until their groundbreaking effort in the period preceding the release of DSM-IV (American Psychiatric Association 1994), we were collectively left in the embarrassing position of having to label normative spiritual and religious experiences, which are readily accepted in many contemporary cultures and which are experienced by a significant percentage of members of all cultures, as being grossly pathological if not outright psychotic. Such an assessment amounted to a collective assertion on the part of our profession that certain cultures, because they validated these experiences as nonpathological, were at best wrong and badly confused and at worst riddled with psychotic thinking. This current chapter is a further development and refinement of that ongoing effort and a worthy one. It cannot be stressed too strongly that religious and spiritual experiences are not in and of themselves pathological. Indeed, if there is one significant oversight in this chapter, it is the omission of the clear statement that all the problems discussed become problems only when the spiritual or religious experiences of the subject are not well metabolized psychologically but instead become the cause of some conflict, either within the subject or with the surrounding world. The spiritual or religious experience is not a problem; a disequilibrium resulting from that experience may be one.

The definition of *spirituality* could be improved over that given in this chapter. It is defined, quoting Walker (1991), as "degree of involvement or state of awareness or devotion to a higher being or life philosophy. Not always related to conventional religious beliefs." Much of the difficulty in the dialogue between those identifying themselves as believers in science and those believing in spirituality or religion arises because the former group does not recognize and therefore can or will not engage in discourse about a higher power. The current definition immediately invokes that problem. A better definition would be as we suggested in our *Textbook of Transpersonal Psychiatry and Psychology* (Scotton et al. 1996): "Spiritual refers to the realm of the human spirit, that part of humanity that is not limited to bodily experience" (p. 4). That definition should be elaborated, stating that "Spirit is the classical term for what we now call consciousness, a sense of self-awareness capable of observing both itself and things outside." Thus, without needing to invoke a higher power, we can begin to discuss experiences of consciousness that extend beyond the individual self and beyond the body that usually contains that self. Such experiences, it turns out, are widespread across cultures and time, are not at all confined to the pathological, and are the fundamental substance of religion and spirituality. This definition of spirituality seen from the bottom up—man developing beyond the individual, as opposed to from the top down—man being elevated by some higher power, further fosters dialogue between the scientifically minded and the spiritually minded by taking a concept employed by the former group, evolution, and suggesting it applies to spirituality. The growth of spirituality is based on the ongoing evolution of human consciousness toward higher, beyond the self, functioning.

An area of interest in the chapter is the inclusion of alien abduction experiences in the list of potential causes of spiritual problems. At first glance it would appear that the authors had committed a category error, that such an experience would not be spiritual but an encounter with another biological form if real, and evidence of psychopathology and therefore lack of eligibility for inclusion as part of a nonpathological V code entry, if imagined. However, amending the definition of spirituality, as suggested here, clarifies the reason for the inclusion of alien encounters. If the pursuit of spirituality boils down to the attempt to foster the ongoing development of human beings, an encounter with a more developed species would be an encounter with a spiritually evolved entity. We can profitably view such reports, and the worldwide fascination with UFOs, as the widespread and often involuntary attempts of individuals to grapple with the slowly dawning awareness, due to increasingly disseminated scientific knowledge of other solar systems, that we are probably not alone in the universe and likely not the most advanced beings in the universe. Jung (1958/1970) suggested a similar interpretation 50 years ago.

References

American Psychiatric Association: Diagnostic and Statistical Manual of Mental Disorders, 4th Edition. Washington, DC, American Psychiatric Association, 1994

Jung C: Flying saucers: a modern myth of things seen in the skies (1958), in Collected Works, Vol 10. Princeton, NJ, Princeton University Press, 1970, pp 307–433

Scotton B, Chinen A, Battista J: Textbook of Transpersonal Psychiatry and Psychology. New York, Basic Books, 1996

Walker A (ed): Thesaurus of Psychological Terms, 2nd Edition. Washington, DC, American Psychological Association, 1991

Commentary 8B

COMMENTARY ON "DSM-IV RELIGIOUS AND SPIRITUAL PROBLEMS"

Edward P. Shafranske, Ph.D., ABPP

The inclusion of "religious or spiritual problem" as a V code in DSM-IV (American Psychiatric Association 1994) marked an important milestone in the contemporary recognition of the role religious and spiritual beliefs, practices, and affiliations play in mental health. Although the origins of psychiatric care are deeply rooted in early religious tradition, and modern therapeutic practices are embedded with elements common to spiritual forms of healing, such as catharsis (Jackson 1999), religion has to a great extent been a forgotten factor, excluded from medicine. A resurgence of interest, marked by an exponential increase in empirical research in recent decades (Miller and Kelley 2005; Oman and Thoresen 2005) as well as deepening appreciation of the influence of culture, now requires consideration of religion and spirituality as clinical variables. Understanding the religious or spiritual sources of psychological conflict or mental distress serves as an important locus within clinical practice and contributes to the larger examination of associations between spirituality (in its many forms), coping, impairment, and health.

The chapter authored by Drs. Lukoff and Lu (who contributed significantly to the development of the V code) and Yang provides an in-depth discussion of the existing categories of religious and spiritual problems and proposes additional areas to consider in clinical assessment. Drawn from a systematic review of the theoretical and empirical literature, enhanced with perspectives from anthropological, theological, and religious sources, the chapter presents a cogent and practical orientation to religious and spiritual factors through which accurate diagnosis with the use of the V code can be made. The discussion is nuanced and ecumenical, considering traditional forms of institutional religious expression as well as idiosyncratic and anomalous spiritual experiences.

The types of religious and spiritual problems included in DSM-IV and DSM-IV-TR (American Psychiatric Association 2000) are restricted to loss or questioning of faith and conversion to a new faith. The authors usefully expand the typology to encompass not only loss of faith, explicit questioning, and conversion but also the challenges faced within and between these categories of experiences. For example, problems may ensue when changes within a local faith community serve to alienate an individual or differences arise in the faith commitments of partners within a marriage or intimate relationship. Although fundamental beliefs or tenets of faith may not be questioned, strains may occur in the practice of faith and affiliation to the community, leading to impairment of the individual's use of spiritual resources. Intensification of faith, the authors point out, may also place the individual in conflict with family members, or heightened religious fervor may be misdiagnosed as psychiatric disorder. As discussed in the chapter, this may be particularly the case when a person "radically departs" from traditional religious involvement in their family of origin's faith and converts to a cult, a New Religious Movement, or a charismatic group. The sometimes ecstatic states of conversion and the altered states of consciousness frequently associated with mystical or intense religious experience need to be differentiated from mania and require sophisticated skill by the clinician to parse disorder from authentic spiritual experience, taking into consideration the normative and anomalous, as well as potentially dangerous, consequences or concomitant psychiatric illness that may be associated with such experience. Also, more commonly seen, problems may develop (and psychiatric symptoms may appear, such as anxiety) when the religious or spiritual mooring of global life meaning is shaken by trauma, injury, disability, loss, or other hardships (Exline and Rose 2005; Pargament 2007; Park 2005). Patients may seek out psychiatric care to manage symptoms, which are associated with such challenges to meaning. Efforts to conserve or transform religious or spiritual coping may take shape in the consulting room in which the psychotherapeutic task essentially involves finding or constructing spiritual or ontological solutions (Pargament 2007) rather than employing medically defined procedures. Interview guidelines and areas of exploration culled from the research literature furnish clinicians with tools to assist in diagnosis that are sensitive to religious and spiritual cultural forms (see, e.g., Puchalski 2006 and Shafranske 2005).

Religious and spiritual involvement appears to be especially valuable in stressful situations that push people to their limits (Pargament 2002). Problems with terminal and life-threatening illness, as pointed out, can influence the ways that people cope with serious illness. Psychiatric consultation in the medical or hospice setting, with the patient, family members, or loved ones, must take into consideration the resources that religious or spiritual coping offers, the threat that serious illness poses to well-established sources of meaning, and the potential negative effects of certain forms of religious beliefs and practices.

The authors sensitively address paranormal phenomena associated with spirituality, such as near-death experiences, psychic experiences, possession, and so on, and provide a context within which to understand the possible meanings of such unusual experiences. Their discussion suggests that such experiences may, in fact, not be significantly outside of normative human experience, as is often assumed. Clinicians must therefore be mindful when assessing the appearance or report of such transitory phenomena (e.g., depersonalization, altered states of consciousness) of the cultural identification of the patient and the effects of certain spiritual practices (such as meditation) in eliciting such experiences as well as the possible involvement of mental illness. Even in clinical situations in which psychiatric illness has been identified, religious and spiritual problems as well as posttraumatic growth may play a role in the progression of a patient's symptoms or his or her recovery. Although anecdotal reports provide potentially useful approaches to address religious and spiritual experience within the context of psychiatric disorder, further investigation is required to establish practice guidelines.

Clinical competence is built upon a foundation of science-informed knowledge, clinical training, and expert supervision. Advances in our ability to provide culturally sensitive assessment and treatment, which considers religious and spiritual problems and integrates, as appropriate, religious and spiritual resources (Pargament 2007; Sperry and Shafranske 2005) in treatment, including spiritual accommodative forms of psychotherapy (e.g., mindfulness-based cognitive behavioral therapy), require ongoing empirical study and systematic consideration in medical and graduate school curricula and training. Indeed, further basic research needs to be conducted to develop measures that more accurately study religion and spirituality as constructs and as clinical variables. The refinement of the V code, as proposed by Lukoff and colleagues, better captures the range of situations in which religious and spiritual problems occur and enhances the usefulness of the code. Although such formal recognition and inclusion of religion and spiritual problems in psychiatric nosology attests to increased sensitivity to this dimension of human experience, more is required to achieve a holistic appreciation of the multiple factors that influence mental health.

References

American Psychiatric Association: Diagnostic and Statistical Manual of Mental Disorders, 4th Edition. Washington, DC, American Psychiatric Association, 1994

American Psychiatric Association: Diagnostic and Statistical Manual of Mental Disorders, 4th Edition, Text Revision. Washington, DC, American Psychiatric Association, 2000

Exline JJ, Rose E: Religious and spiritual struggles, in The Handbook of the Psychology of Religion. Edited by Paloutzian R, Park C. New York, Guilford, 2005, pp 315–330

Jackson SW: Care of the Psyche: A History of Psychological Healing. New Haven, CT, Yale University Press, 1999

Miller L, Kelley BS: Relationships of religiosity and spirituality with mental health and psychopathology, in The Handbook of the Psychology of Religion. Edited by Paloutzian R, Park C. New York, Guilford, 2005, pp 460–478

Oman D, Thoresen CE: Do religion and spirituality influence health?, in The Handbook of the Psychology of Religion. Edited by Paloutzian R, Park C. New York, Guilford, 2005, pp 435–459

Pargament KI: The bitter and the sweet: an evaluation of the costs and benefits of religiousness. Psychol Inq 13:168–181, 2002

Pargament KI: Spiritually Integrated Psychotherapy: Understanding and Addressing the Sacred. New York, Guilford, 2007

Park CL: Religion and meaning, in The Handbook of the Psychology of Religion. Edited by Paloutzian R, Park CL. New York, Guilford, 2005, pp 295–314

Puchalski C: Spiritual assessment in clinical practice. Psychiatr Ann 36:150–155, 2006

Shafranske EP: Psychology of religion in clinical and counseling psychology, in The Handbook of the Psychology of Religion. Edited by Paloutzian R, Park C. New York, Guilford, 2005, pp 496–514

Sperry L, Shafranske EP (eds): Spiritually Oriented Psychotherapy. Washington, DC, American Psychological Association, 2005

9

RELIGIOUS AND SPIRITUAL ISSUES IN THE OUTLINE FOR CULTURAL FORMULATION

David M. Gellerman, M.D., Ph.D.
Francis G. Lu, M.D.

The inclusion of the Outline for Cultural Formulation and culturally relevant information was a progressive step in DSM-IV (American Psychiatric Association 1994) and DSM-IV-TR (American Psychiatric Association 2000). The DSM classification system is used in the diagnosis and management of diverse cultural populations, not just in the United States but internationally as well, and the Outline provides a standardized assessment tool that clinicians may utilize to describe cultural information relevant to the differential diagnosis and management of mental disorders:

> A clinician who is unfamiliar with the nuances of an individual's cultural frame of reference may incorrectly judge as psychopathology those normal variations in behavior, belief, or experience that are particular to the individual's culture....It is hoped that these new features will increase sensitivity to variations in how mental disorders may be expressed in different cultures and will reduce the possible effect of unintended bias stemming from the clinician's own cultural background. (American Psychiatric Association 2000, p. xxxiv)

Examples of increasing sensitivity to cultural variations in DSM-IV-TR are included in the "Specific Culture, Age, and Gender Features" sections of the narrative descriptions of 79 mental disorders. For example, in the narrative description of brief psychotic disorder, it is stated that hearing voices in a religious ceremony may not necessarily represent a symptom of psychosis (American Psychiatric Association 2000, p. 330). Similarly, voluntarily induced depersonalization or derealization as a part of trance or meditative practices that are prevalent in many religions and cultures should not be confused with depersonalization disorder (p. 531). In addition, utilizing the Outline may increase the awareness of heterogeneity within cultural and sub-ethnic groups (Lewis-Fernandez and Diaz 2002), such that even when there are no obvious cultural differences between a patient and clinician, the Outline may reveal hidden assumptions and biases by the clinician. As such, the American Psychiatric Association's *Practice Guidelines for the Psychiatric Evaluations of Adults,* 2nd Edition, incorporates the Outline for Cultural Formulation and specifically comments on potential cultural, religious, and spiritual factors that may be important to consider in psychiatric assessments (American Psychiatric Association 2006a).

The Outline for Cultural Formulation provides a concise clinical method to incorporate religious and spiritual information within the broad framework of culture. Although religion is mentioned explicitly only once in the Outline (in DSM-IV-TR in section C), religion and spirituality can be important for all five sections. For example, religion and spirituality could be the primary variable in one's culture identity and heritage (Lukoff et al. 1995). It is the purpose of this chapter to explore means in which information about religion and spirituality could be included in all sections of the Outline so that it can help the clinician with differential diagnosis and treatment planning. This discussion includes the concepts of spirituality as well as religion, and although we recognize the nuances between the transcendent relationships of the former and formalized experiences of the latter (Josephson and Wiesner 2004), the two terms are not further differentiated in the rest of the chapter.

The Outline for Cultural Formulation

As described in Appendix I of DSM-IV-TR, the Outline for Cultural Formulation contains five sections of information that are important in clinical care: 1) cultural identity of the individual, 2) cultural explanations of the individual's illness, 3) cultural factors related to the psychosocial environment and levels of functioning, 4) cultural elements of the relationship between the individual and the clinician, and 5) the overall cultural assessment as it relates to diagnosis and care (American Psychiatric Association 2000, pp. 897–898). Although defined briefly in DSM-IV-TR, these sections are expounded upon by Lewis-Fernandez and Diaz (2002), the Group for the Advancement of Psychiatry (2002), and Lim (2006).

CULTURAL IDENTITY OF THE INDIVIDUAL

The influences of various cultural groups upon the individual's sense of self as well as self-described affiliations are documented and described in this category. Although factors such as ethnicity, acculturation, and language are explicitly stated in the Outline, religion and spirituality can offer meaning and purpose in an individual's life, and religious or spiritual affiliation can be an essential part of one's individual identity.

Although predominantly a Christian country, the United States is also home to a diversity of religious faiths (Koenig 2002; Richards and Bergin 2005). Many Americans endorse a belief in a God, pray, and regularly attend a church, temple, or other religious institution. Religious and spiritual belief systems and faith communities can play an important part in transmitting culturally held values, social behavior, and meaning even in early stages of psychological development (Shafranske 1992). Such beliefs and values may be challenged when one's perceived identity is threatened or distorted at times of crisis or transition (Peteet 2004), contributing significantly to one's existential suffering. In the past two decades, the importance of religious faith and identity in patients with mental disorders has been increasingly recognized for how it impacts on cultural explanation of illness and cultural stressors and supports.

Neeleman and Lewis (1994) examined the religious and spiritual beliefs and attitudes of several groups of psychiatric patients compared with nonpsychiatric control subjects. Patients with psychiatric disorders identified themselves as religious and placed importance on religious faith significantly more than the nonpsychiatric control patients. Baetz et al. (2002) examined religious and spiritual commitment in 88 patients admitted to a psychiatric hospital, most having been diagnosed with a major depressive episode. They found that the frequency of worship attendance and intrinsic religiousness were significantly correlated with lower depressive symptoms at the time of admission. In addition, these variables were also negatively related to current and lifetime alcohol abuse. In a qualitative study of outpatients with psychotic illnesses, 85% endorsed that religion was important in their lives and was "most important" in almost half of the participants (Mohr et al. 2006). A majority of participants in the study endorsed that their religious faith was important in giving meaning to their lives as well as to their illness, attributing their ability to cope and gain some control in their lives to their faith.

It is important to remember that one's religious or spiritual identity may also be subject to change in response to significant events in one's life. For example, the experience of trauma in individuals with posttraumatic stress disorder (PTSD) was more likely to predict changes in spiritual or religious beliefs compared with those individuals without PTSD (Falsetti et al. 2003). Of the group meeting criteria for PTSD, 30% described becoming less religious after trauma, compared with only 6% of the non-PTSD group. Additionally, 20% of the PTSD group described an increase in their religious faith, compared with 9% of the non-PTSD group. Fontana and Rosenheck (2004) studied more than 1,000 combat veterans evaluated for PTSD regarding their views of religion as a "source of comfort" prior to service in the military compared with the time of the evaluation. Although 24% of the combat veterans reported that religion had become a greater source of comfort, 29% indicated the opposite. Thus, although religious or spiritual faith may be utilized as a source of coping with trauma, the experience of trauma, and development of PTSD, it can also affect the degree to which patients consider themselves religious or spiritual persons.

When including spiritual and religious factors in this section of the Outline for Cultural Formulation, the clinician may wish to consider the following information:

1. Does the patient identify him- or herself as a "religious" or "spiritual" person, and if so, how?
2. Was the patient raised with a particular religious faith?
3. Does the patient currently belong to a particular church, temple, mosque, or other faith community?
4. How has the patient's faith or spirituality evolved during the patient's childhood and adult development?
5. What brings meaning to the patient's life?

CULTURAL EXPLANATIONS OF THE INDIVIDUAL'S ILLNESS

The section of the Outline on cultural explanations asks the clinician to explore those cultural factors that contribute to the patient's and family's experience and understanding of illness. These factors are noted as idioms of distress and explanatory models, respectively. Such factors not only impact the relationship between the clinician and the individual and family, and hence the diagnosis and treatment, but also the relationships among the patient, the family, and the community at large. This section includes beliefs regarding causation of suffering: perceived severity and impairment as well as help-seeking choices, preferences, and expectations regarding treatment. The individual or family may describe or explain the illness experience from a religious or spiritual framework that the clinician should assess for the possible diagnosis of religious or spiritual problem (discussed further in the fifth section of the Outline, "Overall Cultural Assessment for Diagnosis and Care").

Although the concept of religious coping is discussed in the next section, Pargament et al. (2000) categorized various ways that patients utilize religious or spiritual beliefs to find meaning in times of suffering or illness. For example, "benevolent religious reappraisal" strategies interpret a stressor or illness as a potentially valuable spiritual experience, "punishing God reappraisal" strategies interpret stress and suffering as a punishment from God, and "demonic reappraisal" strategies attribute suffering to the Devil or an evil entity. Religious and spiritual beliefs do not have to be thought of as mutually exclusive of secular explanations of illness. For example, a patient diagnosed with hepatitis C and in need of interferon treatment may understand and accept that infection was likely a result of sharing intravenous needles, but at the same time he or she may understand and believe that the infection was a punishment from God. Therefore, such patients may also seek comfort and counseling from their religious or spiritual leaders in the community either in addition to, or even prior to, seeking help from healthcare professionals. Such patients might benefit from referral for further assessment from a pastoral counselor or chaplain associated with a healthcare organization as part of the treatment plan.

Within the United States, clergy have been described as *de facto* mental health counselors for some individuals, offering a significant amount of time providing pastoral counseling (Weaver 1998). For example, a study of 99 African American clergy in metropolitan New Haven, Connecticut, revealed that participants averaged more than 6 hours per week doing pastoral counseling; 22 pastors, or just more than 20%, spent more than 8 hours a week in counseling (Young et al. 2003). In this study, two-thirds of pastors endorsed counseling individuals who were suicidal or believed to be potentially dangerous to others. In addition to religious or spiritual problems, other problems indicated by pastors as being "very often" or "fairly often" encountered included grief, marital or family problems, and alcoholism and drug addiction.

Similarly, a study of Moslem imams in the United States found that 50% endorsed spending up to 5 hours a week in counseling, whereas 30% endorsed spending 6–10 hours a week (Ali et al. 2005). After spiritual and religious problems, relationship or marital problems and parent–child concerns were described as "often" or "very often" reasons individuals came for counseling. The investigators also inquired about changes in congregants' needs for counseling after September 11, 2001; participants in the study indicated an increased need for counseling for either feared or actual discrimination, financial concerns, and anxiety.

When including spiritual and religious factors in this section of the Outline for Cultural Formulation, clinicians may consider the following questions:

1. Does the patient or family present idioms of distress that use religious or spiritual language or terms?
2. Does the patient or family describe phenomena consistent with a culture-bound syndrome that may use religious or spiritual language or terms?
3. Does the patient or family attribute religious or spiritual etiologies to his or her distress—that is, do religious or spiritual beliefs play a role in the patient's or family's explanatory model? How does this affect the clinical management of the patient?

4. How do religious or spiritual explanatory models affect the patient's choices in help-seeking (including medical and psychiatric care) history, preferences, and expectations? (See the chapters on "Patients and Their Traditions" in Josephson and Peteet 2004.)
5. Has the patient sought aid from a spiritual or religious leader or chaplain? If not, what are the barriers perceived by the patient in seeking religious or spiritual help?
6. Is collaboration with the patient's religious or spiritual leader important and feasible in the patient's care?

CULTURAL FACTORS RELATED TO PSYCHOSOCIAL ENVIRONMENT AND LEVELS OF FUNCTIONING

The psychosocial environment includes both stressors as well as supports related to the patient's cultural identity. Religious beliefs and practices can be among several important factors providing emotional, instrumental, and informational support as explicitly stated in this section of the Outline for Cultural Formulation (American Psychiatric Association 2000). Spiritual beliefs and practices can also play a similar role. Such support may include religious or spiritual coping styles to manage psychosocial stressors.

An early study of religious coping strategies in medical illness used the three-item Religious Coping Index, which includes an open-ended item on coping and specifically asks the degree to which the patient uses religion or spirituality as a mean to cope (Koenig et al. 2001). When administered to hospitalized veterans and patients in an academic hospital, 20% of veterans and 42% of the patients in the academic hospital spontaneously reported that religious beliefs and practices were "most important" to enable coping. Seventy percent of veterans and 90% of the private hospital patients endorsed "moderate" use of religion to help cope in general, whereas 55% and 75%, respectively, indicated religion was used more than a "large extent" to cope with illness. In both self-rated and observer-rated depression scores in a veteran population, religious coping was inversely correlated with depressive symptoms. More interesting, the extent of the use of religion to cope predicted lower depressive scores 6 months later in a follow-up study of 201 readmitted patients.

The degree to which religious coping strategies are effective or harmful for individuals has been studied extensively by Pargament and his colleagues. In cross-sectional studies examining the relationship between different means of religious coping and psychological adjustment to a variety of health stressors and trauma, some specific types of coping were found to be relatively healthy, whereas others appeared to be generally harmful. Examples of helpful or positive coping strategies included perceptions of spiritual support and guidance, congregational support, and attributions of negative life events to the will of God or a loving God. Negative coping strategies related to poorer outcomes included spiritual discontent, either with the congregation or with God, and perceiving negative life events as God's punishment (Pargament and Brant 1998).

A comprehensive self-report tool, the RCOPE (Pargament et al. 2000), was developed to more thoroughly measure religious coping strategies and examine how they may relate to healthcare outcomes. The RCOPE, which incorporated a variety of subscales representing different proposed purposes of religion, was found to relate well with measures of physical, emotional, and spiritual health in samples of both relatively young, healthy college students and elderly hospitalized patients. Factor analysis revealed factors that were consistent with the conceptualization of the subscales exploring both positive as well as negative religious coping strategies. A longitudinal study utilizing the RCOPE and its short version, the Brief RCOPE, was used to explore religious coping and changes in medical, psychological, and spiritual health in a sample of medically ill hospitalized patients over a 2-year period. Negative religious coping strategies in the form of spiritual discontent and demonic reappraisal predicted greater mortality in hospitalized, medically ill elderly adults over a 2-year period, independent of variables related to demographics, physical and mental health, and church attendance (Pargament et al. 2001). In a related study, positive religious coping strategies were predictive of increases in stress-related growth, spiritual outcomes, and cognitive functioning at follow-up, whereas negative coping methods predicted declines in spiritual outcomes and quality of life as well as increased depressed mood and decreased independence in daily activities (Pargament et al. 2004). Interestingly, some of the negative religious coping methods were related to improvements in health measures as well as declines in other measures, suggesting that the relationships between spiritual coping and healthcare outcomes were more complicated than initially envisioned. Thus, although some forms of religious coping may be protective and healthy, some forms of religious coping may contribute to poor spiritual and health outcomes. Such "religious struggle" could contribute to increased physical and psychological stress as well as social isolation (Pargament et al. 2001).

In addition, religious and spiritual beliefs and practices may be a source of suffering and distress in themselves. For example, in a study of African-American women who had experienced an abusive relationship, many described being disappointed by the advice of clergy who recommended that they remain in the relationship or try harder to be a "good wife" (Potter 2007). Religious values can also be manipulated to encourage domestic violence and disrupt psychiatric care, as described by Stotland (2000) in her poignant case description.

Religious or spiritual stressors can also be included in this section. "Religious or spiritual problem" (see Chapter 8 by Lukoff and colleagues) can be the diagnostic category for distress due to intrapsychic, interpersonal, family, or community stressors related to religion and spirituality. For example, relevant religious or spiritual stressors could be related to personal identity conflicts; intergenerational family conflicts due to value clashes related to evolving differences in the cultural identities of family members; or religious conflict in communities such as seen in Iraq, Northern Ireland, or Bosnia. A clinician might want to list the stressors first and then the supports.

When evaluating spiritual and religious stressors and supports, including coping, for this section of the Outline for Cultural Formulation, clinicians may consider the following questions:

1. To what extent are there religious or spiritual stressors?
2. Does the patient consider his or her religious or spiritual faith and community as a source of strength or a source of stress?
3. What spiritual or religious coping strategies does the patient utilize?
4. Are these strategies contributing to the patient's healthy adjustment to illness or to further impairment and suffering?

CULTURAL ELEMENTS OF THE RELATIONSHIP BETWEEN THE INDIVIDUAL AND THE CLINICIAN

Cultural differences and similarities can have a significant influence on the relationship between the patient and the clinician, and this section encourages the clinician to consider these factors as part of the Outline for Cultural Formulation. In addition, the setting of the clinical encounter, such as an outpatient office or an intensive care unit hospital room, may also accentuate cultural differences and challenges. Even without obvious perceived differences in cultural backgrounds, including race/ethnicity, religious and spiritual differences between the patient and clinician may play an important role in psychiatric care, regardless of whether clinicians feel it is appropriate or are confident in their ability to address the spiritual and religious aspects of their patients. Awareness of the patient's religious or spiritual beliefs and practices allows the therapist to accommodate such beliefs in the overall case formulation of the patient, including the patient's struggle to find meaning, his or her means of relating to others, their impact on the transference relationship between the patient and therapist, and the clinician's capacity to make appropriate referrals when religious or spiritual questions extend beyond his or her expertise (Lomax et al. 2002).

Several studies have suggested that many patients desire their physicians to be accepting and attentive to their religious or spiritual beliefs. For example, one qualitative study using moderated focus groups of patients who experienced a life-threatening illness found that patients generally desired their physicians to inquire into coping and means of social support and wanted their physicians to be willing to participate in a spiritually oriented discussion when relevant (Hebert et al. 2001). A large survey of 456 patients revealed that two-thirds of the participants felt that physicians should be aware of their patients' religious and spiritual beliefs (MacLean et al. 2003). Patient preferences regarding three different spiritual interventions (asking about beliefs, silent prayer, and prayer with the patient) varied depending on the medical seriousness as well as the medical setting. Only one-third expressed a preference for physicians to inquire about their religious beliefs during a routine office visit, but in the context of dying, patient preference for physician inquiry increased to 70%. Likewise, only a minority endorsed a preference for prayer with their physician during a routine office visit, but up to half of the participants endorsed a desire to pray with their physician if they were dying. One Canadian study compared the attitudes, expectations, and practices of psychiatrists with those of patients regarding incorporation of spiritual inquiry in mental healthcare. More than 50% of patients indicated that their spiritual or religious issues should be addressed in psychiatric treatment, and 24% endorsed that spiritual or religious faith played an important part in their selection of a psychiatrist (Baetz et al. 2004).

Several studies have suggested a "religion gap" between the extent of religious beliefs among psychiatrists and psychologists and that of the general public; this "gap" could contribute to clinician–patient misunderstandings and missed therapeutic opportunities when spiritual or religious topics are approached. The American Psychiatric Association poll in 1975 revealed that less than half of psychiatrists endorsed a belief in God, compared with more than 90% of Americans (American Psychiatric Association 1975). In comparison, a more recent survey of psychiatric residents in five residency training programs in the mid-1990s reported that more than 75% of psychiatric residents endorsed a belief in God, and almost half endorsed that their religious beliefs affected their decision to enter medicine as a career (Waldfogel et al. 1998). Meanwhile, the Canadian study comparing psychiatrists' and patients' religious attitudes and practices noted that Canadian psychiatrists endorsed significantly lower rates of religiousness than Canadian patients or the general public, as measured by reports of religious attendance and private spiritual or religious activity (Baetz et al. 2004). The American Psychiatric Association's (2006b) resource document, "Religious/Spiritual Commitments and Psychiatric Practice," emphasizes that psychiatrists should inquire into and respect their patient's worldviews and religious/spiritual beliefs and includes several examples of clinical problems that may arise when psychiatrists are unaware of or violate treatment boundaries around religious and spiritual beliefs and practices. At the same time, clinicians should reflect on their own religious and spiritual development so they can effectively understand and empathize with the individual's beliefs and practices as well as not inadvertently adversely affect the relationship.

The following are examples of information for consideration in this section of the Outline for Cultural Formulation:

1. Is the religious or spiritual background of the clinician important to the patient in deciding whether to engage in mental health treatment?

2. How does the clinician's religious or spiritual belief influence his or her understanding of the patient's suffering in making a diagnosis and treatment recommendations?

3. Are there topics or issues that might not be fully addressed and explored due to either differences or similarities between the patient and the clinician's spiritual or religious beliefs?

4. How do the similarities and differences in cultural identity, including religion and spirituality, between clinician and patient affect rapport, communication (verbal and nonverbal), transference, and countertransference?

OVERALL CULTURAL ASSESSMENT FOR DIAGNOSIS AND CARE

The final component of the Outline for Cultural Formulation summarizes the information regarding the patient's cultural identity, explanatory models and help-seeking behavior, psychosocial stressors and supports including coping strategies, and impact upon the clinician–patient relationship with the goal of recognizing those cultural factors that contribute to the differential diagnosis and treatment planning and management. Lewis-Fernandez and Diaz (2002) asserted that regular utilization of the Outline not only teaches providers how to use this information for these clinical responsibilities but also exposes clinicians over time to a wealth of information regarding cultural perspectives and knowledge. The differential diagnosis includes assessing the degree to which religious and spiritual phenomena may be either normative for the person within that person's cultural reference group, a manifestation of a culture-bound syndrome, a religious or spiritual problem, a sign or symptom of a mental disorder, or a combination of these possibilities. This process can be aided by consulting with the patient's family, friends, and others, including indigenous healers, pastoral counselors, chaplains, or clergy. Under such circumstances, pastoral counselors, chaplains, or clergy may be considered "spiritual or religious brokers" similar to the "cultural brokers" described by Kirmayer et al. (2003). Although a religious or spiritual "match" between the clinician and patient may minimize misunderstandings regarding beliefs, practices, and experiences, such a match also potentially risks violating ethical and role boundaries, displacing religious authority, and incorrectly assuming shared values (Richards and Bergin 2005).

Although a knowledge base of various cultures, religions, and spiritual beliefs and practices is helpful to the clinician, comprehensive information is not always available to provide spiritually or religiously competent care. Rather, a knowledge of the differential diagnosis of religious and spiritual phenomenology as described here, an ability to listen for and be aware of religious and spiritual themes, and an ability to comfortably perform a cultural and spiritual assessment may allow clinicians to incorporate religious or spiritually relevant information into the overall clinical assessment and treatment plan of the patient (Blass 2007; Miller and Thoresen 1999).

Actively listening for religious, spiritual, or existential themes may reveal the use of metaphors and narratives by the patient to describe experiences and ideas that are otherwise difficult to articulate (Griffith and Griffith 2001).

By routinely obtaining religious and spiritual information as part of the Outline, the clinician can better understand the patient's personal coping and sociocultural resources as well as allow the patient to express and explore religious, spiritual, and existential issues that may contribute to his or her suffering. Considering the prominent role of religion and spirituality in the values, attitudes, and beliefs of different cultures and ethnicities, this information can easily be organized using the Outline for Cultural Formulation in DSM-IV-TR.

Recommendations for DSM-V

The Outline for Cultural Formulation should be revised to include religious and spiritual factors (in italics):

Cultural identity of the individual. Note the individual's ethnic or cultural reference groups, *including religious/spiritual affiliations, changes or development in religious or spiritual faiths, and the relative importance of religion/spirituality to the individual.* For immigrants and ethnic minorities, note separately the degree of involvement with both the culture of origin and the host culture (where applicable). Also note language abilities, use, and preference (including multilingualism).

Cultural explanations of the individual's illness. The following may be identified: the predominant idioms of distress through which symptoms or the need for social support are communicated (e.g., "nerves," possessing spirits, somatic complaints, inexplicable misfortune, *testing or punishment from God),* the meaning and perceived severity of the individual's symptoms in relation to norms of the cultural, *religious, and/or spiritual* reference group, any local illness category used by the individual's family and community to identify the condition[...], the perceived causes or explanatory models that the individual and the reference group use to explain the illness, and current preferences for and past experiences with professional and popular sources of care. *Note if a cultural, religious, or spiritual leader has been consulted regarding the symptoms, the degree to which this was found helpful, and the potential value of collaboration with such leaders.*

Cultural factors related to psychosocial environment and levels of functioning. Note culturally, *religiously, or spiritually* relevant interpretations of social stressors, available social supports, and levels of functioning and disability, *as well as the use of religious or spiritual coping strategies which may provide relief from or contribute to suffering.* This would include stresses in the local social environment and the role of religion and kin networks in providing emotional, instrumental, and informational support.

Cultural elements of the relationship between the individual and the clinician. Indicate differences in culture, *religion/spirituality,* and social status between the individual and the clinician and problems that these differences may cause in diagnosis and treatment (e.g., difficulty in communicating in the individual's first language, in eliciting symptoms or understanding their cultural significance, in negotiating an appropriate relationship or level of intimacy, in determining whether a behavior is normative or pathological).

Overall cultural assessment for diagnosis and care. The formulation concludes with a discussion of how cultural, *religious, and spiritual* considerations specifically influence comprehensive diagnosis and care.

References

Ali OM, Milstein G, Marzuk PM: The imam's role in meeting the counseling needs of Muslim communities in the United States. Psychiatr Serv 56:202–205, 2005

American Psychiatric Association: Psychiatrists' Viewpoints on Religion and Their Services to Religious Institutions and the Ministry. Task Force Report 10. Washington, DC, American Psychiatric Press, 1975

American Psychiatric Association: Diagnostic and Statistical Manual of Mental Disorders, 4th Edition. Washington, DC, American Psychiatric Association, 1994

American Psychiatric Association: Diagnostic and Statistical Manual of Mental Disorders, 4th Edition, Text Revision. Washington, DC, American Psychiatric Association, 2000

American Psychiatric Association: Practice Guidelines for the Psychiatric Evaluation of Adults, 2nd Edition, Text Revision. Washington, DC, American Psychiatric Association, 2006a. Available at: http://www.psychiatryonline.com/pracGuide/pracGuideChapToc_1.aspx. Accessed September 4, 2007.

American Psychiatric Association: Religious/Spiritual Commitments and Psychiatric Practice: Resource Document. Washington, DC, American Psychiatric Association, 2006b. Available at: http://www.psych.org/Departments/EDU/Library/APAOfficialDocumentsandRelated/ResourceDocuments/200604.aspx. Accessed September 4, 2007.

Baetz M, Larson DB, Marcoux G, et al: Canadian psychiatric inpatient religious commitment: an association with mental health. Can J Psychiatry 47:159–166, 2002

Baetz M, Griffin R, Bowen R, et al: Spirituality and psychiatry in Canada: psychiatric practice compared with patient expectations. Can J Psychiatry 49:265–271, 2004

Blass DM: A pragmatic approach to teaching psychiatric residents the assessment and treatment of religious patients. Acad Psychiatry 31:25–31, 2007

Falsetti SA, Resick PA, Davis JL: Changes in religious beliefs following trauma. J Trauma Stress 16:391–398, 2003

Fontana A, Rosenheck R: Trauma, change in strength of religious faith, and mental health service use among veterans treated for PTSD. J Nerv Ment Dis 192:579–584, 2004

Griffith J, Griffith M: Encountering the Sacred in Psychotherapy: How to Talk With People About Their Spiritual Lives. New York, Guilford, 2001

Group for the Advancement of Psychiatry: Cultural Assessment in Clinical Psychiatry. Washington, DC, American Psychiatric Publishing, 2002

Hebert RS, Jenckes MW, Ford DE, et al: Patient perspectives on spirituality and the patient–physician relationship. J Gen Intern Med 16:685–692, 2001

Josephson AM, Wiesner IS: Worldview in psychiatric assessment, in Handbook of Spirituality and Worldview in Clinical Practice. Edited by Josephson AM, Peteet JR. Washington, DC, American Psychiatric Publishing, 2004, pp 15–30

Josephson AM, Peteet JR (eds): Handbook of Spirituality and Worldview in Clinical Practice. Washington, DC, American Psychiatric Publishing, 2004

Kirmayer LJ, Groleau D, Guzder J, et al: Cultural consultation: a model of mental health service for multicultural societies. Can J Psychiatry 48:145–153, 2003

Koenig HG: Spirituality in Patient Care: Why, How, When and What. Philadelphia, PA, Templeton Foundation Press, 2002

Koenig HG, Larson DB, Larson SS: Religion and coping with serious medical illness. Ann Pharmacother 35:352–359, 2001

Lewis-Fernandez R, Diaz N: The Cultural Formulation: a method for assessing cultural factors affecting the clinical encounter. Psychiatr Q 73:271–295, 2002

Lim R (ed): The Clinical Manual of Cultural Psychiatry. Washington, DC, American Psychiatric Publishing, 2006

Lomax JW, Karff S, McKenny GP: Ethical considerations in the integration of religion and psychotherapy: three perspectives. Psychiatr Clin North Am 25:547–559, 2002

Lukoff S, Lu FG, Turner R: Cultural considerations in the assessment and treatment of religious and spiritual problems. Psychiatr Clin North Am 18:467–485, 1995

MacLean CD, Susi B, Phifer N, et al: Patient preference for physician discussion and practice of spirituality. J Gen Intern Med 18:38–43, 2003

Miller WR, Thoresen CE: Spirituality and health, in Integrating Spirituality into Treatment. Edited by Miller WR. Washington, DC, American Psychological Association, 1999

Mohr S, Brandt P-Y, Borras L, et al: Toward an integration of spirituality and religiousness into the psychosocial dimensions of schizophrenia. Am J Psychiatry 163:1952–1959, 2006

Neeleman J, Lewis G: Religious identity and comfort beliefs in three groups of psychiatric patients and a group of medical controls. Int J Soc Psychol 40:124–134, 1994

Pargament KI, Brant CR: Religion and coping, in Handbook of Religion and Mental Health. Edited by Koenig HG. San Diego, CA, Academic Press, 1998

Pargament KI, Koenig HG, Perez LM: The many methods of religious coping: development and initial validation of the RCOPE. J Clin Psychol 56:519–543, 2000

Pargament KI, Koenig HG, Tarakeswar N, et al: Religious struggle as a predictor of mortality among medically ill elderly patients: a two-year longitudinal study. Arch Intern Med 161:1881–1885, 2001

Pargament KI, Koenig HG, Tarakeswar N, et al: Religious coping methods as predictors of psychological, physical, and spiritual outcomes among medically ill elderly patients: a two-year longitudinal study. J Health Psychol 9:713–730, 2004

Peteet JR: Therapeutic implications of worldview, in Handbook of Spirituality and Worldview in Clinical Practice. Edited by Josephson AM, Peteet JR. Washington, DC, American Psychiatric Publishing, 2004, pp 47–59

Potter H: Battered black women's use of religious services and spirituality for assistance in leaving abusive relationships. Violence Against Women 13:262–284, 2007

Richards PS, Bergin AE: A Spiritual Strategy for Counseling and Psychotherapy, 2nd Edition. Washington, DC, American Psychological Association, 2005

Shafranske EP: Religion and mental health in early life, in Religion and Mental Health. Edited by Schumaker JF. New York, Oxford University Press, 1992

Stotland N: Tug-of-war: domestic abuse and the misuse of religion. Am J Psychiatry 157:696–702, 2000

Waldfogel S, Wolpe PR, Shmuely Y: Religious training and religiosity in psychiatry residency programs. Acad Psychiatry 22:29–35, 1998

Weaver AJ: Mental health professionals working with religious leaders, in Handbook of Religion and Mental Health. Edited by Koenig HG. San Diego, CA, Academic Press, 1998

Young JL, Griffith EEH, Williams DR: The integral role of pastoral counseling by African-American clergy in community mental health. Psychiatr Serv 54:688–692, 2003

Commentary 9A

COMMENTARY ON "RELIGIOUS AND SPIRITUAL ISSUES IN THE OUTLINE FOR CULTURAL FORMULATION"

From Spiritual Assessment to Spiritually Focused Cultural Formulation

Len Sperry, M.D., Ph.D.

Because religious and spiritual factors can significantly affect the course of treatment and its outcomes, it can be useful and efficacious for clinicians to develop cultural formulations that account for such relevant factors and then utilize these formulations to clarify diagnosis and inform treatment planning decisions. Unfortunately, there is relatively little written about how to assess cultural factors and develop cultural formulations. One of the few publications is the Group for the Advancement of Psychiatry Committee on Cultural Psychiatry's (2002) *Cultural Assessment in Clinical Psychiatry*. I recall receiving a request to provide feedback on the manuscript about 2 years before it was published. One of its stated purposes was to amplify the Outline for Cultural Formulation in Appendix I of DSM-IV-TR (American Psychiatric Association 2000) with six extended case examples. I responded that although the wonderfully thick descriptions of the cultural formulations made the Outline come alive, I had two reservations. First, there appeared to be considerable inconsistency in how the various formulations operationalized some of the categories, particularly "cultural explanations of illness" and "cultural elements in the relationship between the clinician and the individual." Second, I was concerned that most clinicians would probably not adopt this method because of the time involved in drafting such detailed formulations—15 or more long paragraphs for each case—for their patients. In short, it seemed that although the book had some theoretical value, it had limited clinical utility because of at least these two reservations.

On the other hand, the superb chapter "Religious and Spiritual Issues in the Outline for Cultural Formulation" by Gellerman and Lu (Chapter 9) offers a method that has considerable clinical utility. The authors make a compelling case and offer a novel method for using the Outline to develop spiritually focused cultural formulations. Following the categories of the Outline for Cultural Formulation, they provide a series of clinician-centered queries or questions to consider in developing a cultural formulation. A total of 19 such questions are provided for categories I–IV of the Outline. Because the questions so clearly articulate and operationalize the meaning of each of the categories, this method can foster a higher level of consistency in cultural formulations based on them than simply using the category descriptors.

It is noteworthy that the authors provide no questions for the fifth category: "overall cultural assessment for diagnosis and care" but rather offer some general observations on religion, spirituality, and culture. Nevertheless, it seems to me that a slight modification in the questions for categories I–IV of the Outline and a single instruction for category V could greatly increase the likelihood that clinicians would develop spiritually focused cultural formulations for at least those patients with religious/spiritual issues.

The modification includes rephrasing the author's questions to make them patient-centered spiritual assessment questions (i.e., questions asked directly of the patient). The instruction for category V is straightforward: write a formulation based on the responses to these 19 spiritual assessment questions. In other words, the clinician elicits specific patient information that will be directly incorporated into the written cultural formulation. Because case formulation involves both obtaining and then organizing information about a patient into a format that clarifies diagnosis and guides treatment (Page and Stritzke 2006), the clinical interview is essentially an iterative process of assessing not only the patient's symptoms and history but also cultural factors including illness experience and explanations and treatment expectations (Sperry 2006). Table 1 includes these spiritual assessment questions for categories I–IV and instructions for drafting the cultural formation in category V.

Concluding Note

Gellerman and Lu's chapter is an important contribution to the spirituality and psychiatry literature. The two suggestions offered simply extend their contribution.

TABLE 1. Developing a spiritually focused cultural formulation based on spiritual assessment

---

I. Cultural identity
  1. Would you consider yourself as a "religious" or "spiritual" person, and if so, how?
  2. Were you raised with a particular religious faith? Which one?
  3. Do you currently belong to a particular church, temple, or faith community?
  4. How has your faith or spirituality evolved during and since your childhood?
  5. How do religious/spiritual beliefs and practices affect your choices about medical and psychiatric care?

II. Cultural explanations of illness and help-seeking pathways
  6. Do you believe that there is a religious/spiritual cause to your distress? Will it affect treatment?
  7. Have you sought help from a spiritual/religious leader or chaplain? If not, what do you see as barriers in getting religious/spiritual help?
  8. Is having your religious/spiritual leader involved in your care important to you?

III. Cultural factors related to the psychosocial environment
  9. Do you consider your religious/spiritual faith and community a source of strength or a source of stress?
  10. To what extent are there religious/spiritual stressors?
  11. What spiritual/religious coping strategies do you utilize?
  12. Do these strategies contribute positively to your adjustment to illness or to further impairment and suffering?

IV. Cultural elements of the relationship between the individual and the clinician
  13. Is the religious/spiritual background of a clinician important in your decision about whether to enter and remain in mental health treatment?
  14. How might a clinician's religious/spiritual beliefs influence his or her understanding of your suffering in making a diagnosis and providing treatment?
  15. Are there topics or issues that you probably would not be comfortable discussing fully because of differences or similarities between your and a clinician's spiritual or religious beliefs?

V. Overall cultural assessment for diagnosis and care
  Based on the responses to the preceding questions draft a brief summary statement consisting of a sentence or phrase from the patient's responses to each of the questions. This summary statement represents the spiritually focused cultural formulation for your patient.

My hope is that the set of spiritual assessment questions and the accompanying instruction will encourage more clinicians to develop spiritually focused formulations. After all, drafting 15 sentences is much less daunting than drafting 15 or more paragraphs.

References

American Psychiatric Association: Diagnostic and Statistical Manual of Mental Disorders, 4th Edition, Text Revision. Washington, DC, American Psychiatric Association, 2000

Group for the Advancement of Psychiatry Committee on Cultural Psychiatry: Cultural Assessment in Clinical Psychiatry. Washington, DC, American Psychiatric Publishing, 2002

Page A, Stritzke W: Clinical Psychology for Trainees: Foundations of Science-Informed Practice. Cambridge, United Kingdom, Cambridge University Press, 2006

Sperry L: Psychological Treatment of Chronic Illness: The Biopsychosocial Therapy Approach. Washington, DC, American Psychological Association, 2006

Commentary 9B

COMMENTARY ON "RELIGIOUS AND SPIRITUAL ISSUES IN THE OUTLINE FOR CULTURAL FORMULATION"

C. Paul Yang, M.D., Ph.D.

In recent years, a growing literature suggests that religion and spirituality may have an important influence on an individual's health (Matthews et al. 1998). Drs. Gellerman and Lu's chapter is a timely contribution that expands on religious and spiritual components in the DSM-IV-TR Outline for Cultural Formulation (American Psychiatric Association 2000). The purpose of this commentary is to critique, highlight, and expand on some of the key issues that were raised in this chapter.

The first category concerns cultural identity. Gellerman and Lu maintain that religion and spiritual affiliation can be an essential part of an individual's identity given that culturally held values, social behaviors, and meaning frequently are transmitted through faith communities. *Spiritual identity* refers to a person's sense of identity and worth in relation to God and his or her place in the universe (Richards and Bergin 2005). It should be noted that religious and/or spiritual identities are subject to change in response to significant life events such as trauma. Many spiritual traditions hold that awakening to a greater identity is a manifestation of spiritual maturity through which an individual gradually relinquishes the private self to achieve a larger self that encompasses the greater community (Fulton and Siegel 2005; Yang 2006). Thus, it is essential to include change in religious and/or spiritual identity over time in the cultural formulation.

The second category pertains to cultural explanations of illness and help-seeking pathways. Many patients resort to religion and spirituality to find meaning in times of illness or suffering. Yalom (1980) distinguished cosmic/divine meaning from secular/personal meaning. Gellerman and Lu assert that religious and spiritual attributions are not necessarily mutually exclusive with secular explanations of illness. Indeed, a patient of mine was hospitalized after failing multiple suicide attempts. When questioned about the meaning of his repeated failure, he was quick to reply that it was an indication for him to utilize more lethal means to complete his suicide task. I asked him whether there was any deeper spiritual meaning behind this. He pondered momentarily and answered with enthusiasm that there was a divine purpose to keep him alive to serve others. Carefully discerning personal from divine meaning in assessing cultural explanations of illness may help to engage the sacred in the healing process.

The third category examines cultural factors related to the psychosocial environment. Based on research evidence and clinical examples, Gellerman and Lu caution that some forms of religious coping and practices may be protective and healthy whereas others may contribute to poor health outcomes and intensify suffering. Griffith and Griffith (2002) proposed that spiritual ways of being that enhance hope, agency, purpose, communion, gratitude, and joy may foster resilience against medical and psychiatric illnesses, whereas existential crises that lead to despair, helplessness, meaninglessness, isolation, resentment, and sorrow may activate or accelerate progression of illnesses. One question that I find useful in inviting a therapeutic conversation is: "What is your inner strength?" Interested readers are referred to Griffith and Griffith (2002, p. 273), Richards and Bergin (2005, p. 219), and Josephson and Wiesner (2004) for further information on spiritual assessment.

The fourth category explores cultural elements in the relationship between the clinician and the individual. Gellerman and Lu point out that differences in religious or spiritual backgrounds between the clinician and the patient may hinder therapeutic processes. For instance, a mismatch in background may contribute to misunderstandings of patient's religious beliefs, spiritual practices, and experiences. Furthermore, Wittine (1993) proposed that the clinician's spiritual worldview is central in shaping the nature, process, and outcome of therapy and that the clinician's ongoing spiritual development facilitates the process of healing and growth in therapy. Parallel to this observation, Richards and Bergin (2005) used the term "meta-empathy" to describe therapists' experiences in which feelings of inspiration and intuitive insights in therapy came from the divine source. Thus, the fourth category of the cultural formulation should consider not only the religious background but also the spiritual maturity of the therapist. It is advisable that clinicians adopt individual spiritual practices or undergo spiritually oriented psychotherapy to further their spiritual development.

The last category, "Overall Cultural Assessment for Diagnosis and Care," allows for a summation of the significant issues discovered in the foregoing cultural categories and modification to be made in the differential diagnosis, treatment planning, and patient management. To enhance cultural competence in religious and spiritual issues, Gellerman and Lu advocate routinely obtaining religious and spiritual information and recommend the Outline for Cultural Formulation as an important instrument to organize the wealth of clinical materials. The information it provides may help clinicians to better understand whether their clients' religiosity or spirituality in some way contributes to problems and disturbances and/or whether they have religious or spiritual resources that could be used in therapy to help promote coping, healing, and change.

The Joint Commission (2005) mandates the routine assessment of spiritual needs and that the spiritual component of a person's life be considered in healthcare. I applaud Gellerman and Lu's effort to help clinicians do so by expanding on religion and spiritual components in the cultural formulation and by making recommendations for DSM-V.

References

American Psychiatric Association: Outline for cultural formulation, in Diagnostic and Statistical Manual of Mental Disorders, 4th Edition, Text Revision. Washington, DC, American Psychiatric Association, 2000, pp 897–898

Fulton PR, Siegel RD: Buddhist and Western psychology: seeking common ground, in Mindfulness and Psychotherapy. Edited by Germer CK, Siegel RD, Fulton PR. New York, Guilford, 2005, pp 28–51

Griffith JL, Griffith ME: Encountering the Sacred in Psychotherapy. New York, Guilford, 2002

The Joint Commission: Comprehensive Accreditation Manual for Hospitals. Oakbrook Terrace, IL, The Joint Commission, 2005

Josephson AM, Wiesner IS: Worldview in psychiatric assessment, in Handbook of Spirituality and Worldview in Clinical Practice. Edited by Josephson AM, Peteet JR. Washington, DC, American Psychiatric Publishing, 2004, pp 15–30

Matthews DA, McCullough ME, Larson DB: Religious commitment and health status: a review of the research and implications for family practice. Arch Fam Med 7:118–124, 1998

Richards PS, Bergin AE: A Spiritual Strategy for Counseling and Psychotherapy, 2nd Edition. Washington, DC, American Psychological Association, 2005

Wittine B: Assumptions of transpersonal psychotherapy, in Paths Beyond Ego: the Transpersonal Vision. Edited by Walsh R, Vaughan F. Los Angeles, CA, Tarcher/Perigee Books, 1993, pp 165–171

Yalom I: Existential Psychotherapy. New York, Basic Books, 1980, pp 419–460

Yang CF: The Chinese conception of the self: towards a person-making perspective, in Indigenous and Cultural Psychology: Understanding People in Context. Edited by Kim U, Yang KS, Hwang KK. New York, Springer, 2006, pp 327–356

MAPPING THE LOGICAL GEOGRAPHY OF DELUSION AND SPIRITUAL EXPERIENCE

A Linguistic-Analytic Research Agenda Covering Problems, Methods, and Outputs

K.W.M. (Bill) Fulford, D.Phil., FRCP, FRCPsych
John Z. Sadler, M.D.

This chapter draws on a branch of analytic philosophy called *linguistic analysis* in order to set out an agenda for research on delusion and spiritual experience. Linguistic analysis, as we will see, suggests 1) a particular way of understanding the *problems* raised by the distinction between delusion and spiritual experience, 2) a particular range of *methods* for investigating these problems, and 3) a particular kind of *output*, namely, the "logical geography" of our title.

The long-standing difficulties in the relationship between psychiatry and religion cited by other contributors to this book come to a sharp focus in psychopathology. This is partly a matter of conflicting worldviews (Fulford 1996). Psychiatry, as a discipline within scientific medicine, is at best uneasy with the received authority and revealed truths of religion. Conversely, many of those within religious and spiritual traditions are at best uneasy with the causal (hence deterministic) models of human experience and behavior that underpin the sciences basic to psychiatry. These conflicting worldviews, in turn, carry different and sometimes contrary implications for treatment. One man's miracle is another man's medication, as it were, and the burden of deciding between them is carried, from the perspective of psychiatry at least, by psychopathology.

In this chapter we do not engage directly with the differences of worldview between psychiatry and religion, relevant as philosophy may be to exploring these differences. Rather, we show how linguistic analysis, as a particular method of conceptual clarification, might contribute to improved understanding of the differences between delusion and spiritual experience, thereby improving mutual understanding between the worldviews of psychiatry and religion and contributing to improved practice at the interface between them.

The plan of the chapter is as follows. First, we outline briefly the "tools" of linguistic analysis as developed in the middle decades of the twentieth century by J.L. Austin and a number of colleagues in what has come to be called the "Oxford school" of philosophy. In three further sections we then apply the tools of linguistic analysis in developing our research agenda as they inform, respectively, the problem, the methods, and the outputs of research into delusion and spiritual experience. Finally, returning to the tension between psychiatry and religion, we conclude with a note on where our research agenda, if carried through, leaves 21st-century medical psychiatry as a discipline that is not only firmly science based but also fully person centered.

What Is Linguistic Analysis, and What Is a Logical Geography?

Linguistic analysis is a method of conceptual clarification that starts from the observation that what we call "higher-level" concepts are easier to use than to define. This key distinction between the *use* and *definition* of concepts is well illustrated by a standard philosophical example of a higher-level concept, that of "time." "Time" is a higher-level concept in the sense that the meanings of many other lower-level concepts depend on the meaning of time: the lower-level concept "wristwatch," for example, can be defined straightforwardly as a "small instrument for measuring *time*"; and as an example of an even lower-level concept, a "watch strap" can be defined straightforwardly as the "part of a *watch* by which it is attached to the wearer's wrist." Yet notice this: whereas we can give definitions straightforwardly enough of the lower-level concepts of "watch" and "watch strap," we are immediately stumped if we try to define the higher-level concept of "time," despite the fact that we have just *used* the concept of time effortlessly and without any difficulty in defining the lower-level concepts.

The early Neo-Platonist philosopher and Bishop of Hippo, St. Augustine, was the first to notice this odd disjunction between definition and use. He put it like this in his *Confessions* (Book 11, Chapter 14, No 17): "What then is time? Provided that no one asks me, I know. If I want to explain it to an enquirer, I do not know"

(Chadwick 1992). "Time," then, is a concept that we use regularly without any difficulty and yet are unable to define. Much the same is true of any higher-level concept; space, object, event, and so forth are all concepts that, in more or less any everyday context, we are able to *use* effortlessly and without any conflict or difficulty, not *because* we can define them but *despite* our persistent *inability* to define them (see section "Conclusions" for an exception).

The kind of *problem* with which linguistic analysis is concerned, then, is clarification of the meanings of higher-level concepts, concepts that are easier to use than to define. It is the facility with which we use higher-level concepts, versus defining them, that is the rationale also for the *method* of linguistic analysis, a method that Austin (1956–1957/1968) called "philosophical field work." As its name implies, philosophical fieldwork is a kind of empirical approach to conceptual clarification. Normally when we fail to understand the meaning of a word, we might look it up in a dictionary or ask someone to define it. The traditional philosophical approach to conceptual clarification, by reflecting carefully on the meaning of a concept like time, is an extension of this approach. Philosophical fieldwork, by contrast, involves actively going out and looking carefully at how concepts are actually used in a given area of discourse. What we get from this, the characteristic *output* of linguistic analysis, is not further or better definitions but a more complete understanding of the meanings of the concepts in that area of discourse. This is what a "logical geography" is: a more complete (although not necessarily fully complete) picture of the meanings of higher-level concepts that is revealed not by attempting to define them but by looking carefully at how the concepts in question are actually used.

We owe the metaphor of a "logical geography" to one of Austin's (near) contemporaries in Oxford, Gilbert Ryle (1980). We can see what Ryle had in mind by extending his metaphor a little. Imagine you are in a darkened room, the walls of which are hung with detailed maps covering a wide geographical area with many different, although connected, terrains. We should not push Ryle's metaphor *too* far, of course. His "map" has no routes on it, for example. It is perhaps better understood as a complex picture or mural. Yet the map, or mural, represents the complex and interconnected meanings of the higher-level concepts in a given area of discourse. Now, attempting to *define* the meanings of these concepts by reflecting on their definitions is like shining a small flashlight at just one tiny part of the picture and imagining that you are seeing the whole thing. This is because, as Austin, Ryle, and others of the "Oxford school" argued, our powers of direct introspection on the definitions of higher-level concepts, whether in everyday or philosophical contexts, are considerably limited (Austin 1956–1957/1968). When we try to define higher-level concepts, therefore, the result is that we end up with only a partial and often distorted view of their meanings. Linguistic analysis, by contrast, as the "philosophical field work" of looking at how these concepts are actually used, is like many people shining many flashlights onto the map. This is why the characteristic output of linguistic analysis is a more complete (although again not necessarily *fully* complete) view of the meanings of the concepts making up the "logical geography" of the area as a whole.

We now have all the key "tools" of linguistic analysis that we need to develop our agenda for research on delusion and spiritual experience. As summarized in Table 10–1, linguistic analysis suggests 1) that the *problems* in this area could perhaps be problems arising from the meanings of higher-level psychopathological concepts; 2) that, if so, philosophical fieldwork could well be the basis of fruitful *methods* for examining these problems; and hence, 3) that the *outputs* from such research will not be new and better definitions but rather a more complete view of the meanings of the relevant higher-level psychopathological concepts making up the logical geography of the interface between delusion and spiritual experience. In the next three sections we explore each of these three parts of our agenda— problems, methods, and outputs—in more detail.

Problems: Higher-Level Concepts

First, then, we consider the kind of problem that is presented by the distinction between delusion and spiritual experience. We review in particular the indications that this could well be a problem involving the meanings not just of psychopathological concepts but of what in linguistic-analytic terminology we have called *higher-level* psychopathological concepts. Our conclusion is that there are in fact rather clear indications that distinguishing between delusion and spiritual experience does indeed involve, at least to an important extent and in key respects, higher-level psychopathological concepts; this conclusion, as we show, has a number of implications for the infrastructure needed for successful linguistic-analytic research in this area. First, however, in order to reach this conclusion, we need to start by considering the difficulties presented by psychopathological concepts in general.

That psychiatric diagnostic classifications, together with their underpinning psychopathologies, are replete with conceptual difficulties is evident from the history of Western psychiatry in the 20th century. Thus, the century opened with the philosopher-psychiatrist Karl Jaspers' attempts to reconcile causal with meaningful accounts of psychosis (Jaspers 1913b/1974) and to establish the phenomenological method (Jaspers 1913c/1968) as the twin conceptual pillars of his foundational *General Psychopathology* (Jaspers 1913a/1963). Midcentury developments included the seminal contributions of Carl Hempel (an American philosopher of science), Sir Aubrey Lewis, Norman Sartorius, Robert Spitzer, John Wing, and others to the crucial shift in the conceptual foundations of psychiatric classifications, from etiology-based to our modern symptom-based categories (Fulford et al. 2006), with corresponding major improvements in the reliability of psychiatric-diagnostic concepts. (We return to this crucial shift in more detail later.) From the 1960s

TABLE 10–1. The tools of linguistic analysis

	Linguistic-analytic formulation
Research problems	Clarification of the meanings of the relevant *higher-level concepts*
Research methods	*Philosophical fieldwork,* i.e., focusing on the *use* of concepts rather than attempting to *define* them
Research outputs	*A more complete view* of the meanings of the relevant higher-level concepts, i.e., what Gilbert Ryle called a "logical geography"

onward there have been wide ranging debates, both within and between mental health disciplines and involving both service users and caregivers as well as professionals, about the very concept of mental disorder (Blashfield 1984; Fulford 2003; Sadler 2005). The launch of DSM-IV (American Psychiatric Association 1994) was paralleled by a seminal publication exploring the conceptual issues raised by psychiatric diagnostic classification and psychopathology, and with a foreword by the Chair of the DSM-IV Task Force, Allen Frances (Sadler et al. 1994). Most recently, in the case of the DSM, we have seen the publication of the American Psychiatric Association's *Research Agenda for DSM-V* (Kupfer et al. 2002), the first chapter of which is entirely taken up with conceptual issues. True, the chapter is titled "Issues of Basic Nomenclature," but the issues actually discussed—the meaning of mental disorder, the relationship between reliability and validity, the criteria for category change, and so forth—are all *conceptual* issues nonetheless.

That the conceptual problems raised by psychiatric diagnostic classification and psychopathology (and these problems particularly as they relate to the distinction between delusion and spiritual experience) are or involve problems specifically with higher-level psychopathological concepts is perhaps not so immediately self-evident. After all, the progress made in the middle years of the 20th century, and associated improvements in the reliability of our classifications, were essentially the result of careful *definition* of diagnostic concepts as the basis of empirical research: John Wing's Present State Examination (Wing et al. 1974) and Robert Spitzer's Research Diagnostic Criteria (Spitzer et al. 1978) are exemplary in this respect. Look more carefully at these midcentury advances, however, and it is clear that the success of this approach, through careful definition, is entirely with *lower*-level rather than higher-level psychopathological concepts. There are direct parallels here with the concept of "time," our earlier example. The lower-level concepts of "watch strap" and "watch" are straightforwardly definable even though the higher-level concept of "time," on which the lower-level definitions depend, is not. Correspondingly then, in psychopathology and psychiatric diagnostic classification, a lower-level concept such as "delusion of guilt" is readily definable even though the (progressively) higher-level concepts of "delusion," "psychosis," and "mental disorder" (on which the lower-level concept of "delusion of guilt" depends) are not.

Understanding midcentury advances in psychopathology and psychiatric-diagnostic classification as advances primarily in understanding *lower*-level psychopathological concepts—and hence as advances *appropriately* based on careful definitions of the concepts in question—has two important consequences for research in this area. First, it endorses and consolidates these advances. Failure to differentiate between lower- and higher-level psychopathological concepts has contributed to a growing loss of confidence in the whole project of psychiatric diagnostic classification, because the meanings of higher-level concepts—delusion, psychosis, mental disorder—remain as contested as ever. As just noted, the closing decades of the 20th century witnessed a rising chorus of disillusionment with psychiatric diagnostic classification both from researchers in the neurosciences (Andreasen 2007; Hyman 2002; Hyman and Fenton 2003) and from patients and caregivers who actually use services (Kutchins and Kirk 1997). The danger with this widespread disillusionment is that we will end up throwing out the baby (advances in understanding lower-level concepts through the appropriate use of careful definition) with the bathwater (the failure of careful definition when applied inappropriately to higher-level concepts). This danger is indeed made explicit by the authors of the *Research Agenda for DSM-V.* Echoing the wider chorus of disillusionment with DSM and ICD, they pointed out in their introduction that despite improvements in reliability, "not one laboratory marker (of a DSM-defined mental disorder) has been found" and hence that "we need to explore the possibility of fundamental changes in the neo-kraepelinian diagnostic paradigm" (Kupfer et al. 2002, p. xviii).

The first consequence, then, of understanding mid-20th-century advances in psychiatric diagnostic classification as advances in understanding lower-level concepts is to allow us to build on, rather than risk throwing away, the hard-won advances in reliability made during this period. It is small wonder, and certainly no grounds for disillusionment and loss of confidence, that a given method of conceptual clarification (careful definition) fails to work when it is transferred from an appropriate application (lower-level concepts) to an application for which it is inappropriate (higher-level concepts). There is a difference here, of course, with our earlier example of "time" in that the concepts of "delusion," "psychosis," and "mental disorder," unlike the concept of "time," are *not* used, as we put it, effortlessly and without any difficulty in most everyday contexts. The concept of "bodily disorder," by being relatively unproblematic in use, is perhaps closer to the concept of "time" in this respect than the concept of "mental disorder." We return to the significance of the difficulties in the use of "mental disorder," and hence to the need for philosophical research in psychiatry, in our conclusions. For the moment, however, the point is that our continuing failure to define the *higher*-level psychopathological concepts of "delusion," "psychosis," and "mental disorder" provides, on the model of linguistic analysis, positive grounds for building on, rather than negative grounds for abandoning, the advances in reliability made in the middle decades of the 20th century with *lower*-level psychopathological concepts.

The second consequence of understanding mid-20th-century advances in psychiatric diagnostic classification in this way is the counterpart of the first: if definition is an inappropriate method of conceptual clarification for higher-level psychopathological concepts, then we need to find other methods. We return in the next section to a number of specific research methods for research on delusion and spiritual experience suggested by the linguistic-analytic approach of philosophical fieldwork. For these methods to be successfully applied, however, a number of essential research infrastructure supports need to be in place. As summarized in the first part of Table 10–2, these infrastructure supports form the first part of our research agenda. Such infrastructure requirements are often neglected in discussions of the role of philosophical research in psychiatry. We believe, to the contrary, that they are of fundamental importance and we briefly consider each of them in turn.

INSTITUTIONAL REPRESENTATION

Despite the key contributions of philosophers, such as Jaspers and Hempel, to the development of modern psychiatric diagnostic classifications, as things currently stand neither the American Psychiatric Association nor the World Health Organization work groups, reviewing the DSM and ICD classifications, respectively, include either a conceptual workgroup as such or philosophical expertise within specific subject areas. Similar arrangements, with workgroups being made up almost entirely of those with expertise mainly in the *empirical* aspects of psychiatric classification, supported the development of earlier editions of both classifications.

Philosophers themselves have been in part to blame for this. To the extent that they have been concerned with problems in areas of "deep" metaphysics—such as freedom of the will, the mind-brain problem, and the nature of consciousness—their work is indeed relevant in principle to the problems of psychiatric diagnostic classification. Work in such areas, moreover, as the American psychiatrist and neuroscientist Nancy Andreasen (2001) argued, has become more, not less, relevant with recent advances in the sciences underpinning psychiatry. Yet work in these areas, nonetheless, has seemed too far from any determinate output to be helpful in practice. Linguistic analysis, by contrast, as a method of conceptual clarification, connects directly with the problems of psychiatric diagnostic classification as identified not by philosophers but by those with direct responsibility for revising the classifications themselves. The problems set out in Chapter 1 of the American Psy-

TABLE 10–2. A linguistic-analytic agenda for research on delusion and spiritual experience

	Linguistic-analytic formulation	Research agenda
Research problems	Clarification of the meanings of the relevant higher-level concepts	Infrastructure for conceptual research • Institutional representation, e.g., on revision workgroups • Dedicated funding • Education and training • Owning (up to) the issues (i.e., acknowledging the conceptual nature of the problems)
Research methods	Built around philosophical fieldwork, i.e., focusing on the use of concepts rather than attempting to define them and employing combined empirical + conceptual methods	Areas for philosophical fieldwork • Clinical cases • DSM text • Psychopathology "tools," e.g., Present State Examination Target clinical concepts • Mental disorder • Criterion B • Clinical significance • Clinical judgment Partner methods • Philosophical (e.g., phenomenology, hermeneutics, existentialism) • Empirical (e.g., from social sciences)

TABLE 10–2.   A linguistic-analytic agenda for research on delusion and spiritual experience *(continued)*

	Linguistic-analytic formulation	Research agenda
Research outputs	A more complete view of the meanings of the relevant higher-level psychopathological concepts, i.e., what Gilbert Ryle called a "logical geography"	Theory • Refocusing the problem on the use of relevant concepts (e.g., of "clinical significance" and "clinical judgment" in Criterion B), versus the definition of symptoms (e.g., in Criterion A) Practice • Service user empowerment • Clarification of key variables in research • Improvements in the process of diagnosis (vs. revision of individual criteria) in particular through an enhanced role for 1) clinical judgment and 2) value judgments

chiatric Association's *Research Agenda for DSM-V,* as we noted earlier, are *conceptual* problems, and *higher-level* conceptual problems at that (i.e., problems of precisely the kind for which linguistic-analytic methods are appropriate). Linguistic-analytic research, however, as Austin anticipated (Warnock 1973), depends critically on *teamwork* and hence on philosophers being full members of the workgroups in question. This is one of the many respects in which linguistic-analytic philosophical fieldwork is closer to the model of empirical research than many other areas of philosophy.

The problem of distinguishing between delusion and spiritual experience provides a particularly sharp illustration of the importance of Austin's model of teamwork in philosophical research. This is because effective fieldwork on the higher-level concepts involved in such distinctions as that between delusion and spiritual experience depends on bringing together a range of different perspectives reflecting different aspects of the concepts in question. Recall our (extended) version of Ryle's metaphor of a logical geography: in order to get a more complete picture of the map on the walls of our (imaginary) darkened room, we needed lots of different flashlights, each picking out different parts of the logical geography. In the case of delusion and spiritual experience, then, an effective workgroup must include the perspectives of at least four key constituencies: those with expertise (clinical and scientific) on delusion, those with expertise in religious experience, those with expertise in linguistic analysis, and crucially, service users (including patients themselves) and others with direct personal experience of the phenomena in question (Sadler and Fulford 2004).

We return in the next section to the importance of teamwork—and of an appropriate team membership—to the methods for linguistic-analytic research on delusion and spiritual experience. Yet as a contribution to the necessary infrastructure for such research, the failure to include philosophical, service user, and other perspectives in the workgroups concerned with revising psychiatric diagnostic classification limits the extent to which 1) appropriate areas for research are identified; 2) relevant literature is included in background reviews; 3) research questions are appropriately framed; and 4) effective research methods are employed.

AVAILABILITY OF FUNDING

Philosophical research, no less than scientific research, depends on appropriate funding. Philosophy does not require expensive equipment (although it may contribute to research involving such equipment, as in brain imaging research), but it is no less time consuming than scientific research and requires dedicated research time to be effectively carried out.

The problem of delusion and spiritual experience illustrates three particular barriers to obtaining research funding for philosophy: the "blue skies" barrier, the "friend in court" barrier, and the "falling between two stools" barrier. Thus,

- The "blue skies" barrier arises from the (entirely appropriate) demand for practical payoff from medical research. The (still novel) philosophy of psychiatry, as "blue skies" research, will inevitably have difficulty competing in this respect in a peer-review competitive process with proposals from already well-established disciplines.
- The "friend in court" barrier arises from the shortage of those who understand the potential contribution of philosophy. The fact that philosophy is not well represented on relevant workgroups and committees is a major barrier to otherwise sound proposals competing on an even playing field with more traditional empirical studies.
- The "falling between two stools" barrier is directly related to funding sources. Although there are funding bodies that support philosophy and those that support psychiatry, and although any of these can sometimes be persuaded to risk cross-disciplinary funding, there is a distinct lack of funding bodies whose remit is specifically to support research in the new cross-disciplinary field of philosophy of psychiatry.

The teamwork approach of philosophical fieldwork on delusion and spiritual experience noted earlier offers particular advantages in overcoming each of these barriers to obtaining research funding. Thus, bringing together different perspectives within a coherent theoretical framework converts the "blue skies" of philosophical fieldwork from a problem into an asset: philosophy, in the form of conceptual clarification (if in no other ways), brings added value to techniques with which referees and committee members will already be familiar. The need for conceptual clarification must be justified, of course, but for research in such areas as delusion and spiritual experience, conceptual difficulties are at the very heart of the problem. For the "friend in court" and the "falling between two stools" barriers, applications for research funding from teams that include philosophical expertise, if carefully prepared within a more traditional research discipline, are readily seen to strengthen rather than compromise the research protocols in question.

EDUCATION AND TRAINING

Medical education in the second half of the 20th century was almost entirely taken up with the scientific aspects of medicine—even ethics, as a late arrival developed in its practical applications more on the model of law than of philosophy (Maehle and Geyer-Kordesch 2002). This has produced a cycle of deprivation. Today's doctors lack, by and large, an understanding of philosophy, so the potential resources of philosophy in clinical and empirical research contexts are not recognized for what they are. As a result, philosophy is excluded from curricular and other key educational structures. Thus doctors will continue to lack an understanding of philosophy, and a self-sustaining cycle of deprivation is established.

Research on delusion and spiritual experience offers an excellent opportunity to break through this cycle of deprivation. Approaching such research as an exercise in metaphysics, intriguing as this may be to those with an interest in philosophy, would be at best irrelevant and at worst a distraction from the hard issues of differential diagnosis in everyday practice. Yet distinguishing between delusion and spiritual experience—not in principle but in everyday practice—turns on conceptual issues to which (among other philosophical approaches) the tools of linguistic analysis are *prima facie* relevant. So this is an area in which linguistic analysis, focusing as it does on the *conceptual* problems embedded in the directly *practical* issues faced by practitioners and service users in day-to-day clinical work, could contribute to and draw on the development of appropriate philosophical expertise in medicine.

OWNING (UP TO) THE ISSUES (ACKNOWLEDGING THE CONCEPTUAL NATURE OF THE PROBLEMS)

None of the aspects of the infrastructure of research described thus far—institutional representation, funding, and education and training—will be effective unless the issues are acknowledged for what they are—that is, as conceptual issues. As one of us (K.W.M.F.) has put it elsewhere, philosophy needs to be brought out of the psychiatric closet (Fulford 1994).

This is nowhere more true than in relation to research on delusion and spiritual experience. It is remarkable that the American Psychiatric Association's *Research Agenda for DSM-V* devotes a whole chapter to conceptual issues—its opening chapter at that—without actually using the words *concept* or philosophy. The effect of this denial of conceptual issues is to cut psychiatry off from the key (conceptual) resources necessary to tackle the (conceptual) issues with which the chapter is concerned. Empirical methods are essential, yet where the issues concerned are conceptual, empirical methods on their own will not be sufficient for tackling them. In the next section we turn to the added value of linguistic analysis as a specifically *philosophical* research method for tackling the conceptual issues raised by the distinction between delusion and spiritual experience.

Methods: Philosophical Fieldwork

In this section we do not attempt to develop a detailed protocol for research on the differences between delusion and spiritual experience. Rather, we extend our agenda for research in this area by indicating the resources for such protocols under the agenda items (summarized in Table 10–2): 1) areas for philosophical fieldwork, 2) target clinical concepts, and 3) potential partner methods, both empirical and philosophical, of proven effectiveness. We look at the first of these (areas for philosophical fieldwork) in some detail to draw out the differences between a traditional empirical approach and the combined empirical-philosophical approach of philosophical fieldwork. We then review more briefly the other two agenda items, target clinical concepts and partner methods, as they relate to research on delusion and spiritual experience.

AREAS FOR PHILOSOPHICAL FIELDWORK

The most immediately relevant area for linguistic-analytic philosophical fieldwork on delusion and spiritual experience is clinical case histories. In Austin's own philosophical fieldwork on the nature of action or agency, he studied the reports of legal cases (Austin 1956–1957/1968). Correspondingly, then, and as with all other research in medicine, the natural starting point for philosophical fieldwork on delusion and spiritual experience is *clinical* case studies—the real stories of real people in real situations. Austin indeed pointed philosophers to clinical (as opposed to legal) case histories, and specifically to cases involving psychopathology, as a rich resource for philosophers; there is "gold in them thar hills!" he said (Austin 1956–1957/1968, p. 24).

CASE EXAMPLE: THE STORY OF SIMON

Simon, age 40, was a senior, black, American professional from a middle-class Baptist family. Before the onset of his symptoms, he reported sporadic, relatively unremarkable psychic experiences. These had led him to seek the guidance of a professional "seer" with whom he occasionally consulted on major life events and decisions.

Approximately 4 years before the first interview, his hitherto successful career was threatened by legal action from his colleagues. Although he claimed to be innocent, mounting a defense would have been expensive and hazardous. He responded to this crisis by praying at a small altar that he had set up in his front room. After an emotional evening's "outpouring," he discovered that the candle wax had left a "seal" (or "sun") on several consecutive pages of his bible, covering certain letters and words. He described his experiences thus: "I got up and I saw the seal that was in my father's Bible and I called X and I said, you know, 'something remarkable is going on over here.' I think the beauty of it was the specificity by which the sun burned through. It was…in my mind, a clever play on words." Although the marked words and letters had no explicit meaning, Simon interpreted this event as a direct communication from God that signified that he had a special purpose or mission.

From this time on, Simon received a complex series of "revelations" largely conveyed through the images left in melted candle wax. He carried photos of these "revelations," and although they left most observers unimpressed, for Simon they were clearly representations of biblical symbols, particularly from the book of Revelations (the bull, the 24 elders, the arc of the covenant, etc.). They signified that "I am the living son of David…and I'm also a relative of Ishmael, and…of Joseph." He was also the "captain of the guard of Israel." He found this role carried awesome responsibilities: "Sometimes I'm saying—'O my God, why did you choose me?' and there's no answer to that." His special status had the effect of "Increasing my own inward sense, wisdom, understanding, and endurance," which would "allow me to do whatever is required in terms of bringing whatever message it is that God wants me to bring."

He expressed these beliefs with full conviction: "The truths that are up in that room are the truths that have been spoken of for 4,000 years." When confronted with skepticism, he commented, "I don't get upset, because I know within myself, what I know." (K.W.M. Fulford, Extract from "A Study of the Relationship Between Spiritual and Psychotic Experience," M.A. in Philosophy and Ethics of Mental Health [PEMH], University of Warwick, Coventry, United Kingdom, 1991)

The value of philosophical fieldwork based on real case histories is illustrated by the story of Simon. This story is one from a number of similar case histories, all of them stories of real people, first published by the British psychologist Mike Jackson (1997). When Jackson collected these case histories, he was working on a doctorate with Gordon Claridge at Magdalen College, Oxford. Claridge, also a psychologist, is an expert on psychosis, and the aim of Jackson's doctoral research was to improve the discrimination between delusion and spiritual experience. Consistent with the empirical methods of the day, he approached this by applying the careful definitions of key symptoms in such diagnostic instruments as the Present State Examination (Wing et al. 1974) to case histories such as Simon's. Simon did indeed have a diagnostically significant symptom, namely a delusional perception developing in the context of being threatened by a damaging legal court case. That this experience was indeed a delusional perception as defined by the Present State Examination was confirmed by blind ratings from people trained in the use of that instrument.

According to ICD, and 100 years of traditional symptom-based psychiatric diagnostic practice, Simon thus had schizophrenia or some related psychotic illness. The difficulty, however—and this is where Jackson's doctoral research appeared to run into trouble—is that far from being ill, Simon was much empowered by his experiences. Moreover, the information he received from these experiences, despite being entirely idiosyncratic, guided him so effectively in the conduct of his court case that he won. His stock as a lawyer (which was his own profession) then rose considerably, he made a great deal of money, and when last heard from he was planning to establish a research fund to support research not on delusion but on spiritual experience.

Jackson thus found himself up against something of a brick wall. His doctoral research depended on using the best of the currently available empirical diagnostic tools. Yet these tools, although firmly based on careful definitions of key symptoms, rather than improving the distinction between delusion and spiritual experience seemed (in a number of cases at least) actually to bring them closer together. How to make progress, then? One approach, following traditional medical thinking, would be to move from a descriptive symptom-based level of diagnosis to diagnosis based on underlying causes (i.e., on etiology). However, even if adequate etiological theories were available, they would only beg the question of differential diagnosis: for unless delusion and spiritual experience can be reliably differentiated in the first place, we have no basis from which to explore their (putatively) different causes (Fulford 1989). A second approach would be to seek to sharpen the requisite descriptive tools for symptom-based diagnosis. For Jackson, this would have involved reexamining and attempting to sharpen up the definitions of the relevant psychopathological terms. The most immediately relevant would have been the concept of delusion, but the definition of delusion was and remains too widely contested to be helpful (Garety and Freeman 1999). Psychosis and related concepts such as "insight," as higher-level concepts, were more contested still (Markova and Berrios 1992), to the point that both ICD and DSM were seeking to exclude them (Fulford 2004a). Falling back on the (still higher-level) concept of "mental disorder" itself would have led into a veritable quagmire of debate, reflecting the (at the time) highly polarized exchange between psychiatrists and a variety of "anti-psychiatrists" about whether the concept of mental disorder had any validity at all (Fulford 2003).

From a linguistic-analytic perspective, we should not now be surprised by such difficulties of definition. The differences between delusion and spiritual experience, as the main focus of Jackson's research, turned on higher-level psychopathological concepts for which the established tools of psychopathological research—carefully defined terms as the basis of empirical studies—were inappropriate (or at any rate insufficient). As an exercise in philosophical fieldwork, on the other hand, Jackson's findings allow an entirely different interpretation, namely that the difficulties of definition in cases such as Simon's arise not from the definitions in question being wrong but rather from the fact that these definitions reflect only a partial and incomplete view of the meanings of the relevant concepts (in this case, the concepts of delusion and spiritual experience). Our response, correspondingly, to the failure of these definitions is not to seek to sharpen the requisite definitions further but rather to broaden the scope of our philosophical fieldwork in an attempt to get a more complete view of the meanings of the concepts in question.

There are a number of directions in which broadening the scope of philosophical fieldwork in this area might take us. One relevant direction would be to look at a wider range of case studies: Jackson did this, extending his series of cases and then undertaking a full epidemiological study (Jackson 1997). This additional research confirmed that Simon was far from being an exceptional case and that, as others have shown (Lukoff 2007), many of the other traditional psychotic "symptoms," in addition to delusional perception, might appear also as features of a spiritual or religious experience. A further area for philosophical fieldwork, beyond actual case histories, is the diagnostic practice of psychiatrists themselves, including the diagnostic manuals (such as DSM) on which they draw. Thus, in Jackson's work, the practices of psychiatrists as reflected in a series of commentaries on his work in the journal *Philosophy, Psychiatry, and Psychology* (Littlewood 1997; Lu et al. 1997; Sims 1997; Storr 1997; all commenting on Jackson and Fulford 1997), suggest that however firmly psychiatrists believe they work with an exclusively symptom-based approach to diagnosis, in practice (i.e., as reflecting their actual *use* of concepts) they actually draw on many significant aspects of the context in which symptoms are set: the psychiatrist and expert on psychopathology, Andrew Sims (1992, 1997), for example, argued that psychopathology is suggested, among other things, by 1) the experiences and behavior of the person concerned conforming to established symptomatology, 2) the presence of related symptoms and signs, 3) a course that is consistent with the natural history of a mental disorder, and 4) independent evidence of disordered personality. These and other relevant contextual factors, including factors derived from "non-Western" traditions of spiritual thought and practice (Brett 2002), have recently been reviewed by Lukoff (2007). Correspondingly, then, in the diagnostic manuals on which psychiatrists draw, we find these contextual factors made explicit: in DSM we find such "criteria of clinical significance" as, for example, Criterion B for schizophrenia—a criterion of "social/occupational dysfunction." In Simon's case, indeed, it was Criterion B, the contextual criterion, that was the key to distinguishing his spiritual experience from a psychotic illness. To the extent at least that his occupational functioning as a lawyer was actually *enhanced* by his experiences, he failed to satisfy Criterion B and hence did not—despite satisfying Criterion A (the symptom-based criterion)—have schizophrenia at all but a spiritual experience.

TARGET CONCEPTS FOR PHILOSOPHICAL FIELDWORK

At first glance, the success of DSM in producing a diagnosis in cases such as Simon's with a good degree of face validity may appear to vindicate the traditional empirical medical-scientific approach based on careful definition of terms. This would be consistent, furthermore, with the fact that DSM is explicitly evidence based (American Psychiatric Association 2000). To repeat, careful definition is an important tool for the conceptual clarification that is often needed to underpin empirical research. For this to be sufficient for the task of distinguishing delusion from spiritual experience, however, the requisite definitions must be capable of unambiguous application, which they are not. Far from it. As we should expect from the distinction between higher-level and lower-level concepts outlined earlier, when we look at the concepts embedded in the definition of Criterion B, and on which the unambiguous application of Criterion B in practice depends, we find these to be more, rather than less, resistant to unambiguous definition.

Thus, to return to Simon's case, it is clear from the way his story turned out that he did not satisfy Criterion B: he actually won his court case, after all, so he could hardly be said to show *impaired* occupational functioning. However, suppose he had lost his case, or had won his case but the messages from his "suns" (the wax marks on his bible) had led him to abandon or abuse his family and friends. How, then, would we balance different aspects of his social and occupational functioning? Again, there are aspects of his functioning that might be regarded as good from some perspectives but as impaired from others (e.g., if his experience had led him to abandon his legal practice and to become a hermit). The DSM text rightly acknowledges such difficulties. The use of its categories, including by implication its criteria of clinical significance such as Criterion B, requires "clinical judgment," but DSM offers neither a definition of clinical judgment nor guidelines on how it should be deployed. We could turn instead to the definition of "mental disorder" in DSM. Again, however, as the attention to this issue in the *Research Agenda for DSM-V* suggests, the definition of mental disorder in DSM is unhelpful in the clinical context. It turns on the presence of "dysfunction," and beyond the exclusion condition that mental disorder should not be attributed on the basis of social value judgments alone, DSM offers no clarification of how "dysfunction" itself, the concept at the heart of Criterion B and other criteria of clinical significance, should be judged. The DSM definition of mental disorder, indeed, deepens the conceptual difficulties for the clinician further by stipulating that the requisite dysfunction should be "in the individual," a phrase opening up the interpretation of DSM to all the deep metaphysical issues arising from how "individuals" should be defined (see, e.g., Strawson 1977).

This series of embedded concepts—clinical significance, clinical judgment, mental disorder, individual—shows the extent of the conceptual difficulties underpinning the practical task of distinguishing between delusion and spiritual experience: in addition to Criterion B itself, which is the critical differential diagnostic criterion in cases such as Simon's, and the concept of "social/occupational dysfunction" on which Criterion B turns, we have found that Criterion B has embedded within it the further problematic (and largely undefined in DSM) concepts of "clinical significance" and "clinical judgment." These concepts are closely related in turn to the wider concept of "mental disorder." The concept of mental disorder is indeed defined in DSM, but in terms that lead us into the deep metaphysical waters of the concept of an "individual." There is worse still to come. The definition of *mental disorder* in DSM is, at least in relation to Criterion B, at best question begging and at worst contradictory. It is question begging to the extent that, as a resource for clarifying the application of Criterion B in a given case, the DSM definition of mental disorder, no less than the DSM definition of Criterion B itself, turns on the (undefined in DSM) concept of dysfunction. The DSM definition of *mental disorder* is contradictory to the extent that, as noted, it requires the presence of dysfunction "*in* the individual," whereas Criterion B, by contrast, requires dysfunction in an individual's social and/or occupational activities, that is, in areas that are *external* to the individual.

Outlining in this way the web of embedded conceptual difficulties revealed beneath the surface of the DSM criteria shows the extent to which the method of careful definition, developed to such good effect in psychiatry in the 20th century and embodied in our modern symptom-based classifications, depends on our ability, in the day-to-day application of these classifications in clinical psychiatry, to *use* the higher-level concepts (of dysfunction, clinical significance, clinical judgment, mental disorder, and so forth) embedded in the terms in which the categories in these classifications are defined. In this respect, as we have seen, diagnostic concepts are no different from concepts in any other area, including physics (remember the example of the concept of time used earlier). The importance of these embedded concepts is more evident in DSM than in ICD; however, this is not because ICD is somehow clearer than DSM. It is rather because DSM spells out more explicitly than ICD the criteria on which its categories depend. DSM, therefore, in making its criteria explicit, is particularly helpful to us in identifying the key target concepts—the target higher-level concepts on which we must focus in taking forward work on delusion and spiritual experience. Austin (1956–1957/1968) noted the critical importance of making conceptual problems explicit as the first step in conceptual research. In the next section, we turn to the potential methods for research on these target concepts within the linguistic-analytic paradigm of philosophical fieldwork.

PARTNER METHODS

Philosophical fieldwork, as noted earlier in this chapter, is a ready philosophical partner to empirical research methods. Austin, as perhaps the founding father of philosophical fieldwork, resisted the idea that linguistic analysis is, in its own right, anything as grand as a method. It is, he is reported as saying by his pupil and literary executor, the late Sir Geoffrey Warnock (1989), at most "something about one way of possibly doing one part of philosophy" (p. 6). Austin speculated on the extent to which philosophical fieldwork would need to be combined with empirical and other methods appropriate to different research problems. Warnock also reported (Warnock 1989, Chapter 1) that Austin, influenced by his experience as a senior intelligence officer in World War II, took the model of empirical science further still, arguing that complex philosophical problems, traditionally explored by lone philosophers working in isolation, could be broken down into smaller and more manageable parts and then distributed across a team of researchers with different resources of knowledge and skills. The combined outputs from this distributed approach, again pursuing the parallels with empirical science, would not be once-and-for-all solutions but modest increments in understanding that, together and with luck, might add up to an occasional major breakthrough.

So far as we are aware, research combining philosophical with other methods has not yet been done in the area of delusion and spiritual experience. There are, however, a number of relevant examples of such research in other areas of the philosophy of psychiatry that show the potential of combined methods approaches.

We illustrate some of these in the following discussion. Before turning to these methods, however, it is important to emphasize that there is already a rich literature in the philosophy of psychiatry to support research on delusion and spiritual experience. Relevant work includes research in the analytic philosophical tradition on values (Fulford 1989, 2002; Sadler 2002, 2005, see also "Outputs" section that follows). There is also important work in the philosophy of science. This includes work by the British philosopher of psychiatry Tim Thornton (2007) on the irreducibility of individual judgment that is directly relevant to our understanding of the concept of "clinical judgment," to this concept as used in DSM in relation to Criterion B, and to the crucial role of Criterion B in distinguishing between delusion and spiritual experience. Also critically relevant to research in this area is contemporary work in various branches of phenomenology: the Italian psychiatrist and phenomenologist Giovanni Stanghellini (2004), for example, has produced a detailed phenomenology of schizophrenia; other examples include Heidegger's phenomenology and trauma (Bracken 2001, 2002), Merleau-Ponty's phenomenology and dyslexia (Philpott 1998), and Sartre's existential phenomenology and body dysmorphophobia (Morris 2003).

Precisely what kind of combined method is adopted for a given research problem will of course depend on the particular requirements of the research in question. Yet the modern history of psychiatry offers a range of helpful exemplars. Jaspers was a psychiatrist first (who did neuroscience research as a young doctor) and a philosopher second. His General Psychopathology, from which modern descriptive psychopathology is derived, was written as a direct philosophical response to the *scientific* challenges of the psychiatry of his day. Less well known, but no less relevant as an example of combined-methods research in this area, is the way in which modern descriptive classifications emerged directly from the two disciplines, philosophy and psychiatry, coming together in a crucial way. A key contribution to the emergence of these classifications came from the work of the American philosopher of science Carl Hempel (Kendell 1975; Zubin 1961), but it was the British psychiatrist Sir Aubrey Lewis, drawing on Hempel's ideas but *reversing* them, who first pushed psychiatry in the direction of descriptive symptom-based classifications, and it was Lewis, working with Norman Sartorius in the World Health Organization, who went on to produce the first symptom-based classification, the Glossary to ICD-8 (World Health Organization 1974), from which DSM-III (American Psychiatric Association 1980), ICD-9 (World Health Organization 1977), and their respective successor editions have all subsequently been derived (Fulford and Sartorius 2009).

Other more recent examples of effective teamwork between philosophy and psychiatry relevant to delusion and spiritual experience include those of the American psychologist Steven Sabat and the Oxford philosopher Rom Harré, who combined their skills to develop a discursive approach to the problems of communication between professionals and people with Alzheimer's disease (Sabat 2001; Sabat and

Harré 1997); the Dutch philosopher and hermeneuticist Guy Widdershoven, working in partnership with staff on a psychogeriatric ward and employing hermeneutic methods to a similar end (Widdershoven and Widdershoven-Heerding 2003); and, as an example of a more formal partnership relevant to research on delusion and spiritual experience, the combined linguistic-analytic and empirical social science study of models of disorder in schizophrenia led by the British social scientist Anthony Colombo (Colombo et al. 2003). Linguistic analysis provided both the underpinning theory for the Colombo study and the mechanisms for translating its results into practice (Fulford and Colombo 2004), and the study was crucially supported by a research "board" that included Peter Campbell (1996), a politically active service user who has written of his own psychotic experiences in terms of spiritual experience rather than psychopathology. A pilot study extending Colombo's work to issues of race and spirituality, and led by an ex-service user, Colin King (2007), with direct personal experience of being misdiagnosed with schizophrenia, is currently being taken forward under the auspices of the Mental Health Foundation, a nongovernmental organization in London that has led the field in developing service user–led approaches to research in mental health (King et al. 2009).

Each kind of combined-methods approach illustrated in this section—the lone researcher with cross-disciplinary experience, informal partnerships, and more formal research teams, including those with personal experience of mental disorder—illustrates the potential of Austin's vision for teamwork as the basis of philosophical fieldwork on delusion and spiritual experience. In the final main section of this chapter we turn to the outputs we may expect from such fieldwork.

Outputs: A More Complete View

As we noted in the opening section of this chapter, Ryle's "logical geography" of our title is very far from the grand metaphysical theories traditionally associated with philosophy. The distinctive output from philosophical fieldwork is rather what Austin called a "more complete view" of the meanings of the relevant higher-level concepts in a given area of discourse. In this section, we outline the value of the more complete view provided by a logical geography of the higher-level psychopathological concepts relevant to the distinction between delusion and spiritual experience, as illustrated by the studies noted in the previous section. As we discuss, and as Table 10–2 indicates, mapping the logical geography of these concepts contributes to psychiatry equally at the levels of theory and of practice.

The relevance of philosophical fieldwork to the problem of differentiating delusion from spiritual experience, at both theoretical and practical levels, is illustrated particularly clearly by Jackson's work, building on the story of Simon. First, as to theory, Jackson's work showed that the medical view of psychosis as being necessarily a form of illness is, as the linguistic analytic model would suggest, indeed an *incomplete* view: some psychotic experience is properly understood as illness, certainly, but other psychotic experiences, although otherwise identical in form, are not.

One practical result of this more complete view of psychotic experiences is that there are now organizations, mostly service user–led, dedicated to affirming the nonpathological and often life-enhancing effects of some forms particularly of hallucinatory experiences (see, e.g., www.hearing-voices.org). The official position of The British Psychological Society (2000), similarly, is now that psychotic experience as such should be understood as one among a number of problem-solving strategies that people have available to them: sometimes the strategy goes seriously wrong (this is psychotic illness); sometimes, as in Simon's case, it goes well; and in many cases, precisely how an individual's experiences develop may be critically influenced by their interactions with others, including professionals. Professional interventions are of course particularly potent in this respect, for good or ill, partly through their resources for management (including neuroleptic medication and cognitive-behavioral approaches) but also through the ways in which professionals help to frame the experiences themselves through their diagnostic processes. Thus reaching a valid diagnostic formulation at the interface between delusion and spiritual experience, one that is as respectful of the service user's perspective as of that of the professionals concerned, is particularly critical (National Institute for Mental Health in England and the Care Services Improvement Partnership 2008). The demonstration by Colombo et al. (2003) of the extent to which the guiding models both of professionals and of service users may be implicit rather than explicit further strengthens the need for a more complete view of the logical geography of the psychopathological concepts relevant to distinguishing delusion from spiritual experience.

A second practical result from the more complete view provided by philosophical fieldwork is that it helps to give us a more complete picture of which variables may be critical in research. There is no magic bullet here. Critical variables may be identified in other ways, both philosophical and empirical (e.g., through development of new instruments, such as new methods of functional brain imaging), yet linguistic analysis is of proven effectiveness in this respect where the variables concerned are defined by the higher-level concepts by which we frame and make sense of the world around us. Thus, much of the effort to improve the validity of psychiatric diagnostic classifications has focused on symptom-based criteria, as in Criterion A for schizophrenia, with the hope that, as in bodily medicine, this will lead directly to disease-like categories based on etiological theories. The more complete view provided by philosophical fieldwork suggests that although this aspect of validity is important, we should attend equally to the higher-level concepts embedded in Criterion B and other criteria of clinical significance, together with their underpinning concepts, such as clinical judgment, dysfunction, and mental disorder, as outlined in the last section.

A third area of practical pay off is in clinical work. At first glance, it may seem that the more complete view provided by philosophical fieldwork merely complicates matters clinically! After all, the traditional (incomplete) view is challenging enough: a valid diagnosis depends on carefully eliciting and identifying presenting symptoms. The more complete view offered by linguistic analysis suggests that, important as identifying the presenting symptoms may be (and they *are* crucially important, remember), even more important may be judgments of clinical significance. As Simon's case illustrates, judgments of clinical significance may differentiate between diagnoses as radically different as delusion and spiritual experience. The implication of this is to focus attention on the crucial role of good process in diagnosis. The pressure for full definition of diagnostic criteria has led to ever-more complex diagnostic manuals supported by rating scales and other devices. As noted earlier, this has led to important improvements in reliability. Push this program of progressive definition too far, however, and as the authors of the *Research Agenda for DSM-V* anticipate, reliability ends up being achieved at the expense of validity. If higher-level concepts, by their very nature, resist full definition, however, then it is no surprise that codification of criteria has turned out to be of limited effectiveness. Our attention, then, within the more complete picture provided by linguistic analysis, must be as much on good *process* in diagnosis as on the careful definition of diagnostic criteria. As just noted, one area where good process is essential is in clinical judgment. The judgment of individual practitioners, therefore, in the more complete view of the logical geography of delusion and spiritual experience to be had from linguistic-analytic philosophical fieldwork, is not an add-on to applying diagnostic criteria. It is of the essence.

We can take this conclusion of the importance and irreducibility of individual clinical judgment in a number of directions. It points us, again, to the significance of tacit as well as explicit knowledge in differential diagnosis. It points us also, and particularly in respect of delusion and spiritual experience, to the importance of value judgments as being integral to clinical judgment. Issues raised by applying Criterion B, as in Simon's case, are all about values, about weighing good and bad aspects of an individual's social and occupational functioning. More wide-ranging philosophical fieldwork on the DSM texts suggests that values are indeed pervasive throughout psychiatric diagnostic classification (Sadler 1996, 2005). Clearly, there is a considerable research agenda just to explore these evaluative elements in the "more complete" view of DSM (and hence of psychiatric classification in general) opened up by linguistic-analytic research. We include an illustration of how the outputs from such research might affect the drafting of DSM's criteria of clinical significance, specifically, as in Table 10–3, Criterion B for schizophrenia.

Again, we do not have space here to explore at length the implications of the values embedded in DSM and other psychiatric-diagnostic texts as a key feature of the logical geography of our diagnostic concepts. Two points, however, stand out from the example in Table 10–3. The first is that it underlines the way in which linguis-

TABLE 10–3.   Illustration of possible amendments (italicized text) to DSM-IV-TR diagnostic criteria for schizophrenia

A. **Characteristic symptoms:** Two (or more) of the following, each present for a *clinically* significant portion of time during a 1-month period (or less if successfully treated):

1) delusions

2) *true* hallucinations

3) disorganized speech (with specific features, e.g., frequent derailment or incoherence)

4) disorganized behavior (with specific features, e.g., catatonia; *note that to be clinically significant, behavior must normally be grossly disorganized*)

5) negative symptoms, i.e., affective flattening, alogia, or avolition

Note: Only one Criterion A symptom is required if delusions are bizarre or hallucinations consist of a voice keeping up a running commentary on the person's behavior or thoughts, or two or more voices conversing with each other.

B. *Deterioration in* **social/occupational function:** For a *clinically* significant portion of the time since the onset of the *disorder,* one or more areas of functioning such as work, interpersonal relations, or self-care are markedly below the level achieved prior to the onset; or, when the onset is in childhood or adolescence, *there is marked* failure to achieve expected level(s) of interpersonal, academic, or occupational *functioning. In either case the deterioration in social/occupational dysfunctioning must be judged to be clinically significant.*

Note: *Clinical judgment is required to decide whether a change in (actual or anticipated) social or occupational functioning is clinically significant (i.e., pathological). A clinically significant change in social or occupational functioning is a change 1) for the worse that 2) arises from, results in, or takes the form of incapacity. The values and capacities against which these two elements of clinical significance are respectively judged should normally (and always in contentious cases) be made explicit. The subject's own values and normal capacities should always be identified and should normally carry particular weight in the determination of this criterion. The subject's and the clinician's perspectives should be balanced by those of others, including, where appropriate, 1) relatives and caregivers, 2) other health professionals in multidisciplinary teams, 3) nonclinical groups (e.g., lawyers, social workers, service user and/or advocacy groups, etc.), in situations involving interagency cooperation).*

TABLE 10–3. Illustration of possible amendments (italicized text) to DSM-IV-TR diagnostic criteria for schizophrenia *(continued)*

Criteria C through F unchanged

Source. Original criteria reprinted with permission from American Psychiatric Association: Diagnostic and Statistical Manual of Mental Disorders, 4th Edition, Text Revision. Washington, DC, American Psychiatric Association, 2000. Copyright 2000, American Psychiatric Association.

A version of these illustrative revised criteria based on the text of the original DSM-IV was first published in Fulford KWM: "Report to the Chair of the DSM-VI Task Force from the Editors of PPP on 'Contentious and Noncontentious Evaluative Language in Psychiatric Diagnosis' (Dateline 2010)," in *Descriptions and Prescriptions: Values, Mental Disorders, and the DSMs.* Edited by Sadler JZ. Baltimore, MD, The Johns Hopkins University Press, 2002, pp. 323–362.

tic-analytic research is a partner to more traditional empirical research on psychiatric diagnosis. Consistently with the "more complete view" that is the characteristic output from linguistic-analytic research, the suggested amendments shown in Table 10–3 simply *make explicit* the evaluative elements that are already there in judgments of clinical significance. From the perspective of a traditional model of medicine, this may seem to run counter to the need for diagnosis to be based firmly on evidence, but it does not. It simply makes explicit that in addition to being firmly evidence-based, diagnosis also depends, in part—but as an important part of making *clinical* judgments—on a series of *value* judgments that are in turn based on the *evidence* presented by individual cases.

The second point made by Table 10–3 follows on from this: that making the evaluative elements in judgments of clinical significance explicit in this way opens up psychiatric diagnosis to a rich resource of what are increasingly being called values-based—alongside the more traditional evidence-based—tools to support improvements in the *processes* of psychiatric diagnosis. Again, we do not have space here to go into this in detail. Briefly, however, the practical tools of *values-based practice* are derived from work in the "Oxford school" of linguistic-analytic philosophy on philosophical value theory, notably by one of Austin's pupils, R.M. Hare (e.g., Hare 1952), and applied by one of us (K.W.M.F.) to the specific context of the "logical geography" of the medical concepts (Fulford 1989, 2004b). Values-based and evidence-based practice both offer practical tools for improving the processes for working with complexity of values and evidence, respectively, in clinical contexts. The tools of values-based practice, already in use to support diagnostic assessment in psychiatry, are currently being developed in the United Kingdom and internationally in a number of ways, ranging from training in specific learnable clinical skills (Woodbridge and Fulford 2004), to policy and service development initiatives (e.g., Department of Health 2004, 2005, 2007; Mezzich and Salloum

2007; National Institute for Mental Health in England and the Care Services Improvement Partnership 2008), to new research on values in psychiatric diagnosis (Fulford 2005; Fulford et al. 2005; Sadler 2005).

Conclusions: A Science at the Cutting Edge

In this chapter we set out an agenda for research on delusion and spiritual experience, drawing particularly on the resources of linguistic-analytic philosophy as developed by the "Oxford school" in the middle decades of the 20th century. As Table 10–2 summarizes, linguistic analysis generates a rich agenda. It reframes the problem of distinguishing delusion from spiritual experience as one involving *higher-level psychopathological concepts;* it suggests a specific methodological approach, Austin's *philosophical fieldwork;* and it produces a characteristic output, a *more complete view* of the meanings of the relevant higher-level concepts, the logical geography of our title.

As we noted at the start of this chapter, there are no grand metaphysical schemes to be had from linguistic analysis. In this respect, linguistic analysis, along with the many other rich philosophical and empirical traditions contributing to the new philosophy of psychiatry (Fulford et al. 2003, 2006), is closely geared to the needs of service users and service providers in day-to-day practice. The outputs of linguistic analysis, because of its central focus on the *use* of concepts by real people in everyday contexts, are particularly well targeted in this respect. In the case of delusion and spiritual experience, as we indicated, the practical outcomes of linguistic-analytic research are more likely to be improvements in the *processes* of psychiatric diagnosis rather than new or different definitions of diagnostic criteria. The need to improve the processes of diagnostic assessment in psychiatry, furthermore, drawing particularly on the resources of values-based practice, will focus attention on the importance of the clinical skills required to apply DSM's criteria of clinical significance appropriately in the particular circumstances presented by each individual person.

The outputs of linguistic-analytic research, then—the more complete view of the logical geography it provides—reinforce the nature of psychiatry as a discipline that is essentially person centered. There will be some, however, for whom the very suggestion that philosophy, let alone values, has any part to play in research on delusion and spiritual experience will be taken as an indication not of the irreducibly person-centered nature of psychiatry but rather of its limitations as a medical science. This is a reflection of the broadly positivist mindset that psychiatry shared with the rest of medicine through much of the previous century (Meares 2003). We owe to this mindset the important improvements in the reliability of psychiatric diagnostic concepts to which we referred earlier. These improvements, in turn, are the basis for advances arising from the new neurosciences, and we have warned against the growing chorus of disillusionment with our current symptom-based classifications. Yet the positivist mindset is itself an aspect of the limited or incomplete view of psychiatry (and indeed of medicine generally) that it is the aim of linguistic-analytic research to remedy. After all, in all sciences properly understood, and in contrast with the incomplete view represented by positivism, there is an interplay between observation and understanding, between the data we obtain from empirical research and the concepts by which we frame and make sense of that data. In many sciences, the relevant concepts are largely unproblematic. Many medical sciences are of this kind. Yet in sciences at the cutting edge, concepts may be as much part of the challenge as the data. This is nowhere more true than at the cutting edge of the physical sciences—the concept of time, to return to our earlier example, although largely unproblematic in most everyday contexts, is at the very heart of some of the deepest difficulties in quantum mechanics.

Underpinning the whole of our research agenda, then, is what we believe is a key pre-condition for success, namely that we reframe the need for philosophical alongside empirical research in psychiatry not as a mark of the limitations of psychiatric science but as a reflection of the true strengths of psychiatry as a discipline that is firmly and irreducibly person centered but also a science at the cutting edge.

References

American Psychiatric Association: Diagnostic and Statistical Manual of Mental Disorders, 3rd Edition. Washington, DC, American Psychiatric Association, 1980

American Psychiatric Association: Diagnostic and Statistical Manual of Mental Disorders, 4th Edition. Washington, DC, American Psychiatric Association, 1994

American Psychiatric Association: Diagnostic and Statistical Manual of Mental Disorders, 4th Edition, Text Revision. Washington, DC, American Psychiatric Association, 2000

Andreasen NC: Brave New Brain: Conquering Mental Illness in the Era of the Genome. Oxford, UK, Oxford University Press, 2001

Andreasen NC: DSM and the death of phenomenology in America: an example of unintended consequences. Schizophr Bull 33:108–112, 2007

Austin JL: A plea for excuses (1956–1957), in The Philosophy of Action. Edited by White AR. Oxford, UK, Oxford University Press, 1968, pp 19–42

Blashfield RK: The Classification of Psychopathology: Neo-Kraepelinian and Quantitative Approaches. New York, Plenum, 1984

Bracken P: Post modernity and post traumatic stress disorder. Soc Sci Med 53:733–743, 2001

Bracken P: Trauma: Culture, Meaning and Philosophy. London, England, Whurr, 2002

Brett C: Psychotic and mystical states of being: connections and distinctions. Philos Psychiatr Psychol 9:321–342, 2002

The British Psychological Society: Recent Advances in Understanding Mental Illness and Psychotic Experiences. Leicester, UK, The British Psychological Society, Division of Clinical Psychology, 2000

Campbell P: What we want from crisis services, in Speaking Our Minds: An Anthology. Edited by Read J, Reynolds J. Basingstoke, England, Macmillan Press Ltd for The Open University, 1996, pp 180–183

Chadwick H (translator): St Augustine Confessions. Oxford, UK, Oxford University Press, 1992

Colombo A, Bendelow G, Fulford KWM, et al: Evaluating the influence of implicit models of mental disorder on processes of shared decision making within community-based multidisciplinary teams. Soc Sci Med 56:1557–1570, 2003

Department of Health: The Ten Essential Shared Capabilities: A Framework for the Whole of the Mental Health Workforce. London, The Sainsbury Centre for Mental Health, the National Health Service University, and the National Institute for Mental Health England, 2004

Department of Health: New Ways of Working for Psychiatrists: Enhancing Effective, Person-Centred Services Through New Ways of Working in Multidisciplinary and Multi-Agency Contexts (Final Report "But Not the End of the Story"). London, Department of Health, 2005

Department of Health: A Learning and Development Toolkit for the Whole of the Mental Health Workforce Across Both Health and Social Care. London, Department of Health, 2007

Fulford KWM: Moral Theory and Medical Practice. Cambridge, UK, Cambridge University Press, 1989

Fulford KWM: Closet logics: hidden conceptual elements in the DSM and ICD classifications of mental disorders, in Philosophical Perspectives on Psychiatric Diagnostic Classification. Edited by Sadler JZ, Wiggins OP, Schwartz MA. Baltimore, MD, Johns Hopkins University Press, 1994, pp 211–232

Fulford KWM: Religion and psychiatry: extending the limits of tolerance, in Psychiatry and Religion: Context, Consensus and Controversies. Edited by Bhugra D. London, Routledge & Kegan Paul, 1996

Fulford KWM: Values in psychiatric diagnosis: executive summary of a report to the chair of the ICD-12/DSM-VI Coordination Task Force (Dateline 2010). Psychopathology 35:132–138, 2002

Fulford KWM: Mental illness: definition, use and meaning, in Encyclopedia of Bioethics, 3rd Edition. Edited by Post SG. New York, Macmillan, 2003, pp 1789–1800

Fulford KWM: Completing Kraepelin's psychopathology: insight, delusion and the phenomenology of illness, in Insight and Psychosis, 2nd Edition. Edited by Amador XF, David AS. New York, Oxford University Press, 2004a

Fulford KWM: Ten principles of values-based medicine, in The Philosophy of Psychiatry: A Companion. Edited by Radden J. New York, Oxford University Press, 2004b, pp 205–234

Fulford KWM: Values in psychiatric diagnosis: developments in policy, training and research. Psychopathology 38:171–176, 2005

Fulford KWM, Colombo A: Six models of mental disorder: a study combining linguistic-analytic and empirical methods. Philos Psychiatry Psychol 11:129–144, 2004

Fulford KWM, Sartorius N: A secret history of ICD and the hidden future of DSM, in Psychiatry as Cognitive Neuroscience: Philosophical Perspectives. Edited by Broome M, Bortolotti L. Oxford, UK, Oxford University Press, 2009, pp 29–48

Fulford KWM, Morris KJ, Sadler JZ, et al: Past improbable, future possible: the renaissance in philosophy and psychiatry, in Nature and Narrative: An Introduction to the New Philosophy of Psychiatry. Edited by Fulford KWM, Morris KJ, Sadler JZ, et al. Oxford, UK, Oxford University Press, 2003, pp 1–41

Fulford KWM, Broome M, Stanghellini G, et al: Looking with both eyes open: fact and value in psychiatric diagnosis? World Psychiatry 4:78–86, 2005

Fulford KWM, Thornton T, Graham G: Natural classifications, realism and psychiatric science, in The Oxford Textbook of Philosophy and Psychiatry. Edited by Fulford KWM, Thornton T, Graham G. Oxford, UK, Oxford University Press, 2006, pp 316–383

Garety PA, Freeman D: Cognitive approaches to delusions: a critical review of theories and evidence. Br J Clin Psychol 38:113–154, 1999

Hare RM: The Language of Morals. Oxford, UK, Oxford University Press, 1952

Hyman SE: Neuroscience, genetics, and the future of psychiatric diagnosis. Psychopathology 35:139–144, 2002

Hyman SE, Fenton WS: Medicine: what are the right targets for psychopharmacology? Science 299:350–351, 2003

Jackson MC: Benign schizotypy? The case of spiritual experience, in Schizotypy: Relations to Illness and Health. Edited by Claridge GS. Oxford, UK, Oxford University Press, 1997, pp 227–250

Jackson M, Fulford KWM: Spiritual experience and psychopathology. Philos Psychiatry Psychol 4:41–66, 1997

Jaspers K: General Psychopathology (1913a). Translated by Hoenig J, Hamilton MW. Chicago, IL, University of Chicago Press, 1963

Jaspers K: Causal and meaningful connexions between life history and psychosis (1913b), in Themes and Variations in European Psychiatry. Edited by Hirsch SR, Shepherd M. Bristol, John Wright and Sons Ltd, 1974, pp 80–93

Jaspers K: The phenomenological approach in psychopathology (1913c) (in translation on the initiative of Curran JN). Br J Psychiatry 114:1313–1323, 1968

Kendell RE: The Role of Diagnosis in Psychiatry. Oxford, UK, Blackwell Scientific, 1975

King C: They diagnosed me a schizophrenic when I was just a Gemini: the other side of madness, in Reconceiving Schizophrenia. Edited by Chung M, Fulford KWM, Graham G. Oxford, UK, Oxford University Press, 2007, pp 11–28

King C, Bhui K, Fulford KWM, et al: Model Values? Race, Values, and Models in Mental Health. London, The Mental Health Foundation, 2009

Kupfer DJ, First MB, Regier DE (eds): A Research Agenda for DSM-V. Washington, DC, American Psychiatric Association, 2002

Kutchins H, Kirk SA: Making Us Crazy: DSM—The Psychiatric Bible and the Creation of Mental Disorder. London, England, Constable, 1997

Littlewood R: Commentary on "Spiritual experience and psychopathology." Philos Psychiatry Psychol 4:67–74, 1997

Lu FG, Lukoff D, Turner RP: Commentary on "Spiritual experience and psychopathology." Philos Psychiatry Psychol 4:75–78, 1997

Lukoff D: Visionary spiritual experiences. South Med J 100:635–641, 2007

Maehle A-H, Geyer-Kordesch J: Introduction, in Historical and Philosophical Perspectives in Biomedical Ethics: From Paternalism to Autonomy? Edited by Maehle A-H, Geyer-Kordesch J. Burlington, VT, Ashgate Publishing, 2002, pp 1–9

Markova IS, Berrios GE: The meaning of insight in clinical psychiatry. Br J Psychiatry 160:850–860, 1992

Meares R: Towards a psyche for psychiatry, in Nature and Narrative: An Introduction to the New Philosophy of Psychiatry. Edited by Fulford KWM, Morris KJ, Sadler JZ, et al. Oxford, UK, Oxford University Press, 2003, pp 43–56

Mezzich JE, Salloum IM: Towards innovative international classification and diagnostic systems: ICD-11 and person-centered integrative diagnosis (guest editorial). Acta Psychiatr Scand 116:1–5, 2007

Morris KJ: The phenomenology of body dysmorphic disorder: a Sartrean analysis, in Nature and Narrative: An Introduction to the New Philosophy of Psychiatry. Edited by Fulford KWM, Morris KJ, Sadler JZ, et al. Oxford, UK, Oxford University Press, 2003, pp 270–274

National Institute for Mental Health in England and the Care Services Improvement Partnership: 3 Keys to a Shared Approach in Mental Health Assessment. London, Department of Health, 2008. Available at: www.3keys.org.uk/downloads/3keys.pdf.

Philpott MJ: A phenomenology of dyslexia: the lived-body, ambiguity, and the breakdown of expression. Philos Psychiatry Psychol 5:1–20 (with commentaries by Komesaroff PA, Wiltshire J, pp 21–24; Rippon G, pp 25–28; Widdershoven GAM, pp 29–32; and author's response to the commentaries, pp 33–36), 1998

Ryle G: The Concept of Mind. London, Penguin, 1980

Sabat SR: The Experience of Alzheimer's Disease: Life Through a Tangled Veil. Oxford, UK, Blackwell, 2001

Sabat SR, Harré R: The Alzheimer's disease sufferer as semiotic subject. Philos Psychiatry Psychol 1:145–160, 1997

Sadler JZ: Epistemic value commitments in the debate over categorical vs. dimensional personality diagnosis. Philos Psychiatry Psychol 3:203–222, 1996

Sadler JZ (ed): Descriptions and Prescriptions: Values, Mental Disorders, and the DSMs. Baltimore, MD, Johns Hopkins University Press, 2002

Sadler JZ: Values and Psychiatric Diagnosis. Oxford, UK, Oxford University Press, 2005

Sadler JZ, Fulford KWM: Should patients and families contribute to the DSM-V process? Psychiatr Serv 55:133–138, 2004

Sadler JZ, Wiggins OP, Schwartz MA (eds): Philosophical Perspectives on Psychiatric Diagnostic Classification. Baltimore, MD, Johns Hopkins University Press, 1994

Sims A: Symptoms and beliefs. J R Soc Health 112:42–46, 1992

Sims A: Commentary on "Spiritual experience and psychopathology." Philos Psychiatry Psychol 4:79–82, 1997

Spitzer RL, Endicott J, Robins E: Research diagnostic criteria: rationale and reliability. Arch Gen Psychiatry 35:773–782, 1978

Stanghellini G: Deanimated Bodies and Disembodied Spirits: Essays on the Psychopathology of Common Sense. Oxford, UK, Oxford University Press, 2004

Storr A: Commentary on "Spiritual experience and psychopathology." Philos Psychiatry Psychol 4:83–86, 1997

Strawson PF: Individuals: An Essay in Descriptive Metaphysics. Oxford, UK, Oxford University Press, 1977

Thornton T: Essential Philosophy of Psychiatry. Oxford, UK, Oxford University Press, 2007

Warnock GJ: Saturday mornings, in Essays on J.L. Austin. Edited by Berlin I. Oxford, UK, Clarendon, 1973, pp 31–45

Warnock GJ: J.L. Austin. London, England, Routledge, 1989

Widdershoven G, Widdershoven-Heerding I: Understanding dementia: a hermeneutic perspective, in Nature and Narrative: An Introduction to the New Philosophy of Psychiatry. Edited by Fulford KWM, Morris KJ, Sadler JZ, et al. Oxford, UK, Oxford University Press, 2003, pp 103–112

Wing JK, Cooper JE, Sartorius N: Measurement and classification of psychiatric symptoms. Cambridge, UK, Cambridge University Press, 1974

Woodbridge K, Fulford KWM: Whose Values? A Workbook for Values-Based Practice in Mental Health Care. London, England, Sainsbury Centre for Mental Health, 2004

World Health Organization: Glossary of Mental Disorders and Guide to their Classification, for Use in Conjunction With the International Classification of Diseases, 8th Revision. Geneva, Switzerland, World Health Organization, 1974

World Health Organization: International Classification of Diseases, 9th Revision. Geneva, Switzerland, World Health Organization, 1977

Zubin J (ed): Field Studies in the Mental Disorders: Discussion, Various Contributors. New York, Grune and Stratton, 1961, pp 23–50

Commentary 10A

COMMENTARY ON "MAPPING THE LOGICAL GEOGRAPHY OF DELUSION AND SPIRITUAL EXPERIENCE"

Derek Bolton, Ph.D.

The question of method is always a difficult one for philosophy, and much the same goes for any science, art, or humanity. How should it be done? What, specifically, does it have to contribute? How is it different from other ways of knowing? Austin's philosophical methodology—linguistic analysis—included consideration of how words used in typical philosophical discourse were actually used in day to day life. Wittgenstein recommended a similar kind of thing at around the same time. This "ordinary language philosophy," as it was sometimes called, was one of the many ways in which the grand tradition of *a priori* philosophical knowledge, metaphysics, was brought down to earth—that is to say, to an end. The main contrast was between the *philosophical* use of words, often involved in more or less profound philosophical problems such as Augustine's paradoxes of time, and our ordinary, mundane use of words, such as in telling the time, where no such problems hold us up.

It is possible that this ordinary language philosophical methodology can be used for other purposes. The present problem is or includes how some kinds of spiritual experience should be or are distinguished from delusion and mental disorder. It may well be that different groups, distinguished by culture, profession, or individual opinion, would not agree on what the distinctions in question are, or on where they should be drawn. Presumably this is the case, or we would all not be engaged in the current exercise. There are significant disagreements over definitions, principles, and cases. So if we were to ask "How are these words used in day to day practice?" the answer is, it depends on who you ask. So far as I can see this relativity did not arise in the philosophical methods of Austin or Wittgenstein; when they recommended attending to the ordinary as opposed to the philosophical use of words, they were not inviting the question: but whose usage?

On the other hand there may be a related aspect of "ordinary language philosophy"—one more apparent perhaps in Austin rather than in Wittgenstein—in which it is applied to any concept of interest, not one that has a role in traditional metaphysics and its problems. By all means both philosophers had meaning defined by ordinary usage (hence the alleged illegitimacy of exclusively philosophical usage that followed different and incompatible rules). "Ordinary usage" here is best understood as including particular judgments using a term, the theory (if any) in which the term is embedded, and associated proposed definitions. In the present case this would mean attending to particular judgments regarding spiritual experience and delusion, systems of religious or atheistic beliefs, and definitions of delusion, mental disorder, and, for example, rationality. Study of ordinary usage in this sense is already evident in discourse and writing on psychiatric case studies, religious experiences, theology, psychiatry, and philosophy. Fulford and Sadler recommend adding to this—or enhancing the use of—multidisciplinary team work. Everything helps, of course, but it is not clear to me that something new would be added to the methodologies that are already in use.

Fulford and Sadler are very helpful in clarifying the critical principles and cases in this area. The case of Simon is interesting because his religious beliefs apparently conform to the criteria for delusion, yet they do him no harm, but rather good, or at least are associated with a good level of functioning and thus do not signify mental disorder or illness according to standard diagnostic practice and the definitions in DSM and ICD. This apparently presents a problem for those who believe that mental disorder in general or delusion in particular can be defined independent of associated harm and detected on some other grounds such as clinical sense or intuition. However, the underlying problem probably goes deeper, because even if an experience does lead to harm for the person having it, he and others of like mind may still regard it as spiritual (as opposed to, e.g., delusion) because they believe it leads to *more good than harm*. Religious martyrdom is an extreme kind of case, and there are secular analogues involving self-sacrifice for some higher political or other moral end. Which way the judgement goes depends on what you believe, and in the kinds of case in question this varies between cultural circles and individuals. To put it simply, if someone does not believe in God, or does not believe that God communicates in the requisite ways, then his or her threshold for construing alleged religious experience as hallucinatory and delusional will be quite low, especially if they are trained to detect mental disorder. Conversely, if a person believes and lives in a religious world and believes that God or His messengers appear to individuals to guide them, then his or her threshold for construing felt religious experience as just that will be relatively low, although details will depend on the details of the background theology. As far as I can see the conclusions of a multidisciplinary team regarding the understanding of spiritual experience and delusion will depend above all on what—in these terms—the participants bring to it.

Commentary 10B

COMMENTARY ON "MAPPING THE LOGICAL GEOGRAPHY OF DELUSION AND SPIRITUAL EXPERIENCE"

Jennifer Radden, D.Phil.

Spiritual, metaphysical, and frankly religious ideas make their way into psychopathology with startling regularity. Yet because it is a vexed and touchy topic, the intersection of disorder and spiritual experience has often been skirted in discussions of psychiatry and psychiatric concepts. Fulford and Sadler's essay, and the earlier work by Jackson to which they refer, are noteworthy exceptions.

Even preliminary attempts to place delusions *in contrast to* spiritual experience readily reveal the ambiguity and controversy incumbent in this set of ideas. The contrast might be expected to rest on what such attitudes and experiences are over or about, their so-called propositional content. In one sense, however, religious delusions and spiritual experiences are over or about the same things, so this reading will be unhelpful. Although grounding the contrast, an alternative, more religious interpretation will be equally unhelpful. Within traditional frames of reference spiritual or religious experience is distinguished by its supernatural qualities or origins. Religious delusions are beliefs that are *natural* as well as in some way false or unwarranted, then, although spiritual experiences coming from God, are *non-natural* and are in that respect perhaps truer, more valid, or more valuable. Because of its theological presuppositions, such an interpretation can have only limited currency in contemporary discussions. On another reading, "delusion" is restricted to beliefs that are the symptoms of mental disorder—whatever their content, delusions

263

are somehow aberrant, abnormal, or dysfunctional, whereas spiritual experiences are normal and healthy. This reading will be increasingly difficult to maintain today (as Fulford and Sadler recognize), when cases like that of Simon, some recent studies, and much recent emphasis suggest that delusion-like (and hallucination-like) experiences may take both pathological and nonpathological forms.

These are serious difficulties. Presupposing a distinction where one may not exist would place the inquiry in logical jeopardy, rendering potentially question-begging any contrast drawn between pathology with religious or spiritual content and nondelusional spiritual experiences. Philosophers have spoken of certain concepts as essentially contested when they are unable to be defined in terms that entirely avoid controversial theoretical and normative presuppositions (Gallie 1955–1956). These ambiguities arise, I suggest, because "religious delusion" may be one of those concepts. Not only is it widely contested, as Fulford and Sadler willingly agree, but it is *essentially contested*.

Granted the daunting complexity of characterizing the boundary between disorder and spiritual experience, Fulford and Sadler's efforts to clarify our understanding of where we want to end up, and of how we might try to get there, are especially, and commendably, courageous.

Much else in Fulford and Sadler's broader discussion makes eminent good sense, in addition, and comports with recent thinking about the drawbacks of narrowly "scientific" and descriptivist approaches to diagnostic classification in psychiatry. The thorough-going attempt to make diagnostic psychiatry descriptive, explicitly voiced in DSM-III (American Psychiatric Association 1980) and staunchly adhered to in subsequent classifications, reflected an admirable effort to enhance diagnostic reliability. This decontextualized, nonetiological approach provided no advantage from the point of view of the *validity* of psychiatric diagnosis. Nonetheless, as these authors stress, the achievements of descriptive psychiatry were not inconsiderable, and although insufficient alone, should be recognized, preserved, and built upon rather than rejected. (*Re*-contextualizing diagnostic concepts returns us to the ambiguous and normative concept of dysfunction. For all its problems, enumerated by Fulford and Sadler, emphasis on dysfunction seems to capture something right: it is difficult to understand how mental disorder can be attributed without some form of dysfunction being implicated. Although necessary, impaired functioning may not be alone sufficient for such ascriptions, however; the clinical significance of Simon's account changes only when we learn that his unimpaired social and occupational functioning came in the absence of other problems and without any indication of a psychiatric history.)

Fulford and Sadler are also surely right in their conviction that "philosophical field work" into linguistic practices can advance our understanding, even when more abstract or theoretical concepts still want for a definition. Whether or not their particular analogy with "time" holds, the general point does that we may be able to make progress in determining clinical significance using mid-level descriptive concepts even while more abstract categories elude adequate definition. This is most evidently true of the broad category of mental illness or disorder, which many judge closer to a "family resemblance," or Roschian, concept and without basis in any features shared by all types of psychopathology. Lacking a satisfactory account of disorder as such, we can still work toward understanding the symptoms of particular disorders.

Their emphasis on the value of diverse perspectives—particularly those of service users and people able to speak directly of the phenomenology of disorder—is another important feature of Fulford and Sadler's program. This position echoes some of the new "standpoint" and "perspectivalist" epistemologies that have been adopted by philosophers during the past few decades. These epistemologies vary in several respects, including their characterization of the goal sought (whether multiple perspectives will, and perhaps will alone, yield *truth*, for example), and involve in some cases more controversial claims. Yet the modest claim made by Fulford and Sadler that several perspectives will yield a fuller understanding of the phenomenon in question seems hard to deny.

I, too, am impressed by what can be gained in understanding symptoms from the multiple perspectives and teamwork approach Fulford and Sadler recommend. At the boundary of spiritual and religious experience, I would stress one particular example. Those familiar with spiritual and religious language and concepts recognize and distinguish metaphorical, allegorical, and other figurative and nonliteral usage—forms of discourse and distinctions needed for the abstract and close to ineffable subject matter of religion. With their refined insights and more subtle distinctions, those attuned to the nuances of nonscientific and nonliteral discourse must provide a substantial contribution to the understanding of symptoms with spiritual and religious presuppositions and propositional content.

The research goal envisioned here may not be easy to realize in its entirety. Yet this is one of the most contested and controversial margins of psychopathology. In confronting and attempting to demarcate it, and in at least sketching an agenda for going forward, Fulford and Sadler's essay represents a significant achievement.

References

American Psychiatric Association: Diagnostic and Statistical Manual of Mental Disorders, 3rd Edition. Washington, DC, American Psychiatric Association, 1980

Gallie WB: Essentially contested concepts. Proceedings of the Aristotelian Society 56:167–198, 1955–1956

INDEX

Page numbers printed in **boldface** *type refer to tables or figures.*